D0072695

Essentials of Epidemiology in Public Health

Essentials of Epidemiology in Public Health

Ann Aschengrau, Sc.D.
Boston University School of Public Health
Department of Epidemiology

George R. Seage III, Sc.D.
Harvard School of Public Health
Department of Epidemiology

JONES AND BARTLETT PUBLISHERS
Sudbury, Massachusetts
BOSTON • TORONTO • LONDON • SINGAPORE

World Headquarters
Jones and Bartlett Publishers
40 Tall Pine Drive
Sudbury, MA 01776
978-443-5000
info@jbpub.com
www.jbpub.com

Jones and Bartlett Publishers Canada
2406 Nikanna Road
Mississauga, ON L5C 2W6
CANADA

Jones and Bartlett Publishers International
Barb House, Barb Mews
London W6 7PA
UK

PRODUCTION CREDITS
Chief Executive Officer: Clayton Jones
Chief Operating Officer: Don W. Jones, Jr.
Executive V.P. & Publisher: Robert W. Holland, Jr.
V.P., Sales and Marketing: William J. Kane
V.P., Design and Production: Anne Spencer
V.P., Manufacturing and Inventory Control: Therese Bräuer
Publisher: Michael Brown
Senior Production Editor: Linda S. DeBruyn
Editorial Assistant: Chambers Moore
Manufacturing and Inventory Coordinator: Amy Bacus
Composition: Bookwrights
Text Design: Bookwrights
Cover Design: Philip Regan
Printing and Binding: Malloy Lithography

Library of Congress Cataloging-in-Publication Data
CIP data unavailable at time of printing

Printed in the United States of America
07 06 05 04 03   10 9 8 7 6 5 4 3 2 1

We dedicate this book to our parents,
Carol and Mendel Aschengrau, in memoriam,
and Lorraine and George R. Seage Jr.

Acknowledgments

Our ideas about the principles and practice of epidemiology have been greatly influenced by many teachers, colleagues, and students. We feel privileged to have been inspired and nurtured by many outstanding teachers and mentors, including Richard Monson, George (Sandy) Lamb, Steve Schoenbaum, Arnold Epstein, Ken Rothman, Brian MacMahon, Julie Buring, Fran Cook, Ted Colton, Bob Glynn, Adrienne Cupples, George Hutchison, and the late Alan Morrison. We are pleased to help spread the knowledge they have given us to the next generation of epidemiologists.

We are also indebted to many colleagues who contributed to this book in various ways, including clarifying our thinking about epidemiology and biostatistics, providing ideas about how to teach epidemiology, reviewing and commenting on early drafts of the text, pilot-testing drafts in their classes, and, last but not least, dispensing many doses of encouragement during the many years it took to write this text. Among these individuals are Lisa Fredman, Bob Horsburgh, Herb Kayne, Dan Brooks, Michael Shwartz, Dave Ozonoff, Tricia Coogan, Meir Stampfer, Lorelei Mucci, Murray Mittleman, Charlie Poole, Tom Fleming, Megan Murray, Marc Lipsitch, Sam Bozeman, Anne Coletti, and Michael Gross. We are particularly grateful to our colleague Sarah Rogers who conducted literature searches, reviewed every single word of the manuscript, and provided us with unflagging and enthusiastic support. Ted Colton also deserves a special acknowledgment for recommending us to the publisher.

We thank our students for graciously reading drafts of this text in their epidemiology courses, and for contributing many valuable suggestions for improvement. We hope that the book will serve as a useful reference as they embark on productive careers in public health. We also recognize Abt Associates, Inc. for providing George Seage with a development and dissemination grant to write the chapter on screening in public health practice. We are very grateful to the staff of Jones and Bartlett Publishers, particularly Linda DeBruyn, for guiding the publication process so competently and so quickly. Finally, we thank our eight-year-old son Gregory for his patience and for providing many interesting and fun diversions along the way.

Contents

Preface

What is epidemiology and how does it contribute to the health of our society? Most people don't know the answers to these questions. This is somewhat paradoxical because epidemiology, one of the basic sciences of public health, affects the daily life of nearly everyone. It impacts both the way that we make personal decisions about our lives and the ways in which governments, public health agencies, and medical organizations make policy decisions that affect how we live.

In recent years the field of epidemiology has expanded tremendously in size, scope, and influence. The number of epidemiologists has grown rapidly, along with the number of epidemiology training programs in schools of public health and medicine. Many subspecialties have arisen to study public health questions from the molecular level to the societal level.

Recent years have also witnessed an important evolution in the theory and methods of epidemiologic research. For example, epidemiologists have changed considerably their views about the appropriate way to conceptualize and design the case-control study. We used to think that the case-control study was a backwards and inferior design but we now realize that it is a valid and efficient design in many settings. In fact, our current conceptualization of the major epidemiologic study designs reveals many more similarities among them than previously thought.

Epidemiologists' thinking about causality has also changed. Where once we used Sir Austin Bradford Hill's guideposts as an uncompromising checklist for "proving" causation, we now acknowledge that Hill's causal guidelines have many exceptions and uncertainties, and that causal relationships can never be proven. Epidemiologists have also begun to use some newer conceptual models of causation, such as the sufficient/component cause model and the counterfactual causal model, as a way to bridge the gap between theories of causation and the practice of epidemiology.

Unfortunately, few of these changes have been taught in introductory epidemiology courses, particularly those for master's-level students. We believe this has occurred mainly because instructors have mistakenly assumed the new concepts were too difficult or too arcane for beginning students. As a consequence, many generations of public health students have received a dated education.

Our desire to change this practice was the main impetus for writing this book. For more than a decade we have successfully taught the traditional and new concepts to our graduate students at Boston University and Harvard University. Not only have our students successfully mastered the material, but they have also found that the new ideas enhanced their understanding of epidemiology and its application.

In addition to providing an up-to-date education, we have taught our students the necessary skills to become knowledgeable consumers of the epidemiologic literature. Gaining competence in the critical evaluation of this literature is particularly important for public health practitioners because they often need to reconcile confusing and contradictory results.

This textbook reflects our educational philosophy of combining theory and practice in our teaching. It is intended for public health students who will be consumers of epidemiologic literature and those who will be practicing epidemiologists. The first five chapters cover basic epidemiologic concepts and data sources. Chapter 1 describes the approach and evolution of epidemiology, including the definition, goals, and historical development of epidemiology and public health. Chapters 2 and 3 describe how epidemiologists measure and compare disease occurrence in populations. Chapter 4 characterizes the major sources of health data on the U.S. population and describes how to interpret these data appropriately. Chapter 5 describes how epidemiologists analyze disease patterns to understand the health status of a population, formulate and test hypotheses of disease causation, and carry out and evaluate health programs.

The next four chapters of the textbook focus on epidemiologic study design. Chapter 6 provides an overview of study designs—including experimental, cohort, case-control, and cross-sectional and ecological studies—and describes the factors that determine when a particular design is indicated. Each of the three following chapters provides a detailed description of the three main analytic designs: experimental, cohort, and case–control studies.

The next five chapters cover the tools students need to interpret the results of epidemiologic studies. Chapter 10 describes bias, including how it influences study results and the ways in which it can be avoided. Chapter 11 explains the concept of confounding, methods for assessing its presence, and methods for controlling its effects. Chapter 12 covers random error, including hypothesis testing, P-value and confidence interval estimation and interpretation, and sample size and power calculations. We believe this chapter provides a balanced view of the appropriate role of statistics in epidemiology. Chapter 13 covers the concept of effect measure modification, an often-neglected topic in introductory texts. It explains the difference between confounding and effect measure modification and describes the methods for evaluating effect measure modification. Chapter 14 pulls together the information from Chapters 10 through 13 by providing a framework for evaluating the literature, as well as three examples of epidemiologic study critiques.

Chapter 15 covers the epidemiologic approach to causation, including the historical development of causation theories, Hill's guidelines for assessing causation, and the sufficient/component cause model of causation. Chapter 16 explains screening in public health practice, including the natural history of disease, characteristics of diseases appropriate for screening, important features of a screening test, and methods for evaluating a screening program. Up-to-date examples from the epidemiologic literature on diseases of public health importance are used throughout the book.

Our educational background and research interests are also reflected in the textbook's outlook and examples. Ann Aschengrau received her doctorate in epidemiology from Harvard School of Public Health in 1987 and joined the Department of Epidemiology at Boston University School of Public Health shortly thereafter. She is currently Professor of Epidemiology and Director of the Master of Science Degree Program in Epidemiology. For the past 15 years she has taught introductory epidemiology to master's level students. Her research has focused on the environmental determinants of disease, including childhood lead poisoning, cancer, and disorders of reproduction and child development.

George R. Seage, III received his doctorate in epidemiology from Boston University School of Public Health in 1992. For more than a decade he served as the AIDS epidemiologist for the city of Boston and as a faculty member at Boston University School of Public Health. For seven years he directed the U.S. HIV Prevention Trials Network. He is currently Associate Professor of Epidemiology at Harvard School of Public Health and Director of the Interdisciplinary Concentration in Infectious Disease Epidemiology. For the past 13 years he has taught courses in HIV epidemiology to master's and doctoral students. His research has focused on the biological and behavioral determinants of HIV-1 transmission and their application to HIV-1 prevention trials, particularly those involving vaccines and microbicidal agents.

1

The Approach and Evolution of Epidemiology

LEARNING OBJECTIVES

By the end of this chapter the reader will be able to:

- Define and discuss the goals of public health.
- Distinguish between basic, clinical, and public health research.
- Define epidemiology and explain its objectives.
- Discuss the key components of epidemiology (population and frequency, distribution, determinants, and control of disease).
- Discuss important figures in the history of epidemiology including John Graunt, James Lind, William Farr, and John Snow.
- Discuss important modern studies including the Streptomycin Tuberculosis Trial, Doll and Hill's studies on smoking and lung cancer, and the Framingham Study.
- Discuss the current activities and challenges of modern epidemiologists.

Introduction

Most people do not know what epidemiology is or how it contributes to the health of our society. This fact is somewhat paradoxical, given that epidemiology pervades our lives. Consider, for example, the following statements that have recently made headline news:

- Mammographic screening for breast cancer does not benefit women aged 40 to 49 years.

- Cellular telephone users who talk on the phone while driving are more likely than other drivers to become involved in a car accident.

- Saint John's wort, a popular alternative medicine, is an ineffective treatment for severe depression.

- Disinfection byproducts in drinking water increase a pregnant woman's risk of miscarriage.

- Premarital screening for human immunodeficiency virus (HIV) infection is ineffective in reducing viral transmission.

The breadth and importance of these topics indicate that epidemiology directly affects the daily lives of most people. It affects the way that individuals make personal decisions about their lives and the way that the government, public health agencies, and medical organizations make policy decisions that affect how we live. For example, the results of epidemiologic studies described by the headlines might prompt a person to request a traditional medication for her depression, to wait until age 50 years to begin regular mammograms, or to install a water treatment device on her kitchen faucet. It might prompt a gynecologist to tailor recommendations about mammographic screening to suit the patient's preferences, a water utility to change its methods for disinfecting drinking water, cell phone manufacturers to design safer phones, or state legislators to vote against laws mandating premarital HIV screening of heterosexual couples and to vote for laws banning cell phone use by drivers.

This chapter helps the reader understand what epidemiology is and how it contributes to important issues affecting the public's health. In particular, it describes the definition, approach, and goals of epidemiology, as well as key aspects of its historical development, current state, and future challenges.

Definition and Goals of Public Health

Public health is a multidisciplinary field whose goal is to promote the health of the population through organized community efforts.[1(pp3–15)] In contrast to medicine, which focuses mainly on treating illness in separate individuals, public health focuses on preventing illness in the community. Key public health activities include assessing the health status of the population, diagnosing its problems, searching for the causes of those problems, and designing solutions for them. The solutions usually involve community-level interventions that control or prevent the cause of the problem. For example, public health interventions include establishing educational programs to discourage teenagers from smoking, implementing screening programs for the early detection of cancer, and passing laws that require automobile drivers and passengers to wear seat belts.

Unfortunately, public health achievements are difficult to recognize because it is hard to identify people who have been spared illness.[1(pp6–7)] For this reason, the field of public health has received less attention and fewer resources than the field of medicine has received. Nevertheless, public health has had a greater impact than medicine on the health of populations. For example, since the turn of the 20th century, the average life expectancy of Americans has increased by almost 30 years from 47.3 to 76.7 years.[2] Of this increase, 25 years can be attributed to improvements in public health and only 5 years can be attributed to improvements in the medical care system.[3] Public health achievements that account for improvements in health and life expectancy include the routine use of vaccinations for infectious diseases, improvements in motor vehicle and workplace safety, control of infectious diseases through improved sanitation and clean water, modification of risk factors for coronary heart disease and stroke (such as smoking cessation and blood pressure control), safer foods from decreased microbial contamination, improved access to family planning and contraceptive services, and the acknowledgment of tobacco as a health hazard and the ensuing antismoking campaigns.[4]

The public health system's activities in research, education, and program implementation have made these accomplishments possible. In the United States this system includes federal agencies such as the Centers for Disease Control and Prevention, state and local government agencies, nongovernmental organizations such as Mothers Against Drunk Driving, and academic institutions such as schools of public health. This complex array of institutions has achieved success through political action and gains in scientific knowledge.[1(pp13–14)] Politics enters the public health process when agencies advocate for resources, develop policies and plans to improve a community's health, and work to ensure that services needed for the protection of public health are available to all. Political action is necessary because the government usually has the responsibility for developing the activities required to protect public health.

Sources of Scientific Knowledge in Public Health

The scientific basis of public health activities mainly comes from (1) the basic sciences such as pathology and toxicology, (2) the clinical or medical sciences such as internal medicine and pediatrics, and (3) the public health sciences such as epidemiology, environmental health science, and health education and behavioral science. Research in these three areas provides complementary pieces of a puzzle that, when properly assembled, provide the scientific foundation for public health action. Other fields such as engineering and economics also contribute to public health. The three main areas approach research questions from different yet complementary viewpoints, and each field has its own particular strengths and weaknesses.

Basic scientists such as toxicologists study disease in a laboratory setting by conducting experiments on cells, tissues, and animals. The focus of this research is often on the disease mechanism or process. Because basic scientists conduct their studies in a controlled laboratory environment, they can regulate all important aspects of the experimental conditions. For example, a laboratory experiment testing the toxicity of a chemical is conducted on genetically similar animals who live in the same physical environment, eat the same diet, and follow the same daily schedule.[5(pp157-237)] Animals are assigned (usually by chance) to either the test group or the control group. Using identical routes of administration, researchers give the chemical under investigation to the test group and an inert chemical to the control group. Thus, the only difference between the two groups is the dissimilar chemical deliberately introduced by the investigator. This type of research provides valuable information on the disease process that cannot be obtained in any other way. However, the results are often difficult to extrapolate to real-life situations involving humans because of differences in susceptibility between species, and differences in the exposure level between laboratory experiments and real-life settings. In general, humans are exposed to much lower doses than those used in laboratory experiments.

Clinical scientists focus their research questions mainly on disease diagnosis, treatment, and prognosis in individual patients. For example, they try to determine if a diagnostic method is accurate or if a treatment is effective. Although clinicians are also involved in disease prevention, this activity has historically taken a back seat to disease diagnosis and treatment. As a consequence, clinical research studies are usually based on people who come to a medical care facility such as a hospital or clinic. Unfortunately, these people are often unrepresentative of the full spectrum of disease in the population at large because many sick people never come to the attention of health care providers.

Clinical scientists contribute to scientific knowledge in several important ways. First, they are usually the first to identify new diseases, the adverse effects of new exposures, and new links between an exposure and a disease. This information is typically published in case reports. For example, the epidemic of acquired immunodeficiency syndrome (AIDS) officially began in the United States in 1981 when clinicians reported several cases of *Pneumocystis carinii* pneumonia and Kaposi's sarcoma (a rare cancer of the blood vessels) among previously healthy, young homosexual men living in New York and California.[6,7] These cases were notable because

Pneumocystis carinii pneumonia had previously occurred only among immunocompromised individuals and Kaposi's sarcoma had occurred mainly among elderly men. We now know that these case reports described symptoms of a new disease that would eventually be called AIDS. Despite their simplicity, case reports provide important clues regarding the causes, prevention, and cures for a disease. In addition, they are often used to justify conducting more sophisticated and expensive studies.

Clinical scientists also contribute to scientific knowledge by recording treatment and response information in their patients' medical records. This information often becomes an indispensable source of research data for clinical and epidemiologic studies. For example, it would have been impossible to determine the risk of breast cancer following fluoroscopic x-ray exposure without patient treatment records from the 1930s through 1950s.[8] Investigators used these records to identify the subjects for the study and gather detailed information about subjects' radiation doses.

Public health scientists study ways to prevent disease and promote health in the population at large. Public health research differs from clinical research in two important ways. First, it focuses mainly on disease prevention rather than disease treatment. Second, the units of concern are groups of people living in the community rather than separate individuals visiting a health care facility. For example, a public health research project called "Lead Free Kids" determined the impact of removing lead-contaminated soil on children's blood lead levels.[9] About 150 healthy, community-dwelling children who were at risk for lead poisoning were targeted for this lead-poisoning prevention project.

The main differences between the three branches of scientific inquiry are summarized in Table 1–1. Although this is a useful way to classify the branches of scientific research, the distinctions between these areas have become blurred. For example, epidemiologic methods are currently being applied to clinical medicine in a field called "clinical epidemiology."

TABLE 1–1 Main Differences Between Basic, Clinical, and Public Health Science Research

Characteristic	Basic	Clinical	Public health
What/who is studied	Cells, tissues, animals in laboratory settings	Sick patients who come to health care facilities	Populations or communities at large
Research goals	Understanding disease mechanisms and the effects of toxic substances	Improving diagnosis and treatment of disease	Prevention of disease, promotion of health
Examples	Toxicology, immunology	Internal medicine, pediatrics	Epidemiology, environmental health science

In addition, newly developed areas of epidemiologic research such as molecular and genetic epidemiology include the basic sciences.

Definition and Objectives of Epidemiology

The term *epidemiology* is derived from the Greek words *epi*, which means "on or upon"; *demos*, which means "the common people"; and *logy*, which means "study."[10(pp484,599,1029)] Putting these pieces together yields the following definition of epidemiology: "the study of that which falls upon the common people." Epidemiology can also be defined as the "branch of medical science which treats epidemics."[11] The latter definition was developed by the London Epidemiological Society, which was formed in 1850 to determine the causes of cholera and other epidemic diseases and methods of preventing them.[12] Over the last century, many definitions of epidemiology have been set forth. Some early definitions reflect the field's initial focus on infectious diseases, and later ones reflect a broader scope encompassing all diseases.[12]

We define epidemiology as follows: *The study of the distribution and determinants of disease frequency in human populations and the application of this study to control health problems.*[13(p1),14(p55)] Our definition is a combination of a popular one coined by MacMahon and Pugh in 1970 and another described by Last in the third edition of the *Dictionary of Epidemiology.*[14(p55),15(p1)] Note that the term "disease" refers to a broad array of health-related states and events including diseases, injuries, disabilities, and death.

We prefer this hybrid definition because it describes both the scope and ultimate goal of epidemiology. In particular, the objectives of epidemiology are to: (1) study the natural course of disease from onset to resolution, (2) determine the extent of disease in a population, (3) identify patterns and trends in disease occurrence, (4) identify the causes of disease, and (5) evaluate the effectiveness of measures that prevent and treat disease. All of these activities contribute scientific knowledge for making sound policy decisions that protect public health.

Our definition of epidemiology has five key words or phrases: (1) population, (2) disease frequency, (3) disease distribution, (4) disease determinants, and (5) disease control. Each term is described in more detail in the following sections.

Population

Populations are at the heart of all epidemiologic activities because epidemiologists are concerned with disease occurrence in groups of people rather than in individuals. The term *population* refers to a group of people with a common characteristic such as place of residence, gender, age, or use of certain medical services. For example, people who reside in the city of Boston are members of a geographically defined population. Determining the size of the population in which disease occurs is as important as counting the cases of the disease, because it is only when the number of cases is related to the size of the population that we know the true frequency of disease. The size of the population is often determined by a census—that is, a complete count—of the population. Sources of these data range from the decennial census, in which the federal government attempts to count every person in the United States every 10 years, to computerized records from medical facilities that provide counts of patients who use the facilities.

Disease Frequency

This phrase refers to quantifying how often a disease arises in a population. Counting, which is a key activity of epidemiologists, includes three steps: (1) developing a definition of disease, (2) instituting a mechanism for counting cases of disease within a specified population, and (3) determining the size of that population.

Diseases must be clearly defined in order to determine accurately who should be counted. Usually disease definitions are based on a combination of physical and pathological examinations, diagnostic test results, and signs and symptoms. For example, a case definition of breast cancer might include findings of a palpable lump during a physical exam and mammographic and pathological evidence of malignant disease.

Currently available sources for identifying and counting cases of disease include hospital patient rosters, death certificates, special reporting systems such as registries of cancer and birth defects, and special surveys. For example, the National Health Interview Survey is a federally funded study that has collected data on the health status of the U.S. population since the 1950s. Its stated purpose is "to secure accurate and current statistical information on the amount, distribution, and effects of illness and disability in the United States."[16] Data are collected on many diseases including cancer; diabetes; and cardiovascular, respiratory, gastrointestinal, and renal disease.

Disease Distribution

Disease distribution refers to the analysis of disease patterns according to the characteristics of person, place, and time. In other words, who is getting the disease, where is it occurring, and how is it changing over time? Variations in disease frequency by these three characteristics provide useful information that helps epidemiologists understand the health status of a population; formulate hypotheses about the determinants of a disease;

and plan, implement, and evaluate public health programs to control and prevent adverse health events.

Disease Determinants

Disease determinants are factors that bring about a change in a person's health—that is, factors that either cause a healthy individual to become sick or cause a sick person to recover.[14(p46)] Thus, determinants include both causal and preventive factors. Determinants also include individual, environmental, and societal characteristics. Individual determinants include a person's genetic makeup, gender, age, immunity level, diet, behaviors, and existing diseases. For example, the risk of breast cancer is increased among women who carry genetic alterations such as BRCA1 and BRCA2, are elderly, give birth at a late age, have a history of benign breast disease, or have a history of radiation exposure to the chest.[17]

Environmental and societal determinants are external to the individual, and thereby encompass a wide range of natural, social, and economic events and conditions. For example, the presence of infectious agents, reservoirs in which the organism multiplies, vectors that transport the agent, poor and crowded housing conditions, and political instability are environmental and social factors that cause many communicable diseases around the world.

Epidemiologic research involves generating and testing specific hypotheses about disease determinants. A hypothesis is defined as "a tentative explanation for an observation, phenomenon, or scientific problem that can be tested by further investigation."[10(p866)] Generating hypotheses is a process that involves creativity and imagination and usually includes observations on the frequency and distribution of disease in a population. Epidemiologists test hypotheses by making comparisons, usually within the context of a formal epidemiologic study. The goal of a study is to harvest valid and precise information about the determinants of disease in a particular population. As described in Chapter 6, epidemiologic research encompasses several types of study designs; each type of study merely represents a different way of harvesting the information.

Disease Control

Epidemiologists accomplish disease control through epidemiologic research, as described above, and through surveillance. The purpose of surveillance is to monitor aspects of disease occurrence that are pertinent to effective control.[18(p507)] For example, since 1985 the Centers for Disease Control and Prevention has collected information on the occurrence of AIDS across the United States.[19] In addition, after the development of serum HIV-antibody tests, states began reporting confirmed cases of HIV infection. For every case of AIDS and HIV infection, the surveillance system gathers data on the individual's demographic characteristics, exposure category (such as injecting drug users or men who have sex with men), and diagnosis date. These surveillance data are essential for formulating and evaluating programs to reduce the spread of AIDS.

Historical Development of Epidemiology

The historical development of epidemiology spans almost 400 years and is best described as slow and unsteady. Only since World War II has the field experienced a rapid expansion. The following sections, which are not meant to be a comprehensive history, highlight several historic figures and studies that made significant contributions to the evolution of epidemiologic thinking. These include John Graunt, who summarized the pattern of mortality in 17th-century London; James Lind, who used an experimental study to discover the cause and prevention of scurvy; William Farr, who pioneered a wide range of activities during the mid-19th century that are still used by modern epidemiologists; John Snow, who showed that cholera was transmitted by fecal contamination of drinking water; members of the Streptomycin in Tuberculosis Trials Committee, who conducted one of the first modern controlled clinical trials; Richard Doll and A. Bradford Hill, who conducted early research on smoking and lung cancer; and Thomas Dawber and William Kannel, who began the Framingham Study—one of the most influential and longest-running studies of heart disease in the world. It is clear that epidemiology has played an important role in the achievements of public health throughout its history.

John Graunt

The logical underpinnings for modern epidemiologic thinking evolved from the scientific revolution of the 17th century.[20(p23)] During this period, scientists believed that the behavior of the physical universe was orderly and could therefore be expressed in terms of mathematical relationships called "laws." These laws are generalized statements based on observations of the physical universe such as the time of day that the sun rises and sets. Some scientists believed that this line of thinking could be extended to the biological universe and reasoned that there must be "laws of mortality" that describe the patterns of disease and death. These scientists believed that the "laws of mortality" could be induced by observing the patterns of disease and death among humans.

John Graunt, a London tradesman and founding member of the Royal Society of London, was a pioneer in this regard. He became the first epidemiologist, statistician, and demographer when he summarized the Bills of Mortality for his 1662 publication *Natural and Political Observations*

Mentioned in a Following Index, and Made Upon the Bills of Mortality.[21] The Bills of Mortality were a weekly count of people who died that had been conducted by the parish clerks of London since 1592 because of concern about the plague. According to Graunt, the Bills were collected in the following manner:

> When any one dies, then, either by tolling, or ringing a Bell, or by bespeaking of a Grave of the Sexton, the same is known to the Searchers, corresponding with the said Sexton. The Searchers hereupon (who are antient matrons, sworn to their office) repair to the place, where the dead Corps lies, and by view of the same, and by other enqueries, they examine by what Disease, or Casualty the Corps did die. Hereupon they make their Report to the Parish-Clerk, and he, every Tuesday night, carries in an Accompt of all the Burials, and Christnings, hapning that Week, to the Clerk of the Hall. On Wednesday the general Accompt is made up, and Printed, and on Thursdays published and dispersed to the several Families, who will pay four shillings per Annum for them.[21(pp25–26)]

This method of reporting deaths is not very different from the system used today in the United States. Like the "searchers" of John Graunt's time, modern physicians and medical examiners inspect the body and other evidence such as medical records to determine the official cause of death, which is recorded on the death certificate. The physician typically submits the certificate to the funeral director, who files it with the local office of vital records. From there, the certificate is transferred to the city, county, state, and federal agencies that compile death statistics. While 17th-century London families had to pay 4 shillings for the Bills of Mortality, these U.S. statistics are available free of charge.

Graunt drew many inferences about the patterns of fertility, morbidity, and mortality by tabulating the Bills of Mortality.[21] For example, he noted new diseases such as rickets, and he made the following observations:

- Some diseases affected a similar number of people from year to year, while others varied considerably over time.
- Common causes of death included old age, consumption, smallpox, plague, and diseases of teeth and worms.
- Many greatly feared causes of death were actually uncommon, including leprosy, suicide, and starvation.
- Four separate periods of increased mortality caused by the plague occurred from 1592 to 1660.
- The mortality rate for men was higher than for women.
- Fall was the "most unhealthful season."

Graunt was the first to estimate the number of inhabitants, age structure of the population, and rate of population growth in London and the first to construct a life table that summarized patterns of mortality and survival from birth until death (see Table 1–2). He found that the mortality rate for children was quite high; only 25 individuals out of 100 survived to age 26 years. Furthermore, even though mortality rates for adults were much lower, very few people reached old age (only 3 of 100 London residents survived to age 66 years).

Graunt did not accept the statistics at face value but carefully considered their errors and ambiguities. For example, he noted that it was often difficult for the "antient matron" searchers to determine the exact cause of death. In fact, by cleverly comparing the number of plague deaths and nonplague deaths, Graunt estimated that London officials had overlooked about 20% of deaths resulting from plague.[22]

Although Graunt modestly stated that he merely "reduced several great confused *Volumes* into a few perspicuous *Tables* and abridged such *Observations* as naturally flowed from them," historians consider his work much more significant. Statistician Walter Willcox summarized Graunt's importance:

> Graunt is memorable mainly because he discovered the numerical regularity of deaths and births, of ratios of the sexes at death and birth, and of the proportion of deaths from certain causes to all causes in successive years and in different areas; or in general terms, the uniformity and predictability of many important biological phenomena taken in the mass. In doing so, he opened the way both for the later discovery of uniformities in many social and volitional phenomena like marriage, suicide and crime, and for a study of these uniformities, their nature and their limits.[21(p xiii)]

TABLE 1–2   Life Table of the London Population Constructed by John Graunt in 1662

Age (years)	Number dying	Number surviving
Birth	0	100
6	36	64
16	24	40
26	15	25
36	9	16
46	6	10
56	4	6
66	3	3
76	2	1
86	1	0

Source: Data from Graunt J. *Natural and Political Observations Made upon the Bills of Mortality,* p. 69. Baltimore, MD: The Johns Hopkins Press; 1932.

James Lind

Only a few important developments occurred in the field of epidemiology during the 200-year period following the publication of John Graunt's *Bills of Mortality*. One notable development was the realization that experimental studies could be used to test hypotheses about the laws of mortality. As described in Chapter 7, these studies involve designed experiments that investigate the role of some factor or agent in the causation, improvement, postponement, or prevention of disease.[23] Their hallmarks are: (1) the comparison of at least two groups of individuals (an experimental group and a "control" group) and (2) the active manipulation of the factor or agent under study by the investigator (that is, the investigator assigns individuals either to receive or not to receive a preventive or therapeutic measure).

In the mid-1700s, James Lind conducted one of earliest experimental studies on the treatment of scurvy, a common disease and cause of death at the time.[24(pp145–148)] Although scurvy affected people living on land, sailors often became sick and died from this disease while at sea. As a ship's surgeon, Lind had many opportunities to observe the "epidemiology" of this disease. His astute observations led him to dismiss the popular ideas that scurvy was a hereditary or infectious disease and to propose that "the principal and main predisposing cause" was moist air and that its "occasional cause" was diet.[24(pp64–67,85,91)] He evaluated his hypothesis about diet with the following experimental study.

> On the 20th of May, 1747 I took twelve patients in the scurvy, on board the *Salisbury* at sea. Their cases were as similar as I could have them. They all in general had putrid gums, the spots and lassitude, with weakness of their knees. They lay together in one place, being a proper apartment for the sick in the fore-hold; and had one diet common to all, *viz*, water-gruel sweetened with sugar in the morning; fresh mutton-broth often times for dinner; at other times puddings, boiled biscuit with sugar, etc.; and for supper barley and raisins, rice and currents, sago and wine, or the like. Two of these were ordered each a quart of cyder a day. Two others took twenty-five gutts of *elixir vitriol* three times a-day. . . . Two other took two spoonfuls of vinegar three times a-day. . . . Two of the worst patients, with the tendons in the ham rigid (a symptom none of the rest had), were put under a course of sea-water. . . . Two others had each two oranges and one lemon given them every day. . . . They continued but six days under this course having consumed the quantity that could be spared. . . . The two remaining patients took bigness of a nutmeg three times a day, of an electuary recommended by an hospital-surgeon made of garlic, mustard seed.[24(pp145–148)]

After 4 weeks, Lind reported the following: "The consequence was, that the most sudden and visible good effects were perceived from the use of the oranges and lemons; one of those who had taken them being at the end of six days fit for duty. . . . He became quite healthy before we came into Plymouth which was on the 16th of June. . . . The other was the best recovered of any in his condition; and being now deem pretty well, was appointed nurse to the rest of the sick."[24(p146)] Lind concluded, "I shall here only observe, that the result of all my experiments was, that oranges and lemons were the most effectual remedies for this distemper at sea. I am apt to think oranges preferable to lemons though perhaps both given together will be found most serviceable."[24(p148)]

Although the sample size of Lind's experiment was quite small by today's standards (12 men divided into six groups of two), Lind followed one of the most important principles of experimental research—ensuring that important aspects of the experimental conditions remained similar for all study subjects. Lind selected sailors whose disease was similarly severe, who lived in common quarters, and who had a similar diet. Thus, the main difference between the six groups of men was the dietary addition purposefully introduced by Lind. He also exhibited good scientific practice by confirming "the efficacy of these fruits by the experience of others."[24(p148)] In other words, Lind did not base his final conclusions about the curative powers of citrus fruits on a single experiment, but rather he gathered additional data from other ships and voyages.

Lind used the results of this experiment to suggest a method for preventing scurvy at sea. Because fresh fruits were likely to spoil and were difficult to obtain in certain ports and seasons, he proposed that lemon and orange juice extract be carried on board.[24(pp155–156)] The British Navy took 40 years to adopt Lind's recommendation; within several years of doing so, it had eradicated scurvy from its ranks.[24(pp377–380)]

William Farr

William Farr made many important advances in the field of epidemiology in the mid-1800s. Now considered one of the founders of modern epidemiology, Farr was the compiler of Statistical Abstracts for the General Registry Office in Great Britain from 1839 through 1880. In this capacity, Farr was in charge of the annual count of births, marriages, and deaths. A trained physician and self-taught mathematician, "Farr pioneered a whole range of activities encompassed by modern epidemiology. He described the state of health of the population, he sought to establish the determinants of public health, and he applied the knowledge gained to the prevention and control of disease."[25(p xi–xii)]

One of Farr's most important contributions involved calculations that combined registration data on births, marriages, and deaths (as the numerator) with census data on the population size (as the denominator). As he stated, "The simple process of comparing the deaths in a given time out of a given number" was "a modern discovery."[25(p170)] His first annual report in 1839 demonstrated the "superior precision of numerical expressions" over literary expressions.[25(p214)] For example, he quantified and arranged mortality data in a manner strikingly similar to modern practice (see Table 1–3). Note that the annual percentage of deaths increased with age for men and women, but for most age groups the percentage was higher for men than for women.

Farr drew numerous inferences about the English population by tabulating vital statistics. For example, he reported the following findings:

- The average age of the English population remained relatively constant over time at 26.4 years.

- Widowers had a higher marriage rate than bachelors.

- The rate of illegitimate births declined over time.

- People who lived at lower elevations had higher death rates resulting from cholera than did those who lived at higher elevations.

- People who lived in densely populated areas had higher mortality rates than did people who lived in less populated areas.

- Decreases in mortality rates followed improvements in sanitation.

Farr used these data to form hypotheses about the causes and preventions of disease. For example, he used data on smallpox deaths to derive a general law of epidemics that accurately predicted the decline of the rinderpest epidemic in the 1860s.[25(p x)] He used the data on the association between cholera deaths and altitude to support the hypothesis that

TABLE 1–3 Annual Mortality per Hundred Males and Females in England and Wales, 1838–1871

Ages (years)	Males	Females
0–4	7.26	6.27
5–9	0.87	0.85
10–14	0.49	0.50
15–24	0.78	0.80
25–34	0.99	1.01
35–44	1.30	1.23
45–54	1.85	1.56
55–64	3.20	2.80
65–74	6.71	5.89
75–84	14.71	13.43
85–94	30.55	27.95
95+	44.11	43.04

Source: Data from Farr W. *Vital Statistics: a Memorial Volume of Selections from the Reports and Writings of William Farr,* p. 183. New York, NY: Academy of Medicine; 1975.

an unhealthful climate was the disease's cause—a theory that was subsequently disproved.

Farr made several practical and methodological contributions to the field of epidemiology. First, he constantly strove to ensure that the collected data were accurate and complete. Second, he devised a categorization system for the causes of death so that these data could be reduced to a usable form. The system that he devised is the antecedent of the modern *International Classification of Diseases,* which categorizes diseases and causes of death. Third, Farr made a number of important contributions to the analysis of data, including the invention of the "standardized mortality rate," an adjustment method for making fair comparisons between groups with different age structures.

John Snow

Another important figure in the development of epidemiologic methods during the mid-1800s was John Snow (see Figure 1–1). A respected physician who was a successful anesthetist and researcher on anesthetic gases, Snow was also interested in the cause and spread of cholera.[26(p xxxiv)] Although Farr mistakenly thought that an unhealthful climate accounted for the variation in cholera mortality by altitude, Snow used these data to support an innovative hypothesis that cholera was an infectious disease spread by fecal contamination of drinking water.

Snow argued, "Cholera must be a poison acting on the alimentary canal by being brought into direct contact with the alimentary mucous surface . . . the symptoms are primarily seated in the alimentary canal and all the after-symptoms of a general kind are the results of the flux from the canal. His inference from this was, that the poison of cholera is taken direct into the canal by mouth. This view led him to consider the media through which the poison is conveyed and the nature of the poison itself. Several circumstances lent their aid in referring him to water as the chief, though not the only, medium, and to the excreted matters from the patient already stricken with cholera, as the poison."[26(p xxxiv–xxxv)]

In 1849 Snow published his views on the causes and transmission of cholera in a short pamphlet titled *The Mode of Communication of Cholera.* During the next few years he continued groundbreaking research testing the hypothesis that cholera was a waterborne infectious disease. The second edition of his pamphlet, published in 1855, describes in greater detail "the whole of his inquiries in regard to cholera."[26(p xxxvi)] The cholera investigations for which Snow is best known are described in the following paragraphs.

One such investigation focused on the Broad Street epidemic. During August and September of 1854, one of the worst outbreaks of cholera occurred in the London neighborhood surrounding Broad Street. Almost

FIGURE 1–1. John Snow investigated the cause and spread of cholera in 19th-century London.

Source: Reprinted with permission from the Wellcome Trust Library, London, England.

500 fatalities from cholera occurred within a 10-day period within 250 yards of the junction between Broad and Cambridge Streets (see Figure 1–2). According to Snow, "The mortality in this limited area probably equals any that was ever caused in this country, even by the plague; and it was much more sudden, as the greater number of cases terminated in a few hours."[26(p38)] Snow continued,

> As soon as I became acquainted with the situation and extent of this irruption of cholera, I suspected some contamination of the water of the much-frequented street-pump in Broad Street, near the end of Cambridge Street; but on examining the water, on the evening of the 3rd of September, I found so little impurity in it of an organic nature that I hesitated to come to a conclusion. Further inquiry, however, showed me that there was no other circumstance or agent common to the cholera occurred, and not extending beyond it, except the water of the above mentioned pump.[26(p39)]

His subsequent investigations included a detailed study of the drinking habits of 83 individuals who died between August 31 and September 2, 1854.[26(pp39–40)] He found that 73 of the 83 deaths occurred among indi-

FIGURE 1–2. Distribution of deaths from cholera in the Broad Street Neighborhood from August 19 to September 30, 1854. "A black mark or bar for each death is placed in the situation of the house in which the fatal attack took place. The situation of the Broad Street Pump is also indicated, as well as that of all the surrounding Pumps to which the public had access."

Source: Reprinted from Snow J. *Snow on Cholera*, Map 1. New York, NY: Hafner Publishers; 1965. With permission from the Commonwealth Fund, New York, NY.

viduals living within a short distance of the Broad Street pump and that 10 deaths occurred among individuals who lived in houses that were near other pumps. According to the surviving relatives, 61 of the 73 individuals who lived near the pump drank the pump water and only 6 individuals did not. (No data could be collected for the remaining 6 because everyone connected with these individuals had either died or departed the city). The drinking habits of the 10 individuals who lived "decidedly nearer to another street pump" also implicated the Broad Street pump. Surviving relatives reported that 5 of the 10 drank water from the Broad Street pump because they preferred it, and 2 drank its water because they attended a nearby school.

Snow also investigated pockets of the Broad Street population that had fewer cholera deaths. For example, he found that only 5 cholera deaths occurred among 535 inmates of a workhouse located in the Broad Street neighborhood.[26(p42)] The workhouse had a pump-well on its premises, and "the inmates never sent to Broad Street for water." Furthermore, no cholera deaths occurred among 70 workers at the Broad Street brewery who never obtained pump water but instead drank a daily ration of malt liquor.

Although Snow never found direct evidence of sewage contamination of the Broad Street pump-well, he did note that the well was near a major sewer and several cesspools. He concluded, "There had been no particular outbreak or increase of cholera, in this part of London, except among the persons who were in the habit of drinking the water of the above-mentioned pump-well."[26(p40)] He presented his findings to the Board of Guardians of St. James's Parish on September 7, and "the handle of the pump was removed on the following day."[26]

Snow's investigation of the Broad Street epidemic is noteworthy for several reasons. First, Snow was able to form a hypothesis implicating the Broad Street pump after he mapped the geographic distribution of the cholera deaths and studied that distribution in relation to the surrounding public water pumps (see Figure 1–2). Second, he collected data on the drinking water habits of unaffected as well as affected individuals, which allowed him to make a comparison that would support or refute his hypothesis. Third, the results of his investigation were so convincing that they led to immediate action to curb the disease—namely, the pump handle was removed. Public health action to prevent disease seldom occurs so quickly.

Another series of Snow's groundbreaking investigations on cholera focused on specific water supply companies. In particular, he found that districts supplied by the Southwark and Vauxhall Company and the Lambeth Company had higher cholera mortality rates than all of the other water companies.[26(pp63–64)] A few years later, a fortuitous change occurred in the water source of several of the south districts of London. As Snow stated, "The Lambeth Company removed their water works, in 1852, from opposite Hungerforth Market to Thames Ditton; thus obtaining a supply of water quite free from the sewage of London."[26(p68)]

Following this change, Snow obtained data from William Farr to show that "districts partially supplied with the improved water suffered much less than the others"[26(p69)] (see Table 1–4). Districts with a mixture of the clean and polluted drinking water (Southwark and Vauxhall and Lambeth Companies combined) had 35% fewer cholera deaths (61 versus 94 deaths per 10,000) than districts with only polluted drinking water (Southwark and Vauxhall Company alone).

TABLE 1–4 Mortality from Cholera in Relation to the Water Supply Companies in the Districts of London, November 1853

Water supply company	Number of cholera deaths	Size of population	Death rate resulting from cholera
Southwark and Vauxhall	111	118,267	94/100,000
Southwark and Vauxhall, Lambeth	211	346,363	61/100,000

Source: Data from Snow J. *Snow on Cholera*, p. 69. New York, NY: Hafner Publishers; 1965. With permission from the Commonwealth Fund, New York, NY.

TABLE 1–5 Mortality from Cholera in Relation to the Water Supply Companies in the Subdistricts of London, 1853

Water supply company	Number of cholera deaths	Size of population	Death rate resulting from cholera
Southwark and Vauxhall alone	192	167,654	114/100,000
Southwark and Vauxhall, and Lambeth combined	182	301,149	60/100,000
Lambeth alone	0	14,632	0/100,000

Source: Data from Snow J. *Snow on Cholera*, p. 73. New York, NY: Hafner Publishers; 1965. With permission from the Commonwealth Fund, New York, NY.

Snow next analyzed the cholera mortality data in smaller geographic units—London subdistricts—in order to make an even clearer distinction between the polluted and clean water supplies. In particular, he examined the death rates in the London subdistricts supplied by: (1) the Southwark and Vauxhall Company alone (heavily polluted water), (2) the Lambeth Company alone (nonpolluted water), and (3) both companies combined (a mixture of polluted and nonpolluted water). The cholera death rates were highest in subdistricts supplied by the heavily polluted water of the Southwark and Vauxhall Company and were intermediate in subdistricts supplied by the mixed water from the Southwark and Vauxhall Company and Lambeth Company combined. No cholera deaths were observed in subdistricts supplied with the nonpolluted water of the Lambeth Company (see Table 1–5).

Although Snow thought that these data provided "very strong evidence of the powerful influence which the drinking of water containing the sewage of a town exerts over the spread of cholera, when that disease is present," he thought that further study of the people living in the subdistricts supplied by both companies would "yield the most incontrovertible proof on one side or another." Snow understood that the differences in cholera deaths rates between the two companies might not have been caused by the water supply itself but rather by differences between the groups such as differences in gender, age, and socioeconomic status. Fortunately for Snow, further study revealed that the two groups were strikingly similar.

Snow made the following observation:

> In the subdistricts enumerated in the above table as being supplied by both companies, the mixing of the supply is of the most intimate kind. The pipes of each Company go down all the street, and into nearly all the courts and alleys. A few houses are supplied by one Company and a few by the other, according to the decision of the owner or occupier at that time when the water companies were in active competition. In many cases a single house has a supply different from that on either side. Each company supplied both rich and poor, both large houses and small; there is no difference either in the condition or occupation of the persons receiving the water of different companies. . . . As there is no difference whatever, either in the houses or the people receiving the supply of the two Water Companies, or in any of the physical conditions with which they are surrounded, it is obvious that no experiment could have been devised which would more thoroughly test the effect of water supply on the progress of cholera than this, which circumstances placed ready made before the observer. The experiment, too, was on the grandest scale. No fewer than three hundred thousand people of both sexes, of every age and occupation, and of every rank and station, from gentlefolks down to the very poor, were divided into two groups without their choice, and, in most cases, without their knowledge; one group being supplied with water containing the sewage of London, and amongst it, whatever might have come from the cholera patients, the other group having water quite free from such impurity.[26(pp74–75)]

Snow's next step was to obtain a listing from the General Register of the addresses of persons dying of cholera in the subdistricts that used water from both suppliers. Then he had the difficult task of going door to door to inquire about the drinking water supplier. According to Snow, "The inquiry was necessarily attended with a good deal of trouble. There were very few instances in which I could get the information I required. Even when the water-rates are paid by the residents, they can seldom remember the name of the Water Company till they have looked for the receipt."[26(p76)] However, Snow found an ingenious solution to this problem:

> It would, indeed, have been almost impossible for me to complete the inquiry, if I had not found that I could distinguish the water of the two companies with perfect certainty by a chemical test. The test I employed was founded on the great difference in the quantity of chloride of sodium contained in the two kinds of water. On adding solution of nitrate of silver to a gallon of water of the Lambeth Company . . . only 2.28 grains of chloride of silver were obtained. . . . On treating the water of Southwark

TABLE 1–6 Mortality from Cholera in Relation to the Water Supply Companies in the Subdistricts of London, July–August 1854

Water supply company	Number of cholera deaths	Number of houses	Death rate resulting from cholera
Southwark and Vauxhall Company	1,263	40,046	315/10,000
Lambeth Company	98	26,107	37/10,000
Rest of London	1,422	256,423	59/10,000

Source: Adapted from Snow J. *Snow on Cholera*, p. 86. New York, NY: Hafner Publishers; 1965. With permission from the Commonwealth Fund, New York, NY.

and Vauxhall Company in the same manner, 91 grains of chloride of silver were obtained.[26(pp77–78)]

Thus, Snow identified the drinking water source of each household and was able to link the death rate from cholera to the water supply companies (see Table 1–6). He concluded, "The mortality in the houses supplied by the Southwark and Vauxhall Company was therefore between eight and nine times as great as in the houses supplied by the Lambeth Company."[26(p86)]

Based on his findings, Snow made a series of recommendations for the prevention of cholera. For example, he recommended, "Care should be taken that the water employed for drinking and preparing food . . . is not contaminated with the contents of cesspools, house-drains, or sewers; or in the event that water free from suspicion cannot be obtained, is [sic] should be well boiled, and if possible, also filtered."[26(pp133–134)] Even though his results and recommendations were reported at once to William Farr and others, it took several years for Snow's theories to be accepted.[27]

Fortunately, over time we have come to recognize the importance of John Snow's contributions to our understanding of infectious diseases, in general, and cholera, in particular. For several reasons, Snow's investigations are considered "a nearly perfect model" for epidemiologic research.[26(pix)] First, Snow organized his observations logically so that meaningful inferences could be derived from them.[20(p29)] Second, he recognized that "a natural experiment" had occurred in the subdistricts of London that would enable him to gather unquestionable proof either for or against his hypothesis. Third, he conducted a quantitative analysis of the data contrasting the occurrence of cholera deaths in relation to the drinking water company.

Modern Experimental Studies

The development and application of epidemiologic methods advanced slowly during the late 1800s and early 1900s. Only during the 1930s and

1940s did physicians begin to realize that it was necessary to refine the methods used to evaluate the effectiveness of disease treatments.[28] Although some physicians still thought that they could assess the usefulness of a treatment merely by observing the patient's response and comparing it to what they expected on the basis of their education and experience, many realized that "modern" experimental studies with comparable treatment and control groups of patients, and comparable methods for assessing the disease changes were needed to yield correct conclusions.[29]

Streptomycin Tuberculosis Trial

In the late 1940s the Streptomycin in Tuberculosis Trials Committee of the British Medical Research Council conducted one of the first modern experimental studies on the use of streptomycin to treat pulmonary tuberculosis.[30] According to the investigators:

> The natural course of pulmonary tuberculosis is in fact so variable and unpredictable that evidence of improvement or cure following the use of a new drug in a few cases cannot be accepted as proof of the effect of that drug. The history of chemotherapeutic trials in tuberculosis is filled with errors due to empirical evaluation of drugs. . . . It had become obvious that . . . conclusions regarding the clinical effect of a new chemotherapeutic agent in tuberculosis could be considered valid only if based on adequately controlled clinical trials.[30(p4582)]

This controlled clinical trial of streptomycin included 107 patients with acute progressive bilateral pulmonary tuberculosis.[30] The investigators decided to include only cases of tuberculosis that were unsuitable for other forms of treatment in order "to avoid having to make allowances for the effect of forms of therapy other than bed-rest." In addition, they excluded cases in which spontaneous regression was likely and cases in which there was little hope of improvement.

One group of 55 patients was treated with bed rest and streptomycin, and a second group of 52 patients was treated with bed rest alone.[30] Patients were assigned to these groups by an innovative method known as randomization, which is defined as "an act of assigning or ordering that is the result of a random process."[23(p220)] As described in Chapter 7, random assignment methods include flipping a coin or using a sequence of random numbers. The exact process used in the Streptomycin Tuberculosis Trial was as follows: "Determination of whether a patient would be treated by streptomycin and bed rest (S case) or by bed rest alone (C case) was made by reference to a statistical series based on random sampling numbers drawn up for each sex at each centre by Professor Bradford Hill; the details of the series were unknown to any of the investigators or to the co-ordinator and were contained in a set of sealed envelopes."[30(p770)]

Patients in the streptomycin group received the drug by injection four times a day.[30] Although investigators observed toxic effects in many patients, these effects were not so severe as to require the termination of treatment. During the 6-month follow-up period, 7% of the streptomycin patients died and 27% of the control patients died. Investigators observed x-ray evidence of considerable pulmonary improvement in 51% of the streptomycin patients and only 8% of the control patients. Clinical improvement was also more common in the streptomycin group. The investigators reached the following conclusion: "The course of bilateral acute progressive disease can be halted by streptomycin therapy. . . . That streptomycin was the agent responsible for this result is attested by the presence in this trial of the control group of patients, among whom considerable improvement was noted in only four (8%)."[30(p780)]

According to Richard Doll, "Few innovations have made such an impact on medicine as the controlled clinical trial that was designed by Sir Austin Bradford Hill for the Medical Research Council's Streptomycin in Tuberculosis Trials Committee in 1946."[29(p343)] Four features of the trial were particularly innovative. First and foremost was its use of randomization to assign patients to the streptomycin and control groups. Although randomization had been used in agriculture and laboratory research, this trial was one of the first instances in which it was used in medical research. As described in Chapter 7, the main advantage of randomization is that the order of future assignments cannot be predicted from that of past ones. Lack of predictability is the key to minimizing bias, which is defined as a systematic error in the study that causes a false conclusion.

The second innovation was the placement of restrictions on the type of patient eligible for the trial.[29] Patients with the type of tuberculosis that was unsuitable for therapies other than bed rest were excluded so that the results would not be obscured by the effects of other treatments. Patients who were likely to get better without any treatment or who were so ill that the streptomycin was unlikely to help were also excluded.

Third, the data collection methods helped ensure that the results would be free of bias.[29] These methods included using a precise and objective endpoint such as death, and masking the investigators who were assessing the radiological improvements. Masking means that the investigators who reviewed the x-rays were unaware of the person's treatment assignment and so the chances of their making a biased judgment were reduced.

Fourth, the investigators considered the ethical issues involved in conducting the trial, including whether it was ethical to withhold the streptomycin treatment from the control group.[29] Before the trial was conducted, researchers had already shown that streptomycin inhibited the tubercle bacillus in vitro and reduced experimental infections of guinea pigs. Preliminary results of clinical studies had also been encouraging. However, only a small amount of the drug was available in Britain, and it was impossible to treat all patients with tuberculosis. Thus, the committee reasoned, "It would . . . have been unethical *not* to have seized the opportunity to design a strictly controlled trial, which could speedily and effectively reveal the value of the treatment."[29(p339)]

Doll and Hill's Studies on Smoking and Lung Cancer

Most epidemiologists consider Richard Doll and A. Bradford Hill's 1950 study on smoking and lung cancer to be one of the major milestones of epidemiology.[31] Doll and Hill undertook the study because of the striking increase in lung cancer death rates in England and Wales following World War I.[32] Some scientists argued that the increase was the result of improvements in lung cancer diagnosis. However, Doll and Hill believed that improved diagnosis could not be entirely responsible, because the number of lung cancer deaths had increased in areas with and without modern diagnostic facilities. Thus, Doll and Hill thought it was "right and proper" to justify searching for an environmental cause. Their work is emblematic of an important shift in epidemiology following World War II that redirected the focus of epidemiologic research from infectious to chronic diseases.[31] The shift was fueled by the idea that chronic diseases were not merely degenerative disorders of old age but rather were potentially preventable diseases with environmental origins.

Doll and Hill's first study was a "case–control study,"[32] an epidemiologic design that is described in more detail in Chapter 9. The study included 709 subjects who had lung cancer (the cases) and 709 subjects who had diseases other than cancer (the controls). Control patients were purposely selected to be of the same sex, within the same 5-year age group, and in the same hospital at approximately the same time as the lung cancer patients.

Patients from each group were interviewed about their smoking habits while they were in the hospital for treatment. In particular, they were asked: "(a) if they had smoked at any period of their lives; (b) the ages at which they had started and stopped; (c) the amount they were in the habit of smoking before the onset of the illness which had brought them to the hospital; (d) the main changes in their smoking history and the maximum they had ever been in the habit of smoking; (e) the varying proportions smoked in pipes and cigarettes; and (f) whether or not they inhaled."[32(p741)]

Doll and Hill found that proportionately more lung cancer patients than noncancer patients were smokers.[32] In particular, 99.7% of male lung cancer patients and 95.8% of male noncancer patients smoked; 68.3% of female lung cancer patients and only 46.7% of female noncancer patients were smokers. Furthermore, a higher proportion of patients with lung cancer described themselves as heavy smokers. For example, 26.0% of the male lung cancer patients and 13.5% of the male noncancer patients reported that they had smoked 25 or more cigarettes per day before their illness began. Although the authors acknowledged that they did not know what carcinogens in tobacco smoke might be responsible, they concluded that "smoking is an important factor in the cause of lung cancer."

Three other case–control studies published in 1950 also showed an association between smoking and lung cancer. However, modern epidemiologists consider the Doll and Hill study to be "a classic exemplar for the investigation of a given outcome and an array of exposures. . . . No previous research paper lays out the essentials of the case–control method with such understanding and meticulous care."[31(p163)] Far in advance of their peers, Doll and Hill considered a wide range of problems in the design and analysis of their study, including errors that may have occurred when they recruited and interviewed their subjects. These topics are described in Chapters 10 and 11.

In the years following the 1950 Doll and Hill study, several more studies were conducted using the case–control approach of comparing the smoking histories of patients with and without lung cancer (such as Wynder and Cornfeld's 1953 study).[33] These studies all found that the proportion of smokers, particularly heavy smokers, was higher among lung cancer patients than among noncancer patients. However, Doll and Hill believed that additional "retrospective" studies were "unlikely to advance our knowledge materially or to throw any new light upon the nature of the association." (Retrospective studies investigate diseases that have already occurred.) They asserted that if there were "any undetected flaw in the evidence that such studies have produced, it would be exposed only by some entirely new approach." The new approach that they proposed was a "prospective" study, a study that follows participants into the future in order to observe the occurrence of disease (see Chapter 8).

Doll and Hill initiated a prospective study in 1951 by inviting 59,600 male and female members of the British Medical Association to complete a short questionnaire about their smoking habits.[34] The investigators then divided the respondents into four groups on the basis of their answers: nonsmokers and light, moderate, and heavy smokers. The investigators obtained information on the causes of death among those who answered the questionnaire from the Registrars-General Office in the United Kingdom.

During the 29-month period following the administration of the questionnaire, 789 deaths were reported among the 24,389 male doctors aged 35 years and older. Of these deaths, 36 were reported to have died of lung cancer as either the direct or contributory cause. After accounting for age differences between the smoking groups, the investigators found that death rates caused by lung cancer increased from 0.0 per 1000 among nonsmokers to 0.48 per 1000 among light smokers, 0.67 per 1000 among moderate smokers, and 1.14 per 1000 among heavy smokers.[34]

The investigators continued to follow the doctors for the next 20 years.[35] During this period they updated the smoking and mortality data. Of the 34,400 men studied, 10,072 were known to have died from November 1951 through October 1971. Among men under the age of 70 years, the death rate was about twice as high among cigarette smokers as among lifelong nonsmokers. The causes of death related to smoking included not only lung cancer but also heart disease, chronic obstructive lung disease, and a variety of vascular diseases.

Because the proportion of doctors who smoked cigarettes declined over the 20-year period, the investigators were also able to examine the death rate among former smokers who had stopped smoking for various lengths of time. They found that, as compared to lifelong nonsmokers, the risk of lung cancer death among ex-smokers steadily declined in relation to the number of years since they had stopped smoking. However, even 15 or more years after quitting, the risk of lung cancer death was still twice as high among former smokers than among lifelong nonsmokers.

Like their first case–control study, Doll and Hill's prospective study broke new ground. First, the study included tens of thousands of subjects, and so it had adequate "power" to examine numerous health effects of several levels of smoking. Second, the investigators followed the subjects for a long period of time. A long follow-up period is particularly important in the study of diseases such as cancer that take decades to develop. Third, Doll and Hill incorporated changes in smoking habits over time, and so were able to examine the health benefits of smoking cessation.

The Framingham Study

Like the work of Doll and Hill, the Framingham Study is notable for bringing about a shift in focus from infectious to noninfectious diseases following World War II. Considered "the epitome of successful epidemiologic research," this study "has become the prototype and model of the cohort study."[31(p157)] The cohort study is one of the three main study designs used in epidemiologic research, and is described in Chapters 6 and 8.

According to Susser, the Framingham Study is "undisputably the foundation stone for current ideas about risk factors in general and the prevention of ischemic heart disease in particular." In addition, it has provided the impetus for solving difficult design and analysis issues in epidemiologic research, including the development of appropriate methods for measuring the major risk factors for coronary heart disease (such as high blood pressure, elevated serum cholesterol levels, physical activity, and life stress) and for solving problems associated with measurements that vary over time.[31(pp157–161)] The study has also served as a stimulus for developing other cohort studies of cardiovascular disease and other topics.

When the Framingham Study was started in 1947, its goal was to develop ways of identifying latent cardiovascular disease among healthy volunteers.[31] Within a few years, investigators expanded the study's purpose to include determining the causes of cardiovascular disease. The study now investigates a wide variety of diseases, including stroke, cerebrovascular disease, diabetes, Alzheimer's disease, and cancer, and it includes the offspring and grandchildren of the original participants.

Initially, the investigators enrolled about 5000 healthy adult residents in Framingham, Massachusetts, a town located about 18 miles west of Boston.[36(pp14–29)] In the late 1940s, Framingham was a self-contained community of about 28,000 residents who obtained their medical care from local physicians and two hospitals near the center of town. Framingham residents were considered an excellent population for a community-based prospective study because (1) the town's population was stable, (2) the investigators could identify a sufficient number of people with and without risk factors for heart disease, and (3) local medical doctors were eager to help recruit study subjects.

For the past 50 years Framingham Study participants have undergone interviews, physical exams, laboratory tests, and other tests every 2 years.[37] The interviews have gathered information on each subject's medical history and history of cigarette smoking, alcohol use, physical activity, dietary intake, and emotional stress. The physical exams and laboratory tests have measured characteristics such as height and weight, blood pressure, vital signs and symptoms, cholesterol levels, glucose levels, and bone mineral density. These data-gathering efforts have left an immeasurable legacy of research findings on numerous topics.

Modern Epidemiology

In recent years the field of epidemiology has expanded tremendously in size, scope, and influence. The number of epidemiologists has grown rapidly along with the number of epidemiology training programs in schools of public health and medicine. Many subspecialties have been established that are defined either by (1) disease, (2) exposure, or (3) population being studied. Disease-specific subspecialties include reproductive, cancer, cardiovascular, infectious disease, and psychiatric epidemiology. Exposure-specific subspecialties include environmental, behavioral, and nutritional epidemiology and pharmaco-epidemiology. Population-specific subspecialties include pediatric and geriatric epidemiology.

In addition, the scope of epidemiologic research has expanded in two divergent directions. First, some epidemiologists examine health determinants at the molecular and genetic level and so combine the basic and public health sciences. For example, genetic epidemiology investigates whether certain diseases cluster in families, whether the clustering is caused by inherited factors or a shared environment, and how genes influence the risk of disease.[38] Molecular epidemiology involves the use of "molecular markers" to improve the measurement of exposure and diseases.[39(pp413–415)] For example, molecular markers such as serum micronutrient levels can determine a person's fruit and vegetable intake more accurately than can personal interviews.

The second new direction of epidemiologic research involves the study of determinants at the biological and societal level.[40] Social epidemiology is the study of exposures and disease susceptibility and resistance at diverse levels including the individual, household, neighborhood, and region. For example, social epidemiologists investigate how neighborhoods, racial discrimination, and poverty influence a person's health.

In addition, the theories and methods of epidemiologic research have evolved during recent years. For example, epidemiologists have developed new views on disease causation such as the "sufficient-component cause model." The theoretical framework underlying epidemiologic study designs has matured, particularly the conceptualization and design of the case–control study. Finally, the availability of high-powered computer hardware and software has facilitated the analysis of large data sets with many risk factors, enabling epidemiologists to explore new public health questions and to assess the effects of multiple risk factors simultaneously.

Not surprisingly, epidemiology is currently being used to investigate a wide range of important public health topics. Noteworthy topics that have been examined recently include the risk of brain cancer among cell phone users,[41] the epidemiology of emerging and re-emerging infectious diseases such as HIV and tuberculosis,[42] unexplained chronic illnesses among Persian Gulf War veterans,[43] molecular epidemiology of Alzheimer's disease,[44] the effectiveness of mammography for women under the age of 50 years,[45] the safety of hormone replacement therapy during menopause,[46] and the effectiveness of alternative medicines in treating disease.[47]

The 21st century poses even more challenging problems for epidemiologists such as "air, water and soil pollution; global warming; population growth; poverty and social inequality; and civil unrest and violence."[48(p5)] A recent editorial on epidemiology in the 21st century noted that, like public health achievements of the past, solutions to these problems will occur through "the complementary contributions of different facets of epidemiology: calculating disease trends and probabilities, communicating findings to the public and policy makers, and designing and implementing interventions based on data."[49(p1154)] The editorialists went on to observe: "Epidemiology's full value is achieved only when its contributions are placed in the context of public health action, resulting in a healthier populace. . . . Like others in epidemiology's rich history, we should keep our eyes on the prizes of preventing disease and promoting health."[49(p1155)] The prospect of preventing disease and death through "analytic prowess" has attracted many great minds to epidemiology throughout its history, and it will undoubtedly continue to attract them in the coming century.

Summary

Disease prevention and health promotion are the main goals of public health, a multidisciplinary field that focuses on populations and communities rather than separate individuals. Epidemiology, one of the basic sciences of public health, is defined as "the study of the distribution and determinants of disease frequency in human populations and the application of this study to control health problems." Epidemiology has played an important role in public health achievements of the last 400 years. Key historic figures and studies have included John Graunt, who summarized the patterns of mortality in 17th-century London; James Lind, who discovered the cause and prevention of scurvy using an experimental study design in the 18th century; William Farr, who originated many modern epidemiologic methods in the 19th century including the combination of numerator and denominator data; John Snow, who demonstrated that contaminated drinking water was the mode of cholera transmission in the 19th century; members of the Streptomycin in Tuberculosis Trials Committee, who conducted one of the first modern controlled clinical trials in the 1940s; Doll and Hill, who conducted case–control studies on smoking and lung cancer in the 1950s; and investigators who have worked on the Framingham Study, a study that was started in 1947 and has become one of the most influential studies of heart disease in the world. In recent years the field of epidemiology has greatly expanded in size, scope, and influence, and epidemiologists currently investigate a wide range of important public health problems. The 21st century will pose even more challenging problems for epidemiologists. Like past public health achievements, the solutions to these problems will be found by placing the contributions of epidemiology in the context of public health action.

References

1. Schneider MJ. *Introduction to Public Health*. Gaithersburg, MD: Aspen Publishers, Inc; 2000.
2. National Center for Health Statistics. *Health, United States, 2000 with Adolescent Health Chart Book*. Hyattsville, MD: Public Health Service; 2000.
3. Bunker JP, Frazier HS, Mosteller F. Improving health: measuring effects of medical care. *Milbank Q*. 1994;72:225–258.
4. Centers for Disease Control and Prevention. Ten great public health achievements—United States, 1900–1999. *MMWR*. 1999;48:241–243.

5. Loomis TA. *Essentials of Toxicology.* 3rd ed. Philadelphia, PA: Lea & Febiger; 1978.
6. Gottlieb MS, Schanker HM, Fan PT, Saxon A, Weisman JD, Pozalski I. *Pneumocystis* pneumonia—Los Angeles. *MMWR.* 1981;30:250–252.
7. Friedman-Kien A, Laubenstein L, Marmor M, et al. Kaposi's sarcoma and *Pneumocystis* pneumonia among homosexual men—New York City and California. *MMWR.* 1981;30:305–308.
8. Boice JD, Monson RR. Breast cancer in women after repeated fluoroscopic examination of the chest. *J Natl Cancer Inst.* 1977;59:823–832.
9. Weitzman M, Aschengrau A, Bellinger D, Jones R, Hamlin JS, Beiser A. Lead-contaminated soil abatement and urban children's blood lead levels. *JAMA.* 1993;269:1647–1654.
10. Pickett JP, ed. *The American Heritage Dictionary of the English Language.* 4th ed. Boston, MA: Houghton Mifflin; 2000.
11. Simpson JA, Weiner ESC, eds. *Oxford English Dictionary.* 2nd ed. Oxford, England: Clarendon Press; 1989. OED Online. Oxford University Press; Accessed 20 July 2001.
12. Lilienfeld D. Definitions of epidemiology. *Am J Epidemiol.* 1978;107:87–90.
13. MacMahon B, Trichopoulos D. *Epidemiology: Principles and Methods.* 2nd ed. Boston, MA: Little, Brown and Co; 1996.
14. Last JM. *A Dictionary of Epidemiology,* 3rd ed. New York, NY: Oxford University Press; 1995.
15. MacMahon B, Pugh TF. *Epidemiology: Principles and Methods.* Boston, MA: Little, Brown and Co; 1970.
16. Centers for Disease Control and Prevention. National Health Interview Survey. Available at: http://www.cdc.gov/nchs/about/major/nhis. Accessed January 2001.
17. Kelsey JL. Breast cancer epidemiology. *Epidemiol Rev.* 1993;15:256–263.
18. Benenson AS, ed. *Control of Communicable Diseases in Man.* 15th ed. Washington DC: American Public Health Association; 1990.
19. Centers for Disease Control and Prevention. *HIV/AIDS Surveillance Rep.* 1999; 11:1–44.
20. Lilienfeld DE, Stolley. *Foundations of Epidemiology.* 3rd ed. New York, NY: Oxford University Press; 1994.
21. Graunt J. *Natural and Political Observations Made upon the Bills of Mortality.* Willcox WF, ed. Baltimore, MD: The John Hopkins Press; 1939.
22. Rothman KJ. Lessons from John Graunt. *Lancet.* 1996;347:37–39.
23. Meinert CL. *Clinical Trials Dictionary, Terminology and Usage Recommendations.* Baltimore, MD: The Johns Hopkins Center for Clinical Trials; 1996.
24. Stewart CP, Guthrie D, eds. *Lind's Treatise on Scurvy. A Bicentenary Volume Containing a Reprint of the First Edition of a Treatise of the Scurvy by James Lind, MD, with Additional Notes.* Edinburgh, Scotland: Edinburgh University Press; 1953.
25. Farr, W. *Vital Statistics: A Memorial Volume of Selections from the Reports and Writings of William Farr.* New York, NY: New York Academy of Medicine; 1975.
26. Snow J. *On the Mode of Communication of Cholera.* 2nd ed. London, England: Churchill, 1855. Reprinted as Snow J. *Snow on Cholera.* New York, NY: Hafner Publishing Co; 1965.

27. Winkelstein W. A new perspective on John Snow's communicable disease theory. *Am J Epidemiol.* 1995;142:S3–S9.
28. Vandenbroucke JP. Second thoughts: a short note on the history of the randomized controlled trial. *J Chron Dis.* 1987;40:985–987.
29. Doll R. Clinical trials: retrospect and prospect. *Stat Med.* 1982;1:337–344.
30. Medical Research Council. Streptomycin in Tuberculosis Trials Committee. Streptomycin treatment of pulmonary tuberculosis. *Br Med J.* 1948;2:769–782.
31. Susser M. Epidemiology in the United States after World War II: the evolution of technique. *Epidemiol Rev.* 1985;7:147–177.
32. Doll R, Hill AB. Smoking and carcinoma of the lung. *Br Med J.* 1950;2:739–748.
33. Wynder EL, Cornfeld J. Cancer of the lung in physicians. *N Engl J Med.* 1953; 248:441–444.
34. Doll R, Hill AB. The mortality of doctors in relation to their smoking habits. *Br Med J.* 1954;1:1451–1455.
35. Doll R, Peto R. Mortality in relation to smoking: 20 years' observations on male British doctors. *Br Med J.* 1976;2:1525–1536.
36. Dawber TR. *The Framingham Study: The Epidemiology of Atherosclerotic Disease.* Cambridge, MA: Harvard University Press; 1980.
37. Kannel WB. The Framingham Study: its 50-year legacy and future promise. *J Atheroscler Thromb.* 2000;6:60–66.
38. Beaty TH, Khoury MJ. Interface of genetics and epidemiology. *Epidemiol Rev.* 2000;22:120–125.
39. Friis RH, Sellers TA. *Epidemiology for Public Health Practice.* 2nd ed. Gaithersburg, MD: Aspen Publishers, Inc; 1999.
40. Kreiger N. Epidemiology and social sciences: towards a critical reengagement in the 21st century. *Epidemiol Rev.* 2000;22:155–163.
41. Hardell L, Nasman A, Pahlson A, Hallquist A, Hanssion Mild K. Use of cellular telephones and the risk for brain tumours: a case–control study. *Int J Oncol.* 1999;15:113–116.
42. Horsburgh CR Jr, Pozniak A. Epidemiology of tuberculosis in the era of HIV. *AIDS.* 1993;7(suppl 1):S109–S114.
43. Centers for Disease Control and Prevention. Leads from the *Morbidity and Mortality Weekly Report,* Atlanta, GA: Unexplained illness among Persian Gulf War veterans in an Air National Guard Unit: preliminary report, August 1990–March 1995. *JAMA.* 1995;274:16–17.
44. Hyman BT, Tanzi R. Molecular epidemiology of Alzheimer's disease. *N Engl J Med.* 1995;333:1283–1284.
45. Smith RA. Breast cancer screening among women younger than age 50: a current assessment of the issues. *CA Cancer J Clin.* 2000;50:312–336.
46. Finkel ML, Cohen M, Mahoney H. Treatment options for the menopausal woman. *Nurse Pract.* 2001;26:5–17.
47. Moyad MA, Hathaway S, Ni HS. Traditional Chinese medicine, acupuncture, and other alternative medicines for prostate cancer: an introduction and the need for more research. *Semin Urol Oncol.* 1999;17:103–110.
48. Winkelstein W. Interface of epidemiology and history: a commentary on past, present, and future. *Epidemiol Rev.* 2000;22:2–6.
49. Koplan JP, Thacker SB, Lezin NA. Epidemiology in the 21st century: calculation, communication, and intervention. *Am J Public Health.* 1999;89:1153–1155.

EXERCISES

1. Define each of the following terms:
   A. Public health
   B. Epidemiology
   C. Population

2. What is the primary difference between public health and medicine?

3. What are the main objectives of epidemiology?

4. How do epidemiologists quantify the disease frequency in a population?

5. State the contribution that was made by each of the following historical figures:
   A. John Graunt
   B. John Snow
   C. Richard Doll and Austin Bradford Hill

2

Measures of Disease Frequency

LEARNING OBJECTIVES

By the end of this chapter, the reader will be able to:

- Define and provide examples of a population.
- Distinguish between a fixed and dynamic (or open) population.
- Explain how epidemiologists create a case definition and discuss how the definition of acquired immunodeficiency syndrome (AIDS) has changed over time.
- Describe the key aspects of measuring disease occurrence.
- Define and distinguish between cumulative incidence, incidence rate, and prevalence.
- Describe the mathematical relationship between the measures of disease frequency.
- Provide examples of commonly used measures of disease frequency in public health.

Introduction

As described in Chapter 1, epidemiologists study the distribution and determinants of disease frequency in human populations in order to control health problems.[1] (p1), [2](p55) Thus, the objectives of epidemiology are to determine the extent of disease in a population, identify patterns and trends in disease occurrence, identify the causes of disease, and evaluate the effectiveness of prevention and treatment activities. Measuring how often a disease arises in a population is usually the first step in achieving these goals.

This chapter describes how epidemiologists quantify the occurrence of disease in a population. Readers will learn that this quantification process involves developing a definition of a particular disease, counting the number of people who are affected by the disease, determining the size of the population from which the diseased cases arose, and accounting for the passage of time.

Definition of a Population

Because epidemiology is concerned with the occurrence of disease in groups of people rather than in individuals, populations are at the heart of epidemiologists' measurements. A population can be defined as a group of people with a common characteristic such as place of residence, religion, gender, age, use of hospital services, or life event (such as giving birth).

Location of residence such as a country, state, city, or neighborhood is one of the most common ways to define a population. For example, the people who reside in the Brooklyn borough of New York City, the city of Boston, the state of Oregon, and the country of Sweden are members of distinct populations defined by geopolitical entities ranging in size from a neighborhood to an entire country. Residence near natural geographic features such as rivers, mountains, lakes, or islands can also be used to define a population. For example, people who live along the 2350-mile length of the Mississippi River, around Mount St. Helens in Washington State, and on Nantucket Island off the coast of Massachusetts are members of populations defined by geographic formations.

Because epidemiology focuses on disease occurrence, populations are commonly defined in relation to a medical facility such as a doctor's office, clinic, or hospital. The service population of a medical facility (also called catchment population) consists of the people who use the facility's services. This population is often difficult to define because an individual's decision to use a facility may depend on how far it is from home, the person's particular medical condition, his or her type of medical insurance, and so forth.

Consider a situation in which a county has only one general hospital, which provides the complete range of medical services including preventive care, birthing services, and diagnostic and therapeutic services for acute and chronic conditions. The catchment population for this general hospital is likely to consist of all people who live in the county where the hospital is located (see Figure 2–1).

Now suppose that this hospital enhances its cardiology department, adding many well-trained clinicians and the latest diagnostic equipment. As the cardiology department's reputation for excellent care grows, patients travel from greater distances to receive care. As a result, the catchment population for the cardiology department expands to the surround-

Single county hospital with local catchment population

County hospital specialty clinic with broad catchment population

Public and private hospitals whose catchment populations vary by socioeconomic status

FIGURE 2–1. Types of Hospital Catchment Areas

ing counties while the catchment population for the other hospital services, particularly those dealing with acute conditions requiring prompt treatment, remains the single county where the hospital is situated (see Figure 2–1).

Socioeconomic status is still another determinant of hospital catchment populations. Consider a city in which there are two hospitals—one public and one private—located within a few miles of each other. The private hospital generally treats patients with medical insurance, and the public hospital mainly treats patients without insurance. Even though each catchment population resides roughly within the same geographic area, the two service groups are distinct in terms of income, and probably many other factors (see Figure 2–1).

Still another way that a population can be defined is by the occurrence of a life event such as undergoing a medical procedure, giving birth to a child, entering or graduating from school, or serving in the military. For

TABLE 2–1   Types of Populations

Type of population	Key element	Example
Fixed	Membership is based on an event and is permanent	Japanese atomic bomb survivors
Dynamic or open	Membership is based on a condition and is transitory	Residents of a city, hospital patients

example, students who graduated from high school in 1995 are members of the population known as the "Class of '95," and the men and women who served in the U.S. military during the Persian Gulf War are members of the population known as Gulf War veterans. Populations are often defined by other characteristics such as age, gender, religion, or type of job.

A unifying framework for thinking about a population is whether its membership is permanent or transient (see Table 2–1). A population whose membership is permanent is called a *fixed population*. Its membership is always defined by a life event. For example, the people who were in Hiroshima, Japan, when the atomic bomb exploded at the end of World War II are members of a fixed population. This population will never gain any new members because only people who were at this historical event can be members.

The opposite of a fixed population is a *dynamic* or *open population*. Its membership is defined by a changeable state or condition, and so is transient. A person is a member of a dynamic population only as long as he or she has the defining state or condition. For example, the population of the city of Boston is dynamic because people are members only while they reside within the city limits. Turnover is always occurring because people enter the city by moving in or by birth, and people leave the city by moving away or by death. The term *steady state* describes a situation in which the number of people entering the population is equal to the number leaving. Dynamic populations include groups defined by geographic and hospital catchment areas, religious groups, and occupations.

Regardless of the way in which it is defined, a population can be divided into subgroups on the basis of any characteristic. For example, men who undergo coronary bypass surgery are a gender subgroup of a fixed population defined by a life event, and all children up to 6 years of age who live along the Mississippi River are an age subgroup of a dynamic population defined by a geographic formation.

Definitions of Health and Disease

In 1948, the World Health Organization defined health as "a state of complete physical, mental and social well-being and not merely the absence of disease or infirmity."[3] More recently, *Healthy People 2000*, a national plan for improving the health of the American people, stated: "The health of a people is measured by more than death rates. . . . It comes from an improved quality of life. Health is best measured by citizens' sense of well-being."[4]

Because measurement is a cornerstone of epidemiology, and "health" and "a sense of well-being" are nonspecific and difficult to quantify, epidemiologists have almost entirely focused their activities on the "absence of health" such as specific diseases, injuries, disabilities, and death. Consequently, epidemiologists must first compose a definition of the "absence of health" or "disease" before they can begin measuring its frequency.

The definition of a disease is usually based on a combination of physical and pathological examinations, diagnostic test results, and signs and symptoms. Which and how many criteria are used to define a "case"—that is, a person who meets the disease definition, has important implications for accurately determining who has the disease.

Consider the various criteria that can be used to define a heart attack "case." One could use the symptoms of chest pain, the results of diagnostic tests such as electrocardiograms, or blood enzyme tests for cardiac damage. What are the implications of using only chest pain to define heart attack cases? Using only this nonspecific symptom will capture most but not all people who have heart attacks because it will miss people who have "silent" heart attacks that occur without chest pain. In addition, it will erroneously include many people who have other conditions that produce chest pain, such as indigestion.

A definition that includes more specific criteria such as the results of diagnostic tests will be more accurate. For example, if positive blood enzyme tests are included, silent heart attacks are likely to be picked up and the other conditions that cause chest pain omitted. In practice, epidemiologists use all available information from physical and pathological examinations and laboratory and other tests to define a case of a disease as accurately as possible.

Changes in Disease Definitions

Even when clear-cut criteria are used, disease definitions often change over time as more is learned about a disease and its various manifestations. For example, the official definition of acquired immune deficiency syndrome (AIDS) has been changed several times as researchers have gained knowledge about the disease's cause and natural course (see Table 2–2).

The story began in the summer of 1981 when the Centers for Disease Control and Prevention (CDC) reported that Kaposi's sarcoma and *Pneumocystis carinii* pneumonia had been observed among previously healthy homosexual men.[5] Previously, Kaposi's sarcoma, a malignant neoplasm of the blood vessels, had been seen primarily among elderly males, and opportunistic infections such as *Pneumocystis carinii* pneumonia had occurred almost exclusively in people with compromised immune systems.

In 1982 the CDC composed the first definition of AIDS for national reporting as "a disease, at least moderately predictive of a defect in cell-mediated immunity, occurring in a person with no known cause for diminished resistance to that disease . . . including Kaposi's Sarcoma, *Pneumocystis carinii* pneumonia, and serious other opportunistic infections."[6] Even then, the CDC acknowledged that the case definition was imperfect because it could possibly miss the full range of AIDS manifestations and falsely include individuals who were not truly immunodeficient. However, because the cause of AIDS was unknown at that time, the definition at least served as a consistent tool for monitoring the epidemic.

The CDC made the first major change in the official AIDS case definition in 1985 after the human immunodeficiency virus (HIV) was determined to be the cause of AIDS and a highly accurate laboratory test was developed to detect the antibody to the HIV virus.[7] Because epidemiologists now knew what to look for and how to find its trail, it was possible to expand the AIDS case definition from a few severe clinical conditions to a wide range of conditions accompanied by laboratory evidence of HIV infection. Conversely, it also became possible to exclude patients who had AIDS-like symptoms but had negative HIV antibody test results.

TABLE 2–2   Changes in the Definition of AIDS over Time

Year	Existing knowledge about AIDS	Conditions included in disease definition
1982	Very limited	Only a few conditions including Kaposi's sarcoma, Pneumocystis carinii pneumonia, and other severe opportunistic infections
1985	HIV virus discovered as cause of AIDS; antibody test developed	23 clinical conditions with laboratory evidence of infection
1993	Discovered importance of CD4 T lymphocytes in monitoring immunodeficiency and disease progression	26 clinical conditions and asymptomatic cases with low CD4 T lymphocyte counts

Sources: Data from Centers for Disease Control. Update on acquired immune deficiency syndrome (AIDS)—United States. *MMWR.* 1982;31:507–514. Centers for Disease Control. Revision of the case definition of acquired immune deficiency syndrome for national reporting—United States. *MMWR.* 1985;34:373–375. Centers for Disease Control. 1993 revised classification system for HIV infection and expanded surveillance case definition for AIDS among adolescents and adults. *MMWR.* 1992;44:1–19.

At the end of 1992, the CDC changed the AIDS case definition again after natural history studies revealed the importance of lymphocytes in the HIV infection.[8] The new definition was expanded to include individuals who had no symptoms of AIDS but had low levels of CD4 T lymphocytes, a type of white blood cell that is responsible for fighting off infections. (These cells are the primary target of HIV and are an excellent marker of disease progression.)

In summary, as epidemiologists discovered the cause of AIDS, learned more about its different manifestations, and developed a test to detect HIV, the AIDS case definition was expanded from a few severe diseases to many varied conditions and the results of sophisticated laboratory tests (see Table 2–2).

What impact did these changes in case definition have on the number of reported AIDS cases? In general, any expansion in the case definition will increase the number of reportable cases and any contraction will decrease that number. With AIDS, the definition changes increased the number of people who were officially counted as AIDS cases in national statistics. Public health officials estimate that the 1985 change produced only small increases in the number of cases, but the 1993 change increased the number of reported AIDS cases in the United States by 75% during the following year.[8] More recent trends in AIDS incidence are no longer affected by the change in the AIDS case definition.[9]

Measuring Disease Occurrence

Epidemiologists must always consider three factors when they measure how commonly a disease occurs in a group of people: (1) the number of people that are affected by the disease, (2) the size of the population from which the cases of disease arise, and (3) the length of time that the population is followed. Failure to consider all three components will give a false impression about the impact of the disease on a population.

Consider the following hypothetical data on the frequency of breast cancer in two counties. In County A, with a population of 50,000, 100 new cases of breast cancer occurred over a 1-year period. In County B, with a population of 5000, 75 new cases occurred over a 3-year period. Which county has a higher frequency of new breast cancer cases? If one considers only the number of new cases, it appears that County A has a higher frequency (100 versus 75). However, simply comparing the number of cases in each town does not provide a full picture because the cases occurred over different lengths of time (1 versus 3 years) and among populations of different sizes (50,000 versus 5000) (see Table 2–3).

In order to make a meaningful comparison between the two counties, it is necessary to convert the data into the same population size and time period. Let us estimate the frequency of breast cancer in the two counties over a 1-year period and as if each population consisted of 100,000 people.

TABLE 2–3 Hypothetical Data on the Frequency of Breast Cancer in Two Counties

Type of data	County A	County B
Number of cases	100	75
Population size	50,000	5,000
Follow-up period	1 year	3 years
Comparable disease frequency	200/100,000/year	500/100,000/year

The frequency of breast cancer in County A is 100 cases/50,000 population/1 year; if the county's population were 100,000, the frequency would double to become 200 cases/100,000 population/1 year.

Two steps are needed to make a similar conversion for County B. (1) Divide the numerator by three to convert the frequency of breast cancer from a 3- to a 1-year period: 25 cases/5000 population/1 year. (2) Multiply both the numerator and denominator by 20 to estimate the frequency for a population of 100,000. Thus, the frequency of new cases in County B is 500 cases/100,000 population/1 year.

Now it is clear that the "rate" at which new cases are occurring is much higher in County B than County A (500 cases/100,000 population/1 year versus 200 cases/100,000 population/1 year), and that examining only the number of new cases gives a false impression. Note that the decision to convert the frequencies to a population size of 100,000 and a 1-year time period, while commonly done, is arbitrary. Other population sizes (such as 1000 or 10,000) and time periods (such as 1 month or 5 years) could be used. The guiding principle is that the same population size and time period should be used for the compared groups.

Types of Calculations: Ratios, Proportions, and Rates

Three types of calculations are used to describe and compare measures of disease occurrence: ratios, proportions, and rates (see Table 2–4). A *ratio* is simply one number divided by another. The entities represented by the two numbers are not required to be related to one another. In other words, the individuals in the numerator can be different from those in the denominator. For example, the "sex ratio" is a ratio of two unrelated numbers: the number of males divided by the number of females, usually expressed as the number of males per 100 females. In the most recent U.S. Census, the sex ratio among U.S. residents aged 65 years and older was 69.9 males per 100 females.[10]

A *proportion* is also one number divided by another, but the entities represented by these numbers are related to one another. In fact, the numerator of a proportion is always a subset of the denominator. Proportions,

TABLE 2–4   Types of Calculations

Type of calculation	Characteristics
Ratio	Division of two unrelated numbers
Proportion	Division of two related numbers; numerator is a subset of denominator
Rate	Division of two numbers; time is always in denominator

also known as fractions, are often expressed as percentages and range from 0 to 1 or 0% to 100%. For example, the proportion of U.S. residents who are black is the number of black residents divided by the total number of U.S. residents of all races. In the most recent U.S. Census, the proportion of black U.S. residents was 0.123 or 12.3%.[10] The remaining proportion included whites (0.751 or 75.1%) and other or multiple races (0.126 or 12.6%). Note that these three proportions add up to 100% because the three groups (black, white, and all other races) are collectively exhaustive.

A *rate* is also one number divided by another, but time is an integral part of the denominator. We are familiar with rates in our daily travels since a rate is a measure of how fast we travel. For example, in many areas of the United States the maximum speed or rate at which cars are permitted to travel is 55 miles per hour. This rate can also be written as 55 miles/ 1 hour. The measure of time in the denominator is what makes this number a rate. The measures of disease occurrence calculated previously for Counties A and B are also rates (200 cases/100,000 population/1 year and 500 cases/100,000 population/1 year, respectively.) Unfortunately, the term *rate* is often incorrectly used to describe ratios and proportions.[11]

Measures of Disease Frequency

There are two basic measures of disease frequency in epidemiology—incidence and prevalence. *Incidence* measures the occurrence of new disease, and *prevalence* measures the existence of current disease. Each measure describes an important part of the natural course of a disease. Incidence deals with the transition from health to disease, and prevalence focuses on the period of time that a person lives with a disease.

Incidence

Incidence is defined as the occurrence of new cases of disease that develop in a candidate population over a specified time period. There are three key ideas in this definition. First, incidence measures *new disease events*. For diseases that can occur more than once, it usually measures the first occurrence of the disease.

Second, new cases of disease are measured in a *candidate population*—a population of people who are "at risk" of getting the disease. Someone is at risk because he or she has the appropriate body organ, is not immune, and so forth. For example, a woman who still has an intact uterus (that is, she has not undergone a hysterectomy) is a candidate for getting uterine cancer, and a child who has not been fully immunized against the polio virus is a candidate for contracting poliomyelitis. Although it is possible to define and measure the incidence of disease in a population not at risk (for example, the incidence of uterine cancer in women who have undergone hysterectomies is, by definition, zero), it is not a particularly interesting pursuit.

Third, incidence takes into account the *specific amount of time* that the members of the population are followed until they develop the disease. Because incidence measures a person's transition from a healthy to a disease state, time must pass for this change to occur and be observed. As described in the following sections, there are two types of incidence measures: cumulative incidence and incidence rate. Although closely related, each measure has different strengths and weaknesses and is used in different settings.

CUMULATIVE INCIDENCE Cumulative incidence is defined as the proportion of a candidate population that becomes diseased over a specified period of time. Mathematically, it is expressed as follows:

$$\frac{\text{Number of new cases of disease}}{\text{Number in candidate population}} \quad \text{Over a specified time period}$$

Note that the numerator (new cases of disease) is a subset of the denominator (candidate population), and so the possible value of cumulative incidence ranges from 0 to 1 or, if expressed as a percentage, from 0 to 100%. Time is not an integral part of this proportion but rather is expressed by the words that accompany the numbers of the cumulative incidence measure. Thus, cumulative incidence is dimensionless (see Table 2–5).

Cumulative incidence can be thought of as the average risk of getting a disease over a certain period of time. (A risk is the probability of getting a disease.) A commonly cited measure of cumulative incidence is the "lifetime risk of breast cancer" among women. Currently estimated at "one in eight" among U.S. women, it means that 13% of women will develop breast cancer sometime during the course of their lives.[12] Cumulative incidence is influenced by the length of time to which it applies. Generally, the cumulative incidence over a long period of time (such as a lifetime) will be higher than that over a few years.

Cumulative incidence is mainly used in fixed populations when there are no or small losses to follow-up. Consider, for example, the estimated 255,000 residents of Hiroshima, Japan, who were present in the city when the atomic bomb was dropped on August 6, 1945 (Figure 2–2). During the blast and in the weeks and months immediately thereafter, an estimated 65,000 people died from physical trauma, burns, and acute radiation sickness resulting in a 25% cumulative incidence of mortality over a 4-month period.[13] Officials estimate that another 21% of the population died during the year following that initial 4-month period. During the subsequent years

TABLE 2–5 Distinguishing Characteristics of Incidence and Prevalence

Measure	Type of number	Units	Range	Type of cases	Major uses
Cumulative incidence	Proportion	None	0 to 1	New	Research on causes, prevention, and treatment of disease
Incidence rate	True rate	1/time or t^{-1}	0 to infinity	New	Research on causes, prevention, and treatment of disease
Prevalence	Proportion	None	0 to 1	Existing	Resource planning

FIGURE 2–2. Dwindling Size of the Hiroshima Atomic Bomb Population over Time: 1945–1991

Source: Data from Liebow AA. *Encounter with Disaster: A Medical Diary of Hiroshima,* pp 175–176. New York, NY: WW Norton and Co; 1970. Committee for the Compilation of Materials on Damage Caused by the Atomic Bombs in Hiroshima and Nagasaki. *Hiroshima and Nagasaki: The Physical, Medical, and Social Effects of the Atomic Bombings.* p 113. New York, NY: Basic Books; 1981. Pierce DA, Shimizu Y, Preston DL, Vaeth M, Mabuchi K. Studies of the mortality of atomic bomb survivors. Report 12, Part 1. Cancer: 1950–1990, *Radiat Res.* 1996;146:6.

and decades, the cumulative incidence of death was much lower, and different causes of death such as cancer predominated.[14,15] The cumulative incidence of death was 46% over the 41-year period from 1950 through 1991 among Hiroshima and Nagasaki survivors who were enrolled in the Life Span Cohort Study of the effects of high-dose radiation on the incidence of disease and death.[15]

Note that the cumulative incidence of death during the first 16 months after the bomb was dropped (25% + 21% = 46%) was identical to that during the 41-year follow-up period of the Life Span Cohort Study. This finding underscores the importance of describing the time period that the measure covers.

Everyone in the Hiroshima atomic bomb population will eventually die, and the cumulative incidence of mortality will ultimately be 100%. In addition, the size of the candidate population dwindles as members die. For example, all 255,000 residents were at risk of dying when the bomb was dropped in August 1945, while approximately 190,000 survivors of the initial period were at risk of dying during the subsequent years (see Figure 2–2).

One critical assumption underlies the cumulative incidence measure. Everyone in the candidate population has been followed for the specified time period. Thus, the estimate that women have a 13% lifetime risk of breast cancer assumes that a population was followed for incidence of breast cancer from birth until death, an average of 70 to 80 years. Complete follow-up is difficult to attain, particularly in a dynamic population where members are continually entering and exiting. Thus, cumulative incidence is usually reserved for fixed populations, particularly when there are no or few losses to follow-up.

INCIDENCE RATE Incidence rate is defined as the occurrence of new cases of disease that arise during person-time of observation. Mathematically, the incidence rate is expressed as follows:

$$\frac{\text{Number of new cases of disease}}{\text{Person-time of observation in candidate population}}$$

Note that the numerator for incidence rate is identical to that of cumulative incidence. The difference between the two measures lies in the denominator. The incidence rate's denominator integrates time (t), and so it is a true rate.[11] Thus, its dimension is $1/t$ or t^{-1}, and its possible values range from zero to infinity (Table 2–5). An incidence rate of infinity is possible if all members of a population die instantaneously.

The concept of person-time can be difficult to understand. Person-time is accrued only among candidates for the disease. Thus, a person contributes time to the denominator of an incidence rate only up until he or she is diagnosed with the disease of interest. However, unlike for cumulative incidence, the incidence rate is not based upon the assumption that everyone in the candidate population has been followed for a specified time period. Person-time is accrued only while the candidate is being followed. Accrual of person-time stops when the person dies or is lost to follow-up (such as when a person moves away from a community). The incidence rate can be calculated for either a fixed or dynamic population. However, because it directly takes into account population changes (such as migration, birth, and death), it is especially useful as a measure of the transition between health and disease in dynamic populations.

Consider the following population of a hypothetical town (Figure 2–3). This dynamic population of five individuals is followed for the 10-year period from 1984 to 1994. Person A moved into town in 1985, was diagnosed with disease in 1989, and so accrued 4 years of person-time. Person B was a resident of the town at the start of the observation period in 1984, died in 1990, and so accrued 6 person-years. Person C moved to town in 1986 and remained healthy until he moved away in 1989. The investigator could not determine where he moved and so could not learn if he became diseased later. Person C was considered lost to follow-up as of the time he moved, and so he accrued 3 person-years. Person D was a resident of the town at the start of the observation period, remained healthy for the

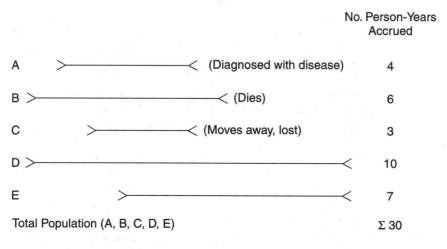

FIGURE 2–3. Measurement of Person–Time in a Hypothetical Population

entire period, and so accrued 10 years of person-time. Person E was born to Person A in 1987, remained healthy for the entire observation period, and so accrued 7 person-years.

The incidence rate in this hypothetical population is 1/30 person-years. Only one person became diseased and 30 person-years of observation were accrued by the population. The denominator of the incidence rate is the sum of person-time accrued by each member of the population at risk.

Now consider an actual population of 1762 women who were studied to determine the relationship between radioactive iodine therapy for hyperthyroidism (an overactive thyroid gland) and the risk of breast cancer.[16] The women were treated from 1946 through 1964 and followed until the end of 1978, the closing date of the study. Each woman's follow-up time began with her thyroid treatment and continued until one of the following events occurred: breast cancer diagnosis, lost to follow-up, or end of follow-up for the study. By 1978, 8% of the women were lost, 32% were deceased, and 60% were still alive. Investigators identified 61 cases of breast cancer among the 30,324 person-years of follow-up, and so the incidence rate was 61/30,324 person-years or 201/100,000 person-years. Although it is most accurate to determine person-time on an individual basis, as was done in this study, this method is very time consuming and labor-intensive. Thus, researchers sometimes use shortcuts such as multiplying the number of people under observation by an estimate of the average follow-up time.

In the hypothetical example portrayed in Figure 2–3, five individuals who were followed for varying amounts of time accrued 30 person-years of follow-up. However, depending on the size of the population and length of follow-up, the 30 person-years could have been accrued in many different ways—five people each contributing 6 years, three people each contributing 10 years, and so forth. Regardless of how the person-time is accrued (for example, from 5 or 50 people), the person-time units are assumed to be equivalent. This assumption is usually reasonable, except in extreme situations where a small number of people are followed for a long period of time.

The particular time unit used to measure person-time can vary, but decisions are guided by how long it takes for the disease to develop. For example, person-years are commonly used for diseases that take many years to develop (such as cancer), and person-months or person-days are used for diseases that develop rapidly (such as infection).

The number of person-time units in the denominator is arbitrary. For example, the same incidence rate can be expressed in terms of 1 person-year, 10 person-years, or 100 person-years. Epidemiologists generally use 100,000 person-years for rare diseases and those that take a long time to develop.

RELATIONSHIP BETWEEN CUMULATIVE INCIDENCE AND INCIDENCE RATE
It is possible to obtain cumulative incidence from an incidence rate. The simplest situation to demonstrate this relationship is in a fixed population with a constant incidence rate and small cumulative incidence (less than 10%). Here, the mathematical relationship is as follows:

$$CI = IR_i \times t_i$$

where CI is cumulative incidence, IR_i is incidence rate, and t_i is the specified period of time.

When the incidence rate is not constant, it is necessary to take into account the different rates that prevail during each time period:

$$CI = \Sigma \, (IR_i \times t_i)$$

For example, the mortality rate (a type of incidence rate) among Hiroshima residents was much higher shortly after the atomic bomb explosion than during subsequent years (see Figure 2–2).

INCIDENCE SUMMARY In summary, two measures of disease frequency—cumulative incidence and incidence rate—focus on measuring the transition from health to disease. These measures have complementary strengths and weaknesses. The cumulative incidence is easy to calculate and understand, although it is less accurate when its assumptions are not met. Although the incidence rate has greater accuracy, its person-time denominator is more difficult to calculate and understand. Finally, the incidence rate is most useful for dynamic populations, and cumulative incidence is usually reserved for fixed populations.

Prevalence

While incidence measures the frequency with which new disease develops, prevalence measures the *frequency of existing disease.* It is simply defined as the proportion of the total population that is diseased. There are two types of prevalence measures—point prevalence and period prevalence—that relate prevalence to different amounts of time. *Point prevalence* refers to the proportion of the population that is diseased at a single point in time and can be thought of as a single snapshot of the population. The point can be either a particular calendar date such as December 1, 2001, or a point in someone's life such as college graduation. *Period prevalence* refers to the proportion of the population that is diseased during a specified duration of time, such as during the year 2001. The period prevalence includes the number of cases that were present at the start of the period (for example, January 1, 2001) as well as the number that developed during the period (for example, January 2 through December 31, 2001).

It may be helpful to think of period prevalence as derived from a series of snapshots.

Mathematically, point prevalence is expressed as follows:

$$\frac{\text{Number of existing cases of disease}}{\text{Number in total population}} \quad \text{At a point in time}$$

Period prevalence can be expressed as follows:

$$\frac{\text{Number of existing cases of disease}}{\text{Number in total population}} \quad \text{During a period of time}$$

Note that the numerator (existing cases) is a subset of the denominator (total population). Unlike the numerator for the two incidence measures, the prevalence numerator includes all currently living cases regardless of when they first developed. The denominator includes everyone in the population—sick, healthy, at risk, and not at risk. Because prevalence is a proportion, it is dimensionless and its possible values range from zero to one, or 0 to 100% (see Table 2–5).

Relationship Between Prevalence and Incidence

Prevalence depends on the rate at which new cases of disease develop (the incidence rate) as well as the duration or length of time that individuals have the disease. The duration of a disease starts at the time of diagnosis and ends when the person either is cured or dies. Mathematically, the relationship between prevalence and incidence is as follows:

$$P/(1 - P) = IR \times D$$

where P is prevalence (the proportion of the total population with the disease), $(1 - P)$ is the proportion of the total population without the disease, IR is incidence rate, and D is the average duration (or length of time) that an individual has the disease.

This equation assumes that the population is in steady state (that is, inflow equals outflow) and that the incidence rate and duration do not change over time. If the frequency of disease is rare (that is, less than 10%), the equation simplifies to:

$$P = IR \times D$$

To better understand this relationship, think of the variables that influence the level of water in a sink (see Figure 2–4). The water level is influenced by both the inflow from the faucet and the outflow down the drain. The water level will be high if the inflow is large, if the outflow is

FIGURE 2–4. Relationship between Incidence, Prevalence, Mortality and Cure

low, or if both occur. The water level will be low if inflow is low, outflow is high, or both. Now consider the water level in the sink as prevalence, the incoming water as incidence, and the outflowing water as diseased people who either are cured or die. The number of cases of people currently living with a disease (prevalence) will be influenced by the rate at which new cases develop as well as by the rate at which they are eliminated through cure or death.

Consider the real-life example of AIDS, whose prevalence has increased steadily during the 1990s (see Figure 2–5).[9,17] In the early 1990s, the prevalence of AIDS increased because the AIDS case definition was expanded and because incidence increased. Thus, prevalence increased because *inflow increased*. In the mid and late 1990s, prevalence increased because improvements in treatment resulted in dramatic reductions in the number of AIDS deaths. Thus, in the latter part of the 1990s, prevalence increased because *outflow decreased*. In fact, prevalence increased despite decreasing incidence during this period.

Uses of Incidence and Prevalence

Epidemiologists and other public health professionals use each measure of disease frequency for specific purposes (see Table 2–5). Incidence is most useful for evaluating the effectiveness of programs that try to prevent disease from occurring in the first place. In addition, researchers who study the causes of disease prefer to study new cases (incidence) over existing ones (prevalence) because they are usually interested in exposures that lead to developing the disease. Prevalence obscures causal relationships because it combines incidence and survival. In addition, many researchers

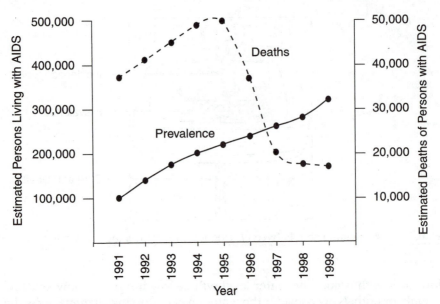

FIGURE 2–5. Estimated Number of Persons Living with AIDS, and Estimated Number of AIDS Deaths, 1991–1999, United States

Source: Data from Centers for Disease Control and Prevention. *HIV/AIDS Surveillance Report.* 1997;19(no 2). Centers for Disease Control and Prevention. *HIV/AIDS Surveillance Report.* 2000:12(no. 1).

prefer to use incidence because the timing of exposures in relation to disease occurrence can be determined more accurately.

On the other hand, prevalence is useful for estimating the needs of medical facilities and for allocating resources for treating people who already have a disease. In addition, researchers who study diseases such as birth defects (where it is difficult to gather information on defects present in miscarried and aborted fetuses) and chronic conditions such as arthritis (whose beginnings are difficult to pinpoint) have no choice but to use prevalence. Unfortunately, results of such studies are difficult to interpret because it is unclear how much the association is influenced by using a group of survivors.

Commonly Used Measures of Disease Frequency in Public Health

There are many measures of disease frequency that are commonly used in the public health disciplines. Some are incidence measures, some are prevalence measures, some are ratios. Descriptions and examples of the major measures follow. Note that the word *rate* is often used incorrectly to describe a proportion or ratio.

Crude mortality (or death) rate: Total number of deaths from all causes per 100,000 population. Usually expressed for a 1-year period. The term *crude* means that the rate is based on raw data. In 1997, 2,314,245 deaths occurred among the estimated 267,636,000 people residing in the United States. Thus, the crude mortality rate was 864.7/100,000 population.[18]

Cause-specific mortality (or death) rate: Number of deaths from a specific cause per 100,000 population. Usually expressed for a 1-year period. In 1997, there were 726,974 deaths from heart disease among U.S. residents resulting in a cause-specific mortality rate of 271.6/100,000.[18]

Age-specific mortality (or death) rate: Total number of deaths from all causes among individuals in a specific age category per 100,000 population in the age category. In 1997, there were 1,728,872 deaths among the 34,076,000 U.S. residents aged 65 and older, resulting in an age-specific death rate of 5,073.6/100,000.[18]

Years of potential life lost: The number of years that an individual was expected to live beyond his or her death. In 1997, 1369 years were lost due to heart disease, 1735 years were lost due to cancer, and 1061 were lost due to unintentional injuries before age 75 per 100,000 population younger than 75 years of age.[18] The number of years of potential life lost reflects both the number of individuals who died of a particular cause and the age at which the death occurred. For example, a cause of death that is more common among children and young adults (such as unintentional injuries) will result in more years of life lost per individual than a cause of death that is common among the elderly (such as heart disease).

Livebirth rate: Total number of livebirths per 1000 population. Usually expressed for a 1-year period. A livebirth is a pregnancy that results in a child who, after separation, breathes or shows any other evidence of life. Sometimes the denominator includes only women of childbearing age. In 1997, approximately 3,880,894 livebirths occurred among U.S. resident women, and the crude livebirth rate was 14.5/1000.[18]

Infant mortality rate: Number of deaths of infants less than 1 year of age per 1000 livebirths. Usually expressed for a 1-year period. This statistic is often divided into neonatal deaths (those occurring during the first 27 days following birth) and postneonatal deaths (those occurring from 28 days through 12 months). In 1996, the infant mortality rate in the United States was 7.3/1000 livebirths, the neonatal mortality rate was 4.8/1000 livebirths, and the postneonatal death rate was 2.5/1000 livebirths.[18]

Birth defect (also called congenital anomaly or malformation) rate: Number of children born with defects per 10,000 births. The numerator and denominator often include both live- and stillbirths. According to a nationwide birth defects monitoring program, the prevalence of spina bifida, a central nervous system malformation, was 4.45/10,000 births from 1986 to 1987.[19]

Morbidity rate: Number of existing or new cases of a particular disease or condition per 1000 population. The time period that is covered and the population size in the denominator vary. *Morbidity* is a general word that can apply to a disease, condition, or event. For example, from 1988 to 1994, the prevalence of hypertension among U.S. adults aged 20 to 74 years was 23.1%.[18]

Attack rate: Number of new cases of disease that develop (usually during a defined and short time period) per the number in a healthy population at risk at the start of the period. This cumulative incidence measure is usually reserved for infectious disease outbreaks. For example, the 24-hour attack rate for food poisoning was 50% among people who ate chicken salad at the banquet.

Case fatality rate: Number of deaths per number of cases of disease. Note that this measure is a type of cumulative incidence, so it is necessary to specify the length of time to which it applies. For example, the 5- and 10-year case fatality rates for breast cancer are approximately 14% and 24% among U.S. women.[20]

Survival rate: Number of living cases per number of cases of disease. This rate is the complement of the case fatality rate; also a cumulative incidence measure. Five-year relative survival rates for cancer compare people with a particular cancer to similar people in the general population. For example, from 1992 to 1997, 5-year relative survival rates for prostate cancer were 97% among whites and 92% among blacks.[20]

Summary

A population is defined as a group of people with a common characteristic such as place of residence, age, or the occurrence of an event. There are two main types of populations, fixed and dynamic (or open). The membership of a fixed population is defined by a life event and is permanent, whereas the membership of a dynamic population is defined by a changeable characteristic and is transient.

Three factors should always be considered when measuring how commonly a disease occurs in a population: (1) the number of affected individuals or cases, (2) the size of the population from which the cases arise, and (3) the amount of time that this population is followed. Before epidemiologists can count the number of affected cases, they must compose a disease definition that is usually based on physical and pathological examinations, diagnostic tests, and signs and symptoms. Disease definitions often change over time, as more is learned about a disease and its manifestations. For example, the official case definition of AIDS expanded when its cause was discovered and improvements in detection were made.

Incidence and prevalence are the two basic measures of disease frequency. Incidence measures the occurrence of new disease and so captures the transition from health to disease. Cumulative incidence and incidence rate are the two main types of incidence measures. Cumulative incidence is defined as the proportion of a candidate population that becomes diseased over a specified time period. It is a dimensionless proportion that measures the average risk of contracting a disease over a certain time period. Incidence rate is the occurrence of new cases of disease that arise during person-time of observation, and so it is a true rate. It is important to remember that person-time accumulates only among candidates for disease. Cumulative incidence and incidence rate are related mathematically. Both measures are most useful for evaluating the effectiveness of disease prevention activities and for etiological studies of disease.

Prevalence measures existing disease and so focuses on the period when a person is ill. Prevalence measures the proportion of the total population that is diseased at a point in time or during a period of time. Its numerator consists of the number of existing cases, and its denominator includes the total population, including sick, healthy, at-risk, and immune individuals. Point prevalence refers to a single point in time and is like a snapshot. Period prevalence refers to a specific duration of time that may be derived from a series of snapshots. Prevalence is typically used for estimating the needs of medical facilities and for allocating resources for treating diseased individuals. The incidence rate and prevalence are mathematically related.

Many measures of disease frequency are commonly used in public health, including the crude, cause-specific, and age-specific mortality rates; morbidity rate; livebirth rate; infant mortality rate; attack rate; case fatality rate; and survival rate. Note that the term *rate* is often incorrectly used to refer to proportions and ratios.

References

1. MacMahon B, Trichopoulos D. *Epidemiology: Principles and Methods*. 2nd ed. Boston, MA: Little, Brown and Co; 1996.
2. Last JM. *A Dictionary of Epidemiology*. 3rd ed. New York, NY: Oxford University Press; 1995.
3. *Preamble to the Constitution of the World Health Organization* as adopted by the International Health Conference, New York, 19–22 June 1946; signed on 22 July by the representatives of 61 States (Official Records of the World Health Organization p. 100) and entered into force on 4 April 1948.
4. *Healthy People 2000: National Health Promotion and Disease Prevention Objectives: Full Report, with Commentary*. Washington DC: U.S. Department of Health and Human Services, Public Health Service; 1992.
5. Centers for Disease Control. Kaposi's sarcoma and Pneumocystis pneumonia among homosexual men—New York City and California. *MMWR*. 1981;30: 305–308.

6. Centers for Disease Control. Update on acquired immune deficiency syndrome (AIDS)—United States. *MMWR*. 1982;31:507–514.

7. Centers for Disease Control. Revision of the case definition of acquired immune deficiency syndrome for national reporting—United States. *MMWR*. 1985;34:373–375.

8. Centers for Disease Control. 1993 Revised classification system for HIV infection and expanded surveillance case definition for AIDS among adolescents and adults. *MMWR*. 1992;41(RR-17):1–19.

9. Centers for Disease Control and Prevention. *HIV/AIDS Surveillance Report*. 1997;9(no 2):1–43.

10. U.S. Census Bureau. Available at: http://www.census.gov/census_2000/datasets/demographic_profile. Accessed July 2001.

11. Elandt-Johnson RC. Definition of rates: some remarks on their use and misuse. *Am J Epidmiol*. 1975;102:267–271.

12. Feuer EJ, Wun LM, Boring CC, Flanders WD, Timmel MJ, Tong T. The lifetime risk of developing breast cancer. *J Natl Cancer Inst*. 1993;85:892–897.

13. Liebow AA. *Encounter with Disaster: A Medical Diary of Hiroshima*. New York, NY: WW Norton and Co; 1970.

14. Shimizu Y, Pierce DA, Preston DL, Mabuchi K. Studies of mortality of atomic bomb survivors. Report 12, part II. Noncancer mortality: 1950–1990. *Radiat Res*. 1999;152:374–389.

15. Pierce DA, Shimizu Y, Preston DL, Vaeth M, Mabuchi K. Studies of the mortality of atomic bomb survivors. Report 12, part I. Cancer: 1950–1990. *Radiat Res*. 1996;146:1–27.

16. Goldman MB, Maloof F, Monson RR, Aschengrau A, Cooper DS, Ridgway EC. Radioactive iodine therapy and breast cancer: a follow-up study of hyperthyroid women. *Am J Epidemiol*. 1988;127:969–980.

17. Centers for Disease Control and Prevention. *HIV/AIDS Surveillance Report*. 2000;2(no 1):1–43.

18. Kramarow E, Lentzer H, Rooks R, Weeks J, Saydah S. *Health and Aging Chartbook. Health, United States, 1999*. Hyattsville, MD: National Center for Health Statistics, 1999.

19. Centers for Disease Control. Temporal trends in the prevalence of congenital malformations at birth based on the Birth Defects Monitoring Program, United States 1979–87. *MMWR*. 1990;39(SS-4):19–23.

20. Ries LAG, Eisner MP, Kosary CL, Hankey BF, Miller BA, Clegg L, Edwards BK, eds. *SEER Cancer Statistics Review, 1973–1998*. Bethesda, MD: National Cancer Institute; 2001.

EXERCISES

1. What measure of disease frequency is each of the following?
   A. The percentage of freshman girls who become pregnant over the course of their high school years
   B. The percentage of senior boys who are fathers at the time of graduation
   C. The number of liveborn babies who die of sudden infant death syndrome during the first year of life per 100,000 baby-years of follow-up
   D. The percentage of infants weighing less than 2500 grams at birth
   E. The lifetime risk of breast cancer

2. Briefly describe the main similarities and differences between each of the following:
   A. Prevalence and incidence
   B. Incidence rate and cumulative incidence
   C. Fixed and dynamic population

3. In 2001, there were 2900 new cases of breast cancer diagnosed among women in Alabama and 200 new cases diagnosed among women in Alaska. Based on these data, is it accurate to say that the incidence rate of breast cancer is higher in Alabama than Alaska. Why or why not?

4. Consider a class with 100 enrolled students. None of the students were ill at the beginning of the school year. On September 30, 5 students reported having gastroenteritis. All continued to be ill on October 1, but all 5 recovered within 3 days. On October 14, 3 more students developed gastroenteritis. All of these students continued to be ill on October 15, but all 3 recovered 5 days later. In this example, assume that a person cannot get gastroenteritis more than once.
   A. Calculate the prevalence of gastroenteritis in the class on October 1.
   B. Calculate the prevalence of gastroenteritis in the class on October 30.
   C. Calculate the cumulative incidence of gastroenteritis in the class during the month of October.

5. The incidence rate of a nonfatal disease is 500/100,000 person-years. People usually have the disease for an average of 3 years, at which time the disease resolves spontaneously. Estimate the prevalence of this disease using this information. Assume that the population is in steady state.

6. A population of 100 healthy men was followed for the development of prostate cancer. After being followed for 5 years, 20 men developed prostate cancer. Ten other men were followed for 1 year and then were lost. The remaining men who never developed the disease were followed for 10 years. Calculate the number of person-years of observation accrued by this population.

7. Consider the following hypothetical data on the occurrence of hepatitis in two cities.

City	New cases	Observation period	Starting population at risk
City A	25	January–December 2001	25,000
City B	30	January–December 2001	50,000

   A. Calculate the cumulative incidence of hepatitis in each city.

   B. Which city has the higher cumulative incidence?

8. Sixty cases of myocardial infarction were reported over a period of 2 years in a city with a population of 100,000 people. Using these data, estimate the incidence rate of myocardial infarction per 100,000 person-years. State any assumptions that are needed.

9. State the type of population (fixed or dynamic) that best describes each of the following:

   A. People who live in New York City

   B. Men who have ever had coronary bypass surgery

   C. Children who were vaccinated against polio in 1955

   D. Women who are practicing physicians

10. An epidemiologic investigation that was started on January 1, 1999, identified a population of 1000 individuals among whom 4 were found to have the disease under study. During the year of the study, 6 new cases were found. Among the total of 10 cases, there were 6 deaths during the year. For the 10 cases, the diagram indicates the time of case recognition, periods of observation during the study, and vital status at the time of the termination of observation. An arrow at the start of the diagram (patients 1, 2, 3, 4) indicates that the start of disease occurred before the study began.

Assume that the 990 remaining individuals in the study did not become ill or die during the year of observation. From the information and diagram given, calculate the following:

A. Prevalence of the disease on January 1, 1999; July 1, 1999; and December 31, 1999

B. Cumulative incidence of disease during 1999

C. Cumulative incidence of death during 1999

1999   2000

| Jan | Feb | Mar | Apr | May | Jun | Jul | Aug | Sep | Oct | Nov | Dec | Jan |

1 ←————————————————————————————————— Alive

2 ←———————————————— Dead

3 ←—————————————————————————— Dead

4 ←— Dead

5 ————————————————————————————————————— Alive

6 ————————————— Dead

7 ————————————————————————————— Alive

8 ———————— Dead

9 ———————————————————————— Alive

10 ————————————————————— Dead

3

Comparing Disease Frequencies

LEARNING OBJECTIVES

By the end of this chapter the reader will be able to:

- Organize disease frequency data into a two-by-two table.
- Describe and calculate absolute and relative measures of comparison, including rate/risk difference, population rate/risk difference, attributable proportion among the exposed and the total population, and rate/risk ratio.
- Verbally interpret each absolute and relative measure of comparison.
- Describe the purpose of standardization and calculate directly standardized rates.

Introduction

Measures of disease frequency are the building blocks epidemiologists use to assess the effects of a disease on a population. Comparing measures of disease frequency organizes these building blocks in a meaningful way that allows one to describe the relationship between a characteristic and a disease and to assess the public health impact of the exposure.

Disease frequencies can be compared between different populations or between subgroups within a population. For example, one might be interested in comparing disease frequencies between residents of France and the United States or between subgroups within the U.S. population according to demographic characteristics such as race, gender, or socioeconomic status; personal habits such as alcoholic beverage consumption or cigarette smoking; and environmental factors such as the level of air pollution. For example, one might compare incidence rates of coronary heart disease between residents of France and those of the United States, or among U.S. men and women, blacks and whites, alcohol drinkers and nondrinkers, and areas with high and low pollution levels.

Usually people who have a particular characteristic (for example, they drink alcoholic beverages) are compared to people who do not share the characteristic. Very often, the characteristic is called the exposure. Those who have it form the *exposed group*, and those who do not have it form the *unexposed group*. The unexposed group can also be called the reference or comparison group. In instances where no group is clearly unexposed, the group with the lowest exposure is used as the reference group. In addition, whenever possible, the exposure is divided into levels such as light, moderate, and heavy. Here, individuals at each exposure level would be compared to the reference group.

For example, to understand the relationship between second-hand tobacco smoke and the risk of childhood asthma, one could compare the frequency (for example, 10-year cumulative incidence) of asthma among children whose parents smoke cigarettes (the exposed group) to that of children whose parents are nonsmokers (the unexposed group). Using detailed data on parental smoking, one could compare the cumulative incidence of asthma among children with two smoking parents (high level of exposure), children with only one smoking parent (low level of exposure), and children of nonsmokers. Depending on the type of comparison made, this analysis could provide information on the degree to which second-hand smoke increases a child's risk of developing asthma and the number of cases of childhood asthma that might be prevented if parents did not smoke.

This chapter describes the various ways that epidemiologists compare measures of disease frequency and the methods they use to ensure that these comparisons are "fair." The chapter focuses not only on mathematical calculations but also on interpretation of these numbers with words.

Data Organization

To compare disease frequencies, epidemiologists first organize the data in a "two-by-two" or "fourfold" table, so called because data are cross-tabulated by two categories of exposure (yes or no) and two categories of disease (yes or no). Table 3–1 depicts a two-by-two table that might be used in a study comparing proportions such as prevalence or cumulative incidence.

Note that the areas outside of the double lines are called the *margins* of the table (for example, a + b) and that the boxes inside the double lines are called the *cells* (a, b, c, d).

Table 3–2 is a two-by-two table that describes data from a cohort study of air pollution and mortality among U.S. residents.[1] The "Six Cities" Study was based on 8111 randomly selected adults who lived in one of six U.S. cities with various levels of air pollution. Investigators followed study participants from the mid-1970s through mid-1991, and then they determined the number and causes of death. The two-by-two table describes the cumulative incidence of mortality for the cities with the highest and lowest pollution levels—Steubenville, Ohio, and Portage, Wisconsin, respectively. A total of 2982 participants resided in these two cities (a + b + c + d). Of these, 1351 lived in Steubenville (a + b) and 1631 lived in Portage (c + d). By the end of the study, 523 deaths had been observed among the participants (a + c). Of the total number of deaths, 291 occurred among residents of Steuben-

TABLE 3–1   General Organization of Cumulative Incidence or Prevalence Data in a Two-by-Two Table

Exposure	Disease		
	Yes	No	Total
Yes	a	b	a + b
No	c	d	c + d
Total	a + c	b + d	a + b + c + d

where: Total number in the study = a + b + c + d
Total number exposed = a + b
Total number unexposed = c + d
Total number diseased = a + c
Total number not diseased = b + d
Number exposed and diseased = a
Number exposed but not diseased = b
Number not exposed but diseased = c
Number neither exposed nor diseased = d

TABLE 3–2   "Six Cities" Study Cumulative Incidence of Mortality Data Arranged in a Two-by-Two Table

Exposure	Dead		
	Yes	No	Total
Lived in most polluted city (Steubenville, Ohio)	291	1,060	1,351
Lived in least polluted city (Portage, Wisconsin)	232	1,399	1,631
Total	523	2,459	2,982

Source: Data from Dockery DW, Pope A, Xu X, Spengler JD, Ware JH, Fay ME, et al. An association between air pollution and mortality in six U.S. cities. *New Engl J Med.* 1993;329:1755.

TABLE 3–3 Organization of Incidence Rate Data in a Two-by-Two Table

	Disease		
Exposure	*Yes*	*No*	*Person-time (PT)*
Yes	a	--	PT exposed
No	c	--	PT unexposed
Total	a + c	--	Total PT

TABLE 3–4 "Six Cities" Study Incidence Rate of Mortality Data Arranged in a Two-by-Two Table

	Dead		
Exposure	Yes	No	Person-Time
Lived in most polluted city (Steubenville, Ohio)	291	--	17,914
Lived in least polluted city (Portage, Wisconsin)	232	---	21,618
Total	523	---	39,532

ville (a) and 232 occurred among residents of Portage (c). Based on these data, the cumulative incidence of mortality was 291/1351 (or 215.4/1000) in Steubenville and 232/1631 (or 142.2/1000) in Portage. The combined cumulative incidence for the two cities was 523/2982 (or 175.4/1000).

The two-by-two table is slightly modified when incidence rates are compared (see Table 3–3). The modifications include omission of the number of people without disease (these data are unnecessary for incidence rate calculations) and substitution of counts with person-time in the margin.

Because the Six Cities investigators also calculated person-time of follow-up for every study subject, it is possible to describe the incidence rate of mortality in a modified two-by-two table (see Table 3–4).

Thus, the incidence rates of mortality were 291/17,914 person-years (or 16.24/1000 person-years) in Steubenville and 232/21,618 person-years (or 10.73/1000 person-years) in Portage. The combined incidence rate of mortality for the two cities was 523/39,532 person-years (or 15.00/1000 person-years).

Measures of Comparison

Measures of disease frequency can be compared in two ways. They can be subtracted from one another or divided by one another. The subtracted measures of disease frequency are termed *absolute comparisons,* and the divided ones are known as *relative comparisons*. Absolute comparisons generally give information about the public health impact of an exposure, and relative comparisons generally give information about the strength of the relationship between an exposure and a disease. Each is described in more detail in the sections that follow.

Absolute Measures of Comparison

An absolute comparison is based on the difference between two measures of disease frequency. A general term for this comparison is the *risk difference* or *rate difference*. More precise terms based on the measure of disease frequency used for the calculation include *incidence rate difference, cumulative incidence difference*, and *prevalence difference*. Although the term *attributable risk or rate* is commonly used, some epidemiologists think that this term should be discarded because it implies a definite causal relationship.[2(p16)]

Absolute comparisons can be calculated either for exposed individuals or for the total population. When exposed individuals are the focus, the absolute difference measure is calculated as follows:

$$RD = R_e - R_u$$

where RD is the rate or risk difference (such as incidence rate difference, cumulative incidence difference, or prevalence difference), R_e is the rate or risk (incidence rate, cumulative incidence, or prevalence) in the exposed group, and R_u is the rate or risk (incidence rate, cumulative incidence, or prevalence) in the unexposed group.

The RD describes the disease burden associated with exposure among the people who are exposed. Interpreted narrowly, the RD is simply the excess number of cases of disease associated with the exposure. However, there is a broader interpretation that makes the assumption of causality. If the exposure is considered a cause of the disease, the RD indicates the number of disease cases among the exposed that would be eliminated if the exposure were eliminated (or reduced to the level of the reference group.)

Let us use the Six Cities data to calculate the mortality incidence rate difference for the least and most polluted cities (see Table 3–4).

Incidence Rate Difference = $IR_{most\ polluted\ city} - IR_{least\ polluted\ city}$
IRD = 16.24/1000 person-years − 10.73/1000 person-years
IRD = 5.51/1000 person-years

Interpreted narrowly, there are 5.51 excess deaths per 1000 person-years among Steubenville residents. Or, more broadly, if pollution caused the deaths, then 5.51 deaths among Steubenville residents (for every 1000 person-years of observation) would be eliminated if the pollution level were reduced to that of Portage.

A population usually consists of exposed and unexposed people. Thus, it is useful to know the impact of the exposure not only on the exposed but also on the total population. A general term used to describe this comparison is the *population risk* or *difference* (or *population rate difference*).

When the total population is of interest, the absolute difference measure is calculated as follows:

$$PRD = R_t - R_u$$

where PRD is the population rate difference (or population risk difference), R_t is the rate or risk (incidence rate, cumulative incidence, or prevalence) in the total population, and R_u is the rate or risk (incidence rate, cumulative incidence, or prevalence) in the unexposed group.

It is also possible to obtain the population rate difference by multiplying the risk or rate difference (RD) by the proportion of the population that is exposed (P_e):

$$PRD = RD \times P_e$$

where RD is the incidence rate difference, cumulative incidence difference, or prevalence difference and P_e is the proportion of population that is exposed.

The disease rate in the total population (R_t) or the proportion exposed (P_e) may be obtained either from the study population or the general population. However, before the study population is used as the source of this information, the study design must be examined carefully. Studies in which the exposed proportion has been arbitrarily set by the investigator will give inaccurate data because the percentage exposed in the study population does not reflect real life. For example, in the Six Cities Study, the investigators arbitrarily included three more and three less polluted cities.

Just as the rate or risk difference describes the public health impact of the exposure among the exposed, the population rate difference (or population risk difference) describes the impact among the total population. The PRD describes the excess number of cases in the total population that is associated with the exposure. Or more broadly, if one believes that there is a causal relationship between the exposure and disease, the PRD identifies the number of cases of disease that would be eliminated in the total population if the exposure were eliminated (or reduced to the level in the reference group). The PRD helps public health officials determine which exposures are most important to a given population and helps prioritize prevention activities.

Note in the second PRD formula that the impact of an exposure on a population is a function of both the rate difference (RD) and the proportion of exposed individuals in the population (P_e). Thus, even if the rate difference is relatively high, the PRD will not be high if the exposure is rare. On the other hand, even if the rate difference is relatively low, the PRD will be high if the exposure is common.

For example, assume that 10% of the U.S. population is exposed to air pollution levels as high as those in Steubenville, Ohio, the most polluted city in the Six Cities Study. Using this information, one would calculate the population rate difference for the United States as follows:

$$PRD = RD \times P_e$$
$$PRD = (5.5/1000 \text{ person-years}) \times (0.10) = 0.55/1000 \text{ person-years}$$

Thus, 0.55 extra deaths for every 1000 person-years of observation in the entire U.S. population can be attributed to pollution. Or, if pollution were the cause of death, then 0.55 deaths for every 1000 person-years of observation in the U.S. population would be eliminated if pollution were reduced.

What would the PRD be if high pollution levels were more common? Let us apply the Six Cities results to the district of Teplice in the Czech Republic, which is considered to be one of the most polluted regions of Europe.[3] If we assume that 40% of the population in Teplice is exposed to air pollution levels as high as those in Steubenville Ohio, population rate difference would be calculated as follows:

$$(5.5/1000 \text{ person-years}) \times 0.40 = 2.2/1000 \text{ person-years}.$$

This means that cleaning up air pollution in this area of Eastern Europe would save even more lives than it would in the United States.

One can see from the formulas that, unless everyone in the population is exposed, the impact of the exposure is always smaller in the total population than in the exposed group, and so the PRD is always smaller than the RD. Also, note that the units and range of the absolute measures of comparison (RD and PRD) depend on the measure of disease frequency that is used for the calculation. For example, if incidence rates are used, then the measure will have person-time units and can range from negative infinity to positive infinity. On the other hand, if one uses cumulative incidence or prevalence, the measure is dimensionless, and can range from -1 to $+1$.

Two parallel measures of comparison that express the public health impact of an exposure as proportions are the attributable proportion among the exposed[4] (also called the etiologic fraction[5]) and the attributable proportion among the total population. The *attributable proportion among the exposed* (AP_e) describes the proportion of disease among the exposed that would be eliminated if the exposure were eliminated. It assumes a causal relationship between the exposure and disease. Mathematically, it is expressed as follows:

$$AP_e = [(R_e - R_u / R_e] \times 100$$

where AP_e is the attributable proportion among the exposed; R_e is the incidence rate, cumulative incidence, or prevalence in the exposed group; and R_u is the incidence rate, cumulative incidence, or prevalence in the unexposed population.

For example, using the Six Cities data,

AP_e = [(16.24/1000 person-years − 10.73/1000 person-years)/16.24/ 1000 person-years] × 100
AP_e = 33.9%

This means that 33.9% of the deaths among participants from Steubenville may be attributed to the high pollution level and, hence, could be eliminated if the pollution level were reduced.

The attributable proportion in the total population (AP_t) describes the proportion of disease among the total population that would be eliminated if the exposure were eliminated. It is expressed as follows:

AP_t = [($R_t − R_u$) / R_t] × 100

where R_t is the incidence rate, cumulative incidence, or prevalence in the total population; and R_u is the incidence rate, cumulative incidence, or prevalence in the unexposed population.

For example, using the Six Cities data,

AP_t = [(12.87/1000 person-years − 10.73/1000 person-years)/12.87/ 1000 person-years] × 100
AP_t = 16.6%

Note that the incidence rate for the total population was derived from the incidence rate among participants in all six of the cities—not just Portage and Steubenville. The AP_t means that 16.6% of the deaths in the total study population may be attributed to high pollution levels and, hence, could be eliminated if the pollution levels were reduced.

The attributable proportion among the total population is very useful for determining priotities for public health action.[6] In the example above, the elimination of the pollution would lead to a substantial reduction in deaths, and so public health policy makers would probably rate it as a priority. On the other hand, if an exposure had a much lower attributable proportion, policy makers would probably not use limited health dollars to eliminate it.

If there is no relationship between the exposure and disease (in other words, the rate or risk of disease among the exposed is exactly the same as that among the unexposed), the numeric value for all of the absolute comparisons (rate difference, population rate difference, attributable proportion among the exposed, and attributable proportion among the total population) is zero.

The attributable proportion is used when an exposure is considered a cause of the disease. When an exposure is thought to protect against the disease, the prevented fraction (PF)[5] can be calculated according to the following formula:

$$PF = [(R_u - R_e)/R_u] \times 100$$

where R_u is the incidence rate, cumulative incidence, or prevalence in the unexposed group and R_e is the incidence rate, cumulative incidence, or prevalence in the exposed group.

For example, the addition of fluoride to drinking water supplies has reduced the incidence of dental caries. The incidence of dental caries in Newburgh, New York, a fluoridated area, is 14.8%; the incidence in Kingston, New York, a nonfluoridated area, is 21.3%.[7] Thus, the preventive fraction is 30.5%. This means that almost 31% of percent of caries in Newburgh were prevented because of fluoridation.

Relative Measures of Comparison

A relative measure of comparison is based on the ratio of two measures of disease frequency. This measure is generally called the *risk ratio, rate ratio, relative rate,* or *relative risk.* More precise terms that are based on the measure of disease frequency used for the calculation include *incidence rate ratio, cumulative incidence ratio,* and *prevalence ratio.*

Mathematically, the relative measure is expressed as follows:

$$RR = R_e/R_u$$

where RR is the rate or risk ratio; R_e is the incidence rate, cumulative incidence, or prevalence in the exposed group; and R_u is the incidence rate, cumulative incidence, or prevalence in the unexposed group.

A relative comparison gives information about the strength of the relationship between the exposure and disease, and is most useful for etiologic research. For example, the relative risk of death in the Six Cities Study is (16.24/1000 person-years)/(10.73/1000 person years) or 1.51. This means that, compared to the residents of Portage, there is a 1.51-fold increased risk of death among residents of Steubenville. Another interpretation is that the death rate in Steubenville is 1.51 times that of Portage.

If there is no relationship between the exposure and disease, the numeric value for the relative measure is 1.0. If there is a positive relationship between the exposure and disease (that is, the exposure increases the risk of disease), the numeric value is greater than 1.0. Another way to express this information is in terms of the *excess relative risk,* which is mathematically equal to $(RR - 1) \times 100$.[4] For example, using the Six Cities relative risk of 1.51, the excess relative risk is $(1.51 - 1) \times 100$ or 51%. Thus, compared to the residents of Portage, the residents of Steubenville have a 51% increased risk of death.

If the exposure prevents disease, the numeric value of the relative comparison measure is less than 1.0. For example, a relative risk of 0.5 means that the exposed group has one half the risk of the unexposed group, or a

50% decreased risk of disease. A relative risk of 0.33 means that the exposed group has one third the risk or a 67% reduction in risk, and so on. For example, the relative risk of dental caries in Newburgh versus Kingston is 0.69.[7] This means that residents of Newburgh have a 31% reduced risk of dental caries (1.0 − 0.69 = 0.31). Note that the relative measure of comparison is always dimensionless and can range from zero to infinity.

Most epidemiologists prefer to use the relative risk method of comparison for etiologic research because of the way it is anchored by a baseline value. In other words, it indicates how many times higher or lower the disease risk is among the exposed as compared to the baseline risk among the unexposed. However, because of this anchoring, interpretation of the relative risk requires caution in several situations. First, when the baseline risk or rate of disease is high, maximum value of the relative risk is limited. For example, if the baseline risk is 50% among the unexposed, then the highest possible value of the relative risk is 2.0 (because disease risk among the exposed cannot exceed 100%). Second, when cumulative incidence or prevalence is used for the comparison, the relative risk will

TABLE 3-5 Absolute and Relative Measures of Comparison

Type of Measure	Formula	Interpretation
Rate or risk difference (RD)	$R_e - R_u$	Excess rate or risk of disease among exposed population
Population rate difference (PRD)	$R_t - R_u$ or $RD \times P_e$	Excess rate or risk of disease in total population
Attributable proportion among exposed (AP_e)	$[(R_e - R_u/R_e] \times 100$	Excess proportion of disease among exposed; if causal, proportion of disease among exposed that would be eliminated if the exposure were eliminated
Attributable proprortion among total population (AP_t)	$[(R_t - R_u)/R_t] \times 100$	Excess proportion of disease in total population; if causal, proportion of disease in total population that would be eliminated if the exposure were eliminated
Rate or risk ratio (RR)	R_e/R_u	Strength of relationship bebetween exposure and disease; the number of times higher or lower the risk is among exposed as compared to risk among unexposed population

approach 1.0 as the disease frequency increases. As the prevalence or cumulative incidence approaches 100% in the exposed and unexposed groups, the ratio (the relative risk) approaches 1.0. This often occurs with cumulative incidence when the population is followed for a long period of time. The ratio of incidence rates is not affected in this manner, because incidence rates can range up to infinity.

The formulas given in this chapter and summarized in Table 3–5 can be used for most types of epidemiologic studies, including cohort studies, experimental studies, and cross-sectional studies. These designs are discussed in detail in Chapters 6, 7, and 8. Other formulas are used for case–control studies because of the way that the subjects are selected. These formulas are discussed in Chapter 9.

Direct Standardization

As was described in Chapter 2, crude rates are summary measures of disease frequency that are based on the raw data. For example, a crude prevalence is calculated by dividing the total number of cases in the population by the total number of individuals in that population at a point in time (point prevalence) or during a period of time (period prevalence). It is difficult to interpret absolute and relative measures of comparison that are based on crude rates when the compared groups differ on a characteristic that affects the rate of disease (such as age, gender, or race). This difference between the groups may result in an unfair comparison and distort the results.

For example, let us compare the crude mortality rates among people living in Alaska to the rates of Florida residents (see Table 3–6). The crude mortality rate among Florida residents (1060.94 per 100,000) is much higher than among Alaska residents (417.91 per 100,000), and the excess crude rate is 643.03 per 100,000 (1060.94 minus 417.91 per 100,000).

What explains the difference between the crude mortality rates of the two states? One possible answer is the different age structures of the populations. Note in Table 3–7 that Florida has relatively fewer residents in the youngest age categories and more residents in the oldest age category. There is a strong association between mortality and age, so it is possible that these age differences account for the mortality differences between the states.

However, let us examine the *age-specific mortality rates* also shown in Table 3–7. Note that Florida has higher mortality rates than Alaska in almost every age group. In fact, individuals aged 5 to 19 are the only group that has a lower mortality rate in Florida. Thus, a side-by-side comparison of the five age-specific mortality rates suggests that the age difference does not account for the difference in the crude mortality rate between the two populations.

Side-by-side comparisons of age-specific rates give a more accurate picture of the mortality rates than do crude rates. However, because there are many age groups to examine, this method results in a cumbersome number of comparisons. Furthermore, comparing age-specific rates can give a confusing picture if, for example, half of the rates are higher in one state and half are higher in the other. For this reason, epidemiologists commonly use an alternative method in which the rates in each state are summarized in a single number that adjusts for the age differences between the populations. These summary rates, which are known as *age-standardized* or *age-adjusted* rates answer the question, "What would the death rate be in each state if the populations had identical age distributions?"

TABLE 3–6   Number of Deaths, Estimated Population Size, and Crude Mortality Rates in Alaska and Florida in 1998

	Alaska	Florida
Number of deaths*	2,571	158,167
Number in population	615,205	14,908,230
Crude mortality rate (per 100,000 persons)**	417.91	1060.94

* From 282 selected causes of death.
** The crude mortality rate is calculated by dividing the number of deaths from 282 selected causes by the number in the population.
Source: Data from National Center for Health Statistics, Division of Data Services. Table III, *Deaths from 282 selected causes, 1998.* Available at http://www.cdc.gov/nchs/data/97gm3_01.pdf. U.S. Census Bureau. Population estimates for the US, regions, divisions, and states, July 1, 1990, to July 1, 1999 (ST-99-8). Available at http://www.census.gov/population/estimates/states/st-99-08.txt.

TABLE 3–7   Census Population Estimates and Age-Specific Mortality Rates for Alaska and Florida in 1998

Age group (years)	Alaska			Florida		
	Number in category	% of total	Death rate per 100,000*	Number in category	% of total	Death rate per 100,000*
Younger than 5	49,602	8.06	149.19	949,845	6.37	181.40
5–19	165,764	26.94	43.44	2,938,824	19.71	36.78
20–44	233,179	37.90	165.97	5,097,349	34.19	178.23
45–64	133,160	21.64	521.18	3,197,475	21.45	725.04
65 and older	33,500	5.45	4,011.94	2,724,737	18.28	4,517.68
Total	615,205	100.00	417.91	14,908,230	100.00	1,060.94

* From 282 selected causes of death
Source: Data from National Center for Health Statistics, Division of Data Services. Table III, *Deaths from 282 selected causes, 1998.* Available at: http://www.cdc.gov/nchs/data/97gm3_01.pdf. U.S. Census Bureau. Population estimates for the US, regions, divisions, and states, July 1, 1990 to July 1, 1999 (ST-99-8). Available at: http://www.census.gov/population/estimates/states/st-99-08.txt.

The two methods for calculating age-standardized rates are known as direct and indirect methods of standardization. This chapter describes only the direct method, which requires the following information: (1) age-specific rates in each group (in this case, each state) and (2) age structure of a "standard" population (see Table 3–8). The choice of the standard population is arbitrary. The total population of the United States is typically used as the standard population for standardization of U.S. rates, and the world standard population is used for standardization of international rates.

Age-standardized rates are weighted averages of the age-specific rates, with the weights equal to the proportion of the standard population in each age category. Thus, the age-standardized rate for Alaska is calculated as follows:

$(0.0700) \times (149.19/100,000) + (0.2173) \times (43.44/100,000) + (0.3734) \times (165.97/100,000) + (0.2118) \times (521.18/100,000) + (0.1272) \times (4011.94/100,000) = 702.56/100,000$

Likewise, the age-standardized rate for Florida is calculated as follows:

$(0.0700) \times (181.40/100,000) + (0.2173) \times (36.78/100,000) + (0.3734) \times (178.23/100,000) + (0.2118) \times (725.04/100,000) + (0.1272) \times (4517.68/100,000) = 815.15/100,000$

Note that the weights used for both of the calculations are the same: the proportion of the entire U.S. population in each age category. Thus, the age-standardized rates are hypothetical rates that would have occurred if each state had the age structure of the entire U.S. population in 1998.

The excess age-adjusted mortality rate is 112.6 per 100,000 (815.15 minus 702.56 per 100,000). This is much smaller than the excess crude mortality

TABLE 3–8 Age-Specific Mortality Rates for Alaska and Florida and U.S. Census Population Estimates for 1998

Age group (years)	Age-specific death rate per 100,00*		1998 U.S. Census population estimates	% of total
	Alaska	Florida		
Younger than 5	149.19	181.40	18,989,257	7.00
5–19	43.44	36.78	58,712,947	21.73
20–44	165.97	178.23	100,919,429	37.34
45–64	521.18	725.04	57,241,131	21.18
65 and older	4,011.94	4,517.68	34,385,239	12.72
Total	417.91	1,060.94	270,248,003	100.00

*From 282 selected causes of death

Source: Data from National Center for Health Statistics, Division of Data Services. Table III, Deaths from 282 selected causes, 1998. Available at: http://www.cdc.gov/nchs/data/97gm3_01.pdf. US Census Bureau. Population estimates for the US, regions, divisions, and states, July 1, 1990 to July 1, 1999 (ST-99-8). Available at: http://www.census.gov/population/estimates/states/st-99-08.txt.

rate of 643.03 per 100,000. This finding suggests that age accounts for most but not all of the difference in the crude mortality rates between the two populations. The remaining difference may be due to other factors such as race, socioeconomic status, and access to heath care.

Summary

Measures of disease frequency are contrasted in either absolute or relative terms, depending on the goals of the epidemiologist. Absolute measures of comparison, which are based in the difference between two measures of disease frequency, describe the public health impact of an exposure. Absolute measures include the rate or risk difference, the population rate or risk difference, and attributable proportion among the exposed and the total population. Relative measures of comparison, which are based on the ratio of two measures of disease frequency, describe the strength of the relationship between the exposure and disease. Relative measures include the rate or risk ratio. Comparing measures of disease frequency in either absolute or relative terms is facilitated by organizing the data into a two-by-two table.

It is often difficult to make fair comparisons of crude measures of disease frequency because of key differences between the groups that affect the disease rates. To overcome this problem, a technique known as direct standardization is used to adjust for these differences. For example, direct standardization for age involves taking a weighted average of age-specific rates with the weights being equal to the proportion of the standard population in each age category. The choice of the standard population is arbitrary, but U.S. population census data are typically used.

References

1. Dockery DW, Pope CA, Xu X, Spengler JD, Ware JH, Fay ME, et al. An association between air pollution and mortality in six U.S. cities. *N Engl J Med*. 1993; 329:1753–1759.
2. Walker AM. *Observation and Inference: An Introduction to the Methods of Epidemiology*. Chestnut Hill, Mass: Epidemiology Resources Inc; 1991.
3. Cerna M, Jelinek R, Janoutova J, Kotesovec F, Benes I, Leixner M. Risk assessment of the common air pollutants in Teplice, Czeck Republic. *Toxicol Lett*. 1998;96–97:203–208.
4. Cole P, MacMahon B. Attributable risk percent in case–control studies. *Br J Prev Soc Med*. 1971;25:242–244.
5. Miettinen OS. Proportion of disease caused or prevented by a given exposure, trait or intervention. *Am J Epidemiol*. 1974;99:325–332.
6. Northridge ME. Annotation: public health methods—Attributable risk as a link between causality and public health action. *Am J Public Health*. 1995;85: 1202–1204.
7. Ast DB, Finn SB, McCaffrey I. The Newburgh-Kingston caries fluorine study. *Am J Public Health*. 1950;40:716–724.

EXERCISES

1. Describe the main similarity and main difference between each of the following:

   A. Incidence rate ratio and incidence rate difference

   B. Risk difference and population risk difference

2. Suppose that an investigation of the association between regular physical activity and ovarian cancer revealed that the incidence rate of ovarian cancer among women who engaged in regular physical activity was 30 per 100,000 woman-years of follow-up while the rate among women who did not engage in regular activity was 45 per 100,000 woman-years of follow-up.

   A. Use these data to compute the incidence rate ratio of ovarian cancer for women who are physically active versus women who are not.

   B. State in words your interpretation of this measure.

   C. Compute the incidence rate difference of ovarian cancer for women who are physically active versus women who are not.

   D. State in words your interpretation of this measure.

   E. If there were no association between regular physical activity and ovarian cancer, what would be the numeric values of the incidence rate ratio and incidence rate difference?

3. State the main difference between an age-specific rate and an age-adjusted rate.

4. Consider the following heart disease mortality data from two hypothetical countries— a developing and a developed country.

Age group (years)	Percentage of population in age group	Death rate from heart disease
Hypothetical developing country		
0–20	30%	2/100,000 person-years
21–50	40%	20/100,000 person-years
51–85	30%	40/100,000 person-years
Hypothetical developed country		
0–20	20%	2/100,000 person-years
21–50	30%	20/100,000 person-years
51–85	50%	40/100,000 person-years

A. Use these data to calculate the overall crude death rates from heart disease in the hypothetical developed and developing countries.

B. Based on these data, do you think that it is better to compare the heart disease death rates in the two countries using the overall crude rate or the age-standardized rate for each country? Briefly justify your answer.

5. The 58th annual convention of the American Legion was held in Philadelphia from July 21 until July 24, 1976. People at the convention included American Legion delegates, their families, and other Legionnaires who were not official delegates. Between July 20 and August 30, some of those who had been present became ill with a type of pneumonia that was subsequently named Legionnaires' disease. No one attending the convention developed the disease after August 30. The numbers of delegates and nondelegates who developed Legionnaires' disease during the period July 20 to August 30 (a 41-day period) are as follows:

Convention Status	Developed Legionnaire's disease		
	Yes	No	Total
Delegate	125	1724	1849
Nondelegate	3	759	762

Source: Data from Fraser DW, Tsai TR, Orenstein W, Parkin WE, Beecham HJ, Sharrar RG, et al. Legionnaires' disease: description of an epidemic of pneumonia. *New Engl J Med.* 1977;297:1189–1197.

A. Compute the cumulative incidence of Legionnaires' disease among delegates and nondelegates.

B. Calculate the cumulative incidence ratio of Legionnaires' disease among delegates compared to nondelegates.

C. State in words the meaning of this measure.

D. Calculate the cumulative incidence difference of Legionnaires' disease among delegates compared to nondelegates.

E. State in words the meaning of this measure.

F. Calculate the attributable proportion of Legionnaires' disease among the delegates.

G. State in words the meaning of this measure.

4

Sources of
Public Health Data

LEARNING OBJECTIVES

By the end of this chapter, the reader will be able to:

- Describe the major sources of health data on the U.S. population.
- Describe the issues involved in appropriately interpreting these data sources.

Introduction

There is a wealth of easily accessible information on the health status of the U.S. population. Most of these public health data are collected by governmental and nongovernmental agencies on a routine basis or by special surveys. Information is obtainable on deaths and a wide variety of diseases and conditions including acute illnesses and injuries, chronic illnesses and impairments, birth defects, and other adverse pregnancy outcomes. Data are also available on characteristics that influence a person's risk of illness (such as ambient air pollution levels; nutritional habits: immunizations; and the use of cigarettes, alcohol, and drugs) and on the impact of these illnesses on the utilization of health services including hospitalizations and visits to office-based physicians and hospital emergency and outpatient departments. Several sources of international data are compiled by the World Health Organization and the United Nations. Although the international data are not as extensive as those about the United States, they include information about births, deaths, and major diseases such as cancer.

This chapter provides short descriptions of the major sources of descriptive public health data including the data collection methods. It is important for epidemiologists to understand data collection methods in order to interpret the information appropriately.[1] In particular, it is important to know the specific population that is covered by a data collection system. For example, although U.S. birth and death data pertain to the whole U.S. population, the target population for most national surveys consists of noninstitutionalized civilians. The latter group excludes members of the armed services and individuals living in institutions such as correctional facilities and nursing and convalescent homes. These groups are usually excluded because of technical and logistical problems.

It is also important to understand the calendar period covered by the data collection system and the frequency with which the data are updated. Generally, the most current available data in the United States lags a year or two behind the present. This is because it takes researchers a long time to collect data, computerize the information, check it for errors, and conduct statistical and epidemiologic analyses.

Every data collection system has some incomplete and inaccurate material. If data come from interview-based surveys, they are limited by the amount and type of information that a respondent can remember or is willing to report. For example, a person may not know detailed information on medical diagnoses and surgeries, or may not want to report sensitive information on sexually transmitted diseases and prior induced abortions.

Census of U.S. Population

The U.S. Constitution requires that a census—that is, a complete count of the U.S. population—be taken every 10 years. The primary purpose of the census is to assign members of the House of Representatives to the states.[1] The decennial census of the population has been conducted since 1790, and a census of housing characteristics has been conducted since 1940. Permanently established in 1902, the U.S. Bureau of the Census currently oversees the population and housing census, compiles relevant statistics, and produces reports and computerized data files that are available to the public.

In recent years, the census has obtained information on certain characteristics (such as race, sex, age, and marital status) from the entire population and information on additional characteristics (such as income, educational level, housing, and occupation) from a representative sample of persons. (About 17% of the U.S. population answers these additional questions.) The Census Bureau uses this approach to obtain the most comprehensive data possible while keeping costs reasonable. The complete population is surveyed on characteristics for which precise data are needed on small geographic areas. For example, accurate data on small areas are needed for congressional apportionments. On the other hand, samples are surveyed when estimates are sufficient for larger geographic areas such as census tracts.

The Census Bureau tabulates complete count and sample population statistics for geographic areas in increasing size from census tracts; to cities, counties, and metropolitan areas; to states; to the entire nation. Information is also collected for Puerto Rico and other areas under U.S. sovereignty. These population counts are crucial components of most public health indicators because they are typically used as the denominators of incidence and prevalence measures.

Although the census attempts to account for every person in the U.S. population, it is well known that some undercounting occurs. An evaluation of the 1990 Census found that undercounting ranged from 1.5 to 2%. However, undercounting was higher for certain racial and ethnic groups including blacks (4.4%), Hispanics (5.0%), and American Indians (4.5%). Analyses of the 2000 Census are currently under way.

Vital Statistics

The National Vital Statistics System of the National Center for Health Statistics (NCHS) compiles and publishes data on births, deaths, marriages, and divorces in the United States.[1] Registration offices in all 50 states, the District of Columbia, and New York City have provided information on births and deaths since 1933. Birth and death registration is considered virtually complete. Most states also provide marriage and divorce registration records.

Most birth and death certificates used in the 50 states correspond closely in content and organization to the standard certificate recommended by NCHS. Although some modifications are made to accommodate local needs, all certificates obtain a minimum amount of information on demographic characteristics. The latest versions of the standard live birth and death certificates appear in Figures 4–1 and 4–2.

Public health data collected currently on birth certificates includes birthweight; gestational age; and adverse pediatric conditions such as the presence of congenital malformations (birth defects), complications during pregnancy, and cigarette smoking. Birth certificates are completed by hospital personnel in consultation with parents. The physician (or other professional) who performs the delivery subsequently verifies the accuracy of the information. Certificates are then sent to the local health departments who, in turn, send them to state health departments and then to the NCHS.

Death certificates collect information on "all conditions that the medical certifier reported as contributing to the death, either directly or indirectly." Thus, the certificate lists the immediate cause of death, any intermediate

STATE USE ONLY

The Commonwealth of Massachusetts
DEPARTMENT OF PUBLIC HEALTH
REGISTRY OF VITAL RECORDS AND STATISTICS
STANDARD CERTIFICATE OF LIVE BIRTH

1. RECORD NUMBER

PLACE OF BIRTH

3. CHILD
3B. COUNTY
3C. CITY/TOWN
3D. REGISTERED NUMBER

1A. CERTIFICATE NUMBER (DPH USE ONLY)
3A. FACILITY NAME-IF NOT IN FACILITY, NUMBER AND STREET

2. FACILITY NUMBER

CHILD
NAME   4A. FIRST   4B. MIDDLE   4C. LAST
5. SEX   6A. PLURALITY   6B. BIRTH ORDER   7. TIME   8. DATE OF BIRTH (Month, Day, Year)

CERTIFIER
9A. SIGNATURE (I Certify that the Child was Born Alive at Date and Time and Place Stated.)   9B. TYPE OR PRINT NAME   9C. LICENSE NUMBER
9D. NO. & STREET   9E. CITY/TOWN   9F. STATE   9G. ZIP CODE   9H. DATE SIGNED (Month, Day, Year)
9I. TYPE   9J. TITLE

MOTHER
NAME   10A. FIRST   10B. MIDDLE   10C. LAST   10D. MAIDEN SURNAME
BIRTHPLACE   11A. CITY/TOWN   11B. STATE/COUNTRY   12. DATE OF BIRTH (Month, Day, Year)
RESIDENCE 13A. NUMBER AND STREET (Do not use mailing address)   13B. CITY/TOWN   13C. COUNTY   13D. STATE   13E. ZIP CODE

FATHER
NAME   14A. FIRST   14B. MIDDLE   14C. LAST
BIRTHPLACE   15A. CITY/TOWN   15B. STATE/COUNTRY   16. DATE OF BIRTH (Month, Day, Year)

INFORMANT
17A. I (WE) CERTIFY THAT THE PERSONAL INFORMATION APPEARING ABOVE IS TRUE AND CORRECT.   17B. RELATIONSHIP TO CHILD
INITIALS
17C. DATE SIGNED (Month, Day, Year)   17D. MAILING ADDRESS (if different from item # 13 above)   NUMBER AND STREET   CITY   STATE   ZIP CODE

CLERK
18. DATE OF RECORD (Month, Day, Year)   19. SUPPLEMENT FILED (Month, Day, Year)   20. CLERK/REGISTRAR
INITIALS

22A. SOCIAL SECURITY CARD
22B. RESIDENT COPY

21. DPH USE ONLY

1. OCCURRENCE

R-3C • 200M • 10-95 • 871201

FIGURE 4–1. Sample of U.S. Standard Certificate of Live Birth

The Commonwealth of Massachusetts
STANDARD CERTIFICATE OF DEATH
REGISTRY OF VITAL RECORDS AND STATISTICS

FIGURE 4–2. Sample of U.S. Standard Certificate of Death

causes, and the underlying cause. For example, respiratory arrest may be the immediate cause of death, pneumonia the intermediate cause, and acquired immune deficiency syndrome (AIDS) the underlying cause of death. Other significant conditions contributing to the death may also be listed.

In order to generate national mortality statistics, "every death is attributed to one underlying condition, based on information reported on the death certificate and utilizing the international rules." These rules, now termed the *International Classification of Diseases (ICD)*, were first developed in 1900 and have been revised about every 10 years by the World Health Organization. The tenth revision of the *ICD* has been used to classify mortality information for statistical purposes since 1999.

Anytime that the *ICD* is revised, a number of artifactual changes in the mortality statistics typically occur. Some revisions have led to small changes, and others have resulted in large ones. For example, male and female breast cancer used to be grouped together but now are classified separately. Because male breast cancer is so rare, comprising 0.5% of all breast cancers,[2] it is unlikely that this change made much of a difference in breast cancer mortality data. On the other hand, the large increase in asthma prevalence and mortality has been attributed, in part, to changes in disease coding in 1979 when the ninth revision of the *ICD* was introduced.[3] Before 1979, deaths due to the condition asthmatic bronchitis were classified bronchitis and not included in asthma mortality statistics. Beginning with the ninth revision of the *ICD*, these cases were classified as asthma deaths. The exact proportion of the increased rate of asthma deaths attributed to this artifact is unclear because of other concomitant changes, including worsened pollution, noncompliance with medications, and poor asthma education of patients and health care providers.

Death record information in the United States has been computerized at a national level since 1979.[4] The National Death Index is administered by the NCHS. Epidemiologists often use this data source to determine if study subjects have died. It is necessary to write to individual state offices to acquire copies of death certificates for information on cause of death.

National data on fetal deaths are kept separately by the NCHS. These data have been reported in the United States and District of Columbia since 1982. However, fetal death reporting depends on state requirements; most states require reporting deaths that occur at 20 or more weeks' gestation. Because most pregnancy losses occur earlier in gestation, the reported data represent only a small proportion of pregnancy losses.

National Survey of Family Growth

The purpose of this survey is to "provide national data on the demographic and social factors associated with childbearing, adoption, and maternal and child health" including information on sexual activity, marriage, contraception, sterilization, infertility, breastfeeding, pregnancy loss, low birthweight, use of medical care for infertility, family planning, and prenatal care.[5] To date, five surveys have been conducted (1973, 1976, 1982, 1988, and 1995).

Over time, the National Survey of Family Growth has expanded in scope and coverage. For example, never married women were excluded from Cycles I and II but were included in Cycles III through V. The 1995 survey was based on a national sample of 10,847 women aged 15 to 44 years from the noninstitutionalized population of all 50 states.[5] Statistical weighting procedures were applied to produce estimates for the entire country. In-person interviews were conducted by trained female interviewers. Questions focused on a woman's ability to become pregnant, pregnancy history, use of contraceptives, family planning, infertility services, breastfeeding, maternity leave, child care, and adoption.

National Health Interview Survey

Mandated by the National Health Survey Act of 1956, the National Health Interview Survey (NHIS) is currently the principal source of information on the health of the civilian noninstitutionalized population of the United States.[6] Administered on a yearly basis since 1957, the NHIS provides data on major health problems, including incidence of acute illnesses and injuries, prevalence of chronic conditions and impairments, and utilization of health services. The data are used to monitor trends in illness and disability and to track progress toward achieving national health objectives.

NHIS uses a stratified, multistage sampling scheme to select a sample of households that form a representative sample of the target population. Each year, approximately 40,000 households including approximately 110,000 people are selected for interview. Participation is voluntary, but more than 90% of eligible households respond each year. Nonresponse stems mainly from refusal or the inability to find eligible individuals in a household. Survey results are statistically weighted and adjusted for nonresponse in order to produce national estimates.

Personal interviews are conducted by the permanent interviewer staff from the Bureau of the Census.[7] All adult household members aged 17 years and older who are home at the time of the survey are invited to participate and respond for themselves. A responsible adult aged 18 and older also responds for adults who are not at home and for children. Every year, basic demographic and health information is collected on age; race; sex; educational level; family income; and acute and chronic conditions and associated disability days, physician visits, and hospital stays. Supplemental data collection on special health topics varies from year to year.

National Health and Nutrition Examination Survey

Since 1960, NCHS has conducted the National Health and Nutrition Examination Survey (NHANES) to gather information on the health and diet of the U.S. population.[8] Participants are selected using a census-based stratified random sample. The survey includes both a home interview and health tests done in a mobile examination center. The current NHANES, the eighth in this series of surveys, was started in 1999 and will continuously survey 15 locations throughout the United States and enroll 5000 people each year.

Behavioral Risk Factor Surveillance System

The Behavioral Risk Factor Surveillance System is a telephone health survey that has been conducted in all 50 states and the District of Columbia since 1994.[9] The purpose of this state-based survey is to monitor a wide variety of health risk behaviors that are related to chronic disease, injuries, and death, including use of screening services, smoking, alcohol use, physical activities, fruit and vegetable consumption, and weight control. Participants are adults from randomly selected households. About 150,000 interviews are conducted annually, making it one of the largest continuous telephone surveys in the world.

National Health Care Survey

NCHS recently merged and expanded four separate record-based surveys into a single integrated survey of health care providers called the National Health Care Survey.[10] The new survey is built upon the National Hospital Discharge Survey, the National Ambulatory Medical Care Survey, the National Nursing Home Survey, and the National Health Provider Inventory. The new survey also incorporates the National Survey of Ambulatory Surgery, the National Hospital Ambulatory Medical Care Survey, and the National Home and Hospice Care Survey. The combined survey provides information on the use and quality of health care, and the impact of medical technology in a wide variety of settings including hospital inpatient and outpatient departments, emergency rooms, hospices, home health agencies, and physician's offices. The following paragraphs describe the component surveys.

The National Hospital Discharge Survey is a national probability survey that has been conducted annually since 1965. Its purpose is to collect information on the characteristics of inpatients who are discharged from nonfederal short-stay hospitals in the United States. The survey collects data on diagnoses, procedures, length of stay, and patient characteristics from a sample of about 270,000 inpatient records from about 500 hospitals.

The National Ambulatory Medical Care Survey, which has been conducted since 1973, collects information on the provision and use of ambulatory medical services in the United States. The survey is based on a sample of visits to nonfederally employed office-based physicians who are primarily engaged in direct patient care. Specialists such as anesthesiologists, pathologists, and radiologists are excluded. Data are collected from the physician—not the patient. Each physician is randomly assigned a 1-week reporting period. Information is obtained on demographic characteristics of patients and services provided for a random sample of visits during the reporting period.

The National Nursing Home Survey is a periodic survey of nursing homes. Four surveys have been conducted to date (1973–1974, 1977, 1985, and 1995). The most recent survey included all freestanding nursing homes in the United States and nursing care units of hospitals, retirement centers, and similar institutions. The survey is based on self-administered questionnaires and interviews with administrators and staff in a sample of about 1500 facilities. Information is collected on the characteristics of the facility such as size; ownership; and the characteristics of the residents such as age, race, health status, and services received.

The National Health Provider Inventory is a national listing of nursing homes, residential care facilities, hospices, and home health agencies that serves as a sampling frame for several surveys and as a source of information on the number, type, and geographic distribution of health providers in the United States. It provides the names, addresses, and other information on more than 7800 home health agencies and hospices and 56,000 facilities (including more than 15,500 nursing homes and more than 31,00 board and care homes).

The National Survey of Ambulatory Surgery began in 1994 to collect information on the use of ambulatory surgical services in the United States. For the purposes of the survey, *ambulatory surgery* refers to surgical and nonsurgical procedures performed on an outpatient basis in a hospital or freestanding center's general operating rooms, dedicated ambulatory surgery rooms, and other specialized rooms such as cardiac catheterization labs. Data on patient characteristics, sources of payment, and medical diagnoses and procedures are available for 1994 through 1996 on about 120,000 sampled visits annually from about 500 facilities.

The National Hospital Ambulatory Medical Care Survey began in 1992 to collect information on the utilization and provision of ambulatory services in hospital emergency and outpatient departments. The annual survey is based on a national sample of visits to the emergency and outpatient departments of noninstitutional general and short-stay hospitals in all 50 states and the District of Columbia. A random sample of visits during a randomly assigned 4-week period is chosen from randomly selected facilities. Data are collected on patient demographic characteristics, source of payment, diagnoses, diagnostic and screening services, medication therapy, procedures, and facility characteristics.

The National Home and Hospice Care Survey is a continuing series of surveys of home and hospice care agencies in the United States. The survey is based on a probability sample of qualifying agencies. Data are collected about the agencies and their current patients and discharges through personal interviews with administrators and staff. In particular, information is collected on the referral and length of service, diagnoses, number of visits, patient charges, health status, reason for discharge, and types of services provided.

National Notifiable Diseases Surveillance System

Managed by the Centers for Disease Control and Prevention (CDC) and the Council of State and Territorial Epidemiologists, the National Notifiable Diseases Surveillance System collects weekly provisional data and compiles annual summaries on the occurrence of 60 notifiable diseases throughout the United States.[11] The CDC's *Morbidity and Mortality Weekly Report* defines notifiable disease as "one for which regular, frequent and timely information regarding cases is considered necessary for the prevention and control of the disease."[12] These diseases include acquired human immune deficiency syndrome (AIDS), human immunodeficiency virus (HIV) infection, botulism, gonorrhea, leprosy, all forms of hepatitis, malaria, plague, paralytic poliomyelitis, human and animal rabies, syphilis, and toxic-shock syndrome. Reports of notifiable diseases are sent to the CDC voluntarily by the 50 states, New York City, the District of Columbia, and five U.S. territories. Completeness of reporting depends on the disease and local notification practices. *Morbidity and Mortality Weekly Report* publishes weekly reports and annual summaries of these diseases.

Surveillance of AIDS and HIV Infection

Since 1985, the CDC has collected information on the occurrence of AIDS cases from all 50 states; the District of Columbia; and U.S. dependencies, possessions, and independent associated countries (such as Puerto Rico).[13] The AIDS surveillance case definition has been modified several times in order to improve the accuracy of reporting. Changes have included broadening the number of indicator diseases and incorporating the results of laboratory tests. Every change in definition has led to artifactual changes in incidence estimates (see Chapter 2 for details). For every person meeting the AIDS case definition, data are gathered on demographic characteristics, exposure category (such as injecting drug users and men who have sex with men), AIDS-indicator conditions (such as Kaposi's sarcoma and *Pneumocystis carinii* pneumonia), and diagnosis date.

Reporting delays between the time of diagnosis of HIV infection and AIDS vary according to geographic area, race, age, sex, and exposure categories. About 50% of all AIDS cases are reported to the CDC within 3 months of diagnosis, but about 20% are reported more than 1 year after diagnosis. Even though completeness of reporting varies according to geographic area and patient population, several studies have found that reporting is about 85% complete. After the development of serum HIV-antibody tests in 1985, states also began reporting confirmed cases of HIV infection.

Induced Abortion Statistics

Since 1969, the CDC has maintained a surveillance system to document the number and characteristics of women obtaining abortions, to monitor unintended pregnancies, and to assist in the effort to eliminate preventable morbidity and mortality associated with abortions.[14] The CDC receives annual reports on the number and characteristics of women obtaining legal abortions from centralized state reporting systems, hospitals, and other medical facilities in all 50 states, the District of Columbia, and New York City. Data are collected on the type of abortion procedure; the number of weeks' gestation when the abortion was performed; and the patient's age, race, and marital status. The Alan Guttmacher Institute, the research and development division of the Planned Parenthood Federation of America, Inc., also conducts annual surveys of abortion providers including hospitals, nonhospital clinics, and physicians.

National Immunization Survey, Survey of Families with Young Children, Survey of Children with Special Health Care Needs

Currently, three surveys—The National Immunization Survey, the Survey of Families with Young Children, and the Survey of Children with Special Health Care Needs—collect information on the immunization coverage and health care of children across the United States.[15] The National Immunization Survey began in 1994 as a continuing survey to provide estimates of vaccination coverage among children aged 19 to 35 months in 78 geographic areas. It includes surveys of households as well as vaccination providers. The latter are identified by parents who respond to the household survey.

The Survey of Families with Young Children, started in 2000, collects data on doctors' visits for children aged 4 to 35 months. Parents are asked about their experiences with pediatricians, family practitioners, and other children's health providers. Parents are also asked about the ways that they keep their children healthy at home, including the use of immunizations.

The Survey of Children with Special Health Care Needs, also started in 2000, collects data on the health care needs and health insurance coverage of children younger than 18 years of age. The survey estimates the prevalence of children with special health care needs in each state, describes the types of services that they require and use, and assesses the need for additional services.

National Occupational Hazard Survey and National Occupational Exposure Survey

In 1972 to 1974, the National Institute for Occupational Safety and Health conducted the National Occupational Hazard Survey, a field survey to describe the "health and safety conditions in the American workplace and to determine the extent of workers' exposure to chemical, physical, and biological agents."[16] This survey included 4636 facilities that were representative of all nonagricultural businesses covered by the 1970 Occupational Safety and Health Act and employing at least eight individuals. Trained staff conducted walk-through inspections and, while doing so, recorded workers' potential exposure to chemical, physical, and trade name products.

A second national survey of the American workplace, the National Occupational Exposure Survey, was conducted in 1981 to 1983. Essentially identical to the first survey, this survey included a sample of 4490 facilities representative of nonagricultural businesses. Data from these two surveys are available in a computerized job exposure matrix that links exposures to industries and job titles. The job exposure matrix can be used to identify jobs and industries in which exposure to a particular chemical was likely to occur at the time of the surveys. Unfortunately, because the survey was last conducted about 20 years ago, the matrix does not include information on current exposures.

National Traumatic Occupational Fatalities Surveillance System

Since 1980, the National Traumatic Occupational Fatalities Surveillance System has been monitoring the number and rates of deaths due to occupational injuries using information from death certificates.[1] The following criteria are needed for a fatal injury to be considered occupational in origin: (1) the decedent must be 16 years or older, (2) the cause of death must be external (that is, resulting from an injury rather than a disease process), and (3) a positive response must be given to the death certificate item "Was the death the result of an injury at work?" Because standardized guidelines for answering the "injury at work" question were not implemented until 1993, data from earlier years should be used with caution.

Annual Survey of Occupational Injuries and Illnesses

Since 1971, the Department of Labor has gathered annual data on occupational injuries and illnesses among employees in the private sector.[1] Data are collected from a national sample of approximately 280,000 establishments where business is conducted, services are provided, or industrial operations occur. Self-employed individuals; small farm employees; and local, state, and federal government employees are excluded. Typically, about 94% of selected employers respond to the survey.

The survey data are based on records of injuries and illnesses that employers are required to maintain under the federal Occupational Safety and Health Act. An occupational injury is defined as "any injury such as a cut, fracture, sprain, or amputation that results from a work accident or from exposure involving a single incident in the work environment." An occupational illness is defined as "any abnormal condition or disorder, other than one resulting from an occupational injury, caused by exposure to environmental factors associated with employment."

National Household Survey on Drug Abuse

Since 1971, the National Household Survey on Drug Abuse has obtained information on the use of alcohol, cigarettes, marijuana, and cocaine.[1] The survey includes civilian, noninstitutionalized individuals living in all 50 states and aged 12 years and older. The survey design and implementation were substantially changed in 1994 in order to improve the quality and timeliness of the data. Because investigators expected these changes to affect the prevalence estimates, the 1994 survey used a multistage probability design that could produce two sets of prevalence figures—one based on 4372 individuals using the same methods used in 1993, and the other based on 17,809 individuals using the new methods. The sample response rates for the two estimates were 77% and 78%, respectively.

Aerometric Information Retrieval System

The federal Clean Air Act of 1970 requires the Environmental Protection Agency to collect data on the levels of certain ambient air pollutants because they pose serious threats to public health.[1] These pollutants include particulates, lead, carbon monoxide, sulfur dioxide, nitrogen dioxide, and ozone. Currently, more than 4000 monitoring sites, located mainly in highly populated urban areas, provide data that are used to determine if a particular geographic area complies with the National Ambient Air Quality Standards. These standards include an adequate margin of safety that protects even the most sensitive members of the population (such as asthmatics) and define a maximum concentration level for each pollutant that cannot be exceeded during a prescribed time period.

Surveillance, Epidemiology and End Results Program

Mandated by the National Cancer Act, the Surveillance, Epidemiology and End Results (SEER) Program has collected data on the prevention, diagnosis, and treatment of cancer in the United States since 1973.[17] In particular, the SEER Program monitors trends in the incidence, mortality, and survival of more than 36 types of cancer according to geographic and demographic characteristics.

Currently, SEER statistics are based on 11 population-based registries—Connecticut, Hawaii, Iowa, New Mexico, Utah, Detroit Standard Metropolitan Statistical Area (SMSA), Atlanta SMSA, San Francisco-Oakland SMSA, Seattle-Puget Sound, and selected rural counties in Georgia and Arizona. These geographic areas were chosen to participate in the SEER registry because of their administrative capabilities and population characteristics. The populations living in these areas cover about 14% of the U.S. population and are considered reasonably representative.

Reporting systems have been set up in each region that gather data on all newly diagnosed cancer cases among area residents. Information is gathered from a variety of sources including medical records, death certificates, laboratories, and radiotherapy units to ensure complete ascertainment of the cancer cases. Data are gathered on the cancer patients' demographic characteristics, primary cancer site (for example, the lung), method of diagnostic confirmation (such as a pathology report), severity of the disease, and first mode of therapy. Patients are actively followed to provide survival information.

Birth Defects Surveillance and Research Programs

From 1970 through 1994, the CDC operated the Birth Defects Monitoring Program (BDMP), the first national system for monitoring occurrence of congenital malformations.[18] The system was launched, in part, in response to the epidemic of limb reduction defects among children whose mothers had taken the sedative thalidomide during pregnancy in the 1960s.

While it was operating, BDMP was the largest single source of uniformly collected data on birth defects in the country. Collected data include dates of birth and discharge, diagnoses and surgical procedures, sex, race, and birthweight. BDMP data were reviewed quarterly to determine if the prevalence of a birth defect had increased. If increases were identified, investigators explored both real and artefactual explanations, sometimes by conducting more detailed studies.

BDMP had several limitations. Because participating hospitals were self-selected and did not serve well-defined geographic areas, these data were not random samples of births occurring in the United States. In addition, BDMP only picked up birth defects discovered during the postpartum hospital stay (usually 2 to 3 days), and so defects diagnosed later in life (such as congenital deafness) were likely to be missed.

In 1996, Congress directed the CDC to establish Centers of Excellence for Birth Defects Prevention Research.[19] The purpose of the centers is to expand and improve existing surveillance systems and to conduct research on etiology and prevention of birth defects. To date, seven centers have been established in California, Iowa, Massachusetts, Arkansas, New York, New Jersey, and Texas. The CDC also operates its own center in Atlanta, Georgia.

In addition, Congress passed the 1998 Birth Defects Prevention Act, which authorizes the CDC to (1) collect, analyze, and make available data on birth defects; (2) operate regional centers for applied epidemiologic research on the prevention of birth defects; and (3) educate the public about the prevention of birth defects.[19] Under this program, the CDC has provided funding to 18 states to initiate and support new surveillance programs or to improve existing ones.

Health, United States

The publication *Health, United States* is one of the most comprehensive sources of information on the current health status of the U.S. population.[20] Published yearly, the report compiles information from various branches of the CDC (including the National Center for Health Statistics, the National Center for HIV, STD, and TB Prevention; and the Epidemiology Program Office), the Substance Abuse and Mental Health Services Administration, the National Institutes of Heath (including the National Cancer Institute), and the Bureau of the Census. A compilation of data from these and other sources, this publication includes the most recent data on mortality, morbidity, health behaviors, reproductive health, health care access and utilization, and substance use. Each edition of *Health, United States* focuses on a major health topic. The 1999 edition highlighted health and aging, because older people are leading consumers of health care and their numbers are rising.

Demographic Yearbook

Since 1948, the Statistical Office of the United Nations has compiled official demographic statistics from countries throughout the world for its annual *Demographic Yearbook*.[21] Currently, data are collected from 233 countries on population size, distribution, and growth; births; deaths (including fetal, infant, and maternal mortality); and marriages and divorces. Because the *Demographic Yearbook* is intended for a broad audience, health data are reprinted for the *World Health Statistics Annual* (described below) to make them more readily accessible to medical and public health professionals. Because definitions of health events vary from country to country, and because some countries provide incomplete or inaccurate vital statistics and population data, the *Yearbook* data should be interpreted carefully.

World Health Statistics Annual

The World Health Organization (WHO) has reported international morbidity and mortality data since 1951.[22] Currently, data are collected on patterns and trends in health status, health care systems, and resources in order to provide information and to facilitate the monitoring and evaluation of the WHO Global Strategy for Health. One section of the *World Health Statistics Annual* summarizes worldwide health and demographic data for health assessment and analysis. Another section focuses on health and demographic data from United Nations member states including presentation of mortality rates by age, sex, and cause. The death rates are based on official statistics sent to the WHO by member nations. The *Annual* includes only those countries that report cause-of-death information in the proper format and whose death registration is regarded as reasonably accurate. Like death registration in the United States, included countries follow the concept of "the underlying cause of death" that is coded according to the rules set forth in the *International Classification of Diseases, Ninth Revision.* However, because the data published in the *Annual* are affected by the same problems as those described for the *Demographic Yearbook,* comparisons between countries should be interpreted with caution.

Cancer Incidence on Five Continents

Since the 1960s, WHO's International Agency for Research on Cancer (IARC) has collected data on cancer incidence and mortality from many countries around the world.[23] Currently, about 170 cancer registries in 50 countries are invited to contribute their data. Most of the registries rely on medical records, laboratory records, and death certificates as their data sources. All registries record the cancer case's name, address, sex, and cancer site. Most registries also collect information on age or date of birth, occupation, and the method of cancer diagnosis. The IARC processes the submitted data, assessing its quality, completeness, and comparability. IARC publishes the information every few years in a monograph titled *Cancer Incidence on Five Continents.* A main goal of the monograph is to allow international comparisons of incidence that will lead to the formulation of hypotheses about the causes of cancer.

Other Resources

A number of additional sources of information are collected by state and local health departments.

■ *State cancer registries:* In addition to the SEER cancer registries, most states currently have population-based cancer registries. For example, the Massachusetts Cancer Registry began operation 1982 and uses a system of hospital-based tumor registrars to collect data on cancer incidence. Compilation of these data has enabled the Massachusetts registry to monitor trends in cancer incidence over time and according to demographic characteristics such as age, gender, race, and geographic area.

■ *Internet resources:* Numerous data sources are available through the Internet. Because the quality of information on the Internet is often unknown, it is best to rely only on resources from the U.S. government and other reliable sources. For example, the home page for the National Center for Health Statistics is located at: http://www/cdc/gov/nchswww/nchshome.htm.

■ *Wide-Ranging Online Data for Epidemiologic Research (WONDER):* One epidemiology resource guide book describes WONDER as "a computerized information system that provides on-line access to epidemiologic and public health data sets." WONDER has data and documentation for many of the data sources listed above including AIDS Public Use Info Data set, Alcohol Abuse and Alcoholism Data, Compressed Mortality Data, SEER cancer incidence data, U.S. Census data, and National Hospital Discharge Data.[4] WONDER can be accessed through the Internet at: http://wonder.cdc.gov.

Summary

Many sources of information are readily available on a wide variety health-related states and events including diseases, injuries, disabilities, and death among individuals living in the United States and around the world. The types and sources of information described in this chapter are summarized in Table 4–1. When interpreting data from these sources it is important to consider: (1) the population about which the information was obtained, (2) the calendar period that was covered, and (3) the level of missing and inaccurate data. It is also important to know about any changes in data collection methods that may have created artifactual changes in the frequency of disease.

TABLE 4–1   Sources of Public Health Data

Type of information	Source of information
Population size and characteristics	U.S. Census, Bureau of Census, Department of Commerce
Births	National Vital Statistics System, National Center for Health Statistics
Deaths	National Vital Statistics System, National Death Index, National Center for Health Statistics
Fetal deaths	Fetal Death Data, National Center for Health Statistics
Childbearing, adoption, maternal and child health, family planning	National Survey of Family Growth, National Center for Health Statistics
Major health problems and utilization of health services	National Health Interview Survey, National Center for Health Statistics
Indicators of nutrition and health	National Health and Nutrition Examination Survey, National Center for Health Statistics

Continued

TABLE 4–1 *Continued*

Type of information	*Source of information*
Use and quality of health care in a wide variety of settings	National Health Care Survey, National Center for Health Statistics
Notifiable diseases	National Notifiable Diseases Surveillance System, Centers for Disease Control and Prevention
HIV and AIDS	AIDS and HIV Surveillance, Centers for Disease Control and Prevention
Cancer incidence, mortality, and survival	Surveillance, Epidemiology, and End-Results Program, National Cancer Institute; state cancer registries
Birth defects	Birth Defects Surveillance, Center for Birth Defects Research and Prevention, Centers for Disease Control and Prevention
Induced abortion	Abortions Surveillance, Centers for Disease Control and Prevention, Alan Guttmaker Institute, Planned Parenthood Federation of America
Immunizations	National Immunization Survey, Survey of Families with Young Children, Survey of Children with Special Needs, National Center for Health Statistics; National Immunization Program
Occupational hazards and exposures	National Occupational Hazard Survey and National Occupational Exposure Survey, National Institute of Occupational Safety and Health
Deaths from occupational injuries	National Traumatic Occupational Fatalities Surveillance System, National Institute of Occupational Safety and Health
Occupational injuries and illnesses in private sector	Annual Survey of Occupational Injuries and Illnesses, U.S. Department of Labor
Behaviors affecting health	Behavioral Risk Factor Surveillance System, Centers for Disease Control and Prevention
Alcohol, cigarette, and drug use	National Household Surveys on Drug Abuse, Substance Abuse and Mental Health Services Administration
Air pollutant levels	Aerometric Information Retrieval System, Environmental Protection Agency

References

1. National Center for Health Statistics. *Health, United States, 1995.* Hyattsville, MD: Public Health Service; 1996.
2. Ries LAG. Rates. In: Harras A, Edwards BK, Blot WJ, Ries LAG, eds. *Cancer Rates and Risks.* NIH pub no 96-691. Bethesda, MD: National Cancer Institute: 1996.
3. Chang CC, Phinney SD, Halpern GM, Gershwin ME. Asthma mortality: another opinion—is it a matter of life and . . . bread? *J Asthma.* 1993;30:93—103.
4. Bernier RH, Mason VM, eds. *Episource: A Guide to Resources in Epidemiology.* 1st ed. Roswell, GA: The Epidemiology Monitor; 1991.
5. Centers for Disease Control and Prevention. Available at http://www.cdc.gov/nchs/nsfg.htm. Accessed January 2001.
6. Centers for Disease Control and Prevention. Available at http://www.cdc.gov/nchs/nhis.htm. Accessed January 2001.
7. Chyba MM, Washington LR. Questionnaires from the National Health Interview Survey, 1985–89. In: *Vital and Health Statistics, Series 1: Programs and Collection Procedures.* No. 31. Hyattsville, MD: National Center for Health Statistics; 1993.
8. Centers for Disease Control and Prevention. Available at: http://www.cdc.gov/nchs/nhanes.htm. Accessed January 2001.
9. Centers for Disease Control and Prevention. Available at: http://www.cdc.gov/nccdphp/brfss/about.htm. Accessed January 2001.
10. Centers for Disease Control and Prevention. Available at: http://www.cdc.gov/nchs/nhcs.htm. Accessed January 2001.
11. Notice to readers: Changes in national notifiable diseases data presentation. *MMWR.* 2000;49:892.
12. Groseclose SL, Knowles CM, Hall PA, et al. Summary of notifiable diseases, United States, 1998. *MMWR.* 1999;47:1–93.
13. Centers for Disease Control and Prevention. *HIV/AIDS Surveillance Report.* 1995;7:1–39.
14. Koonin LM, Strauss LT, Chrisman CE, Parker WY. Abortion surveillance, United States, 1997. *MMWR.* 2000;49:1–44.
15. Centers for Disease Control and Prevention. Available at: http://www.cdc.gov/nis. Accessed January 2001.
16. Seiber WK, Sundin DS, Frazier TM, Robinson CF. Development, use, and availability of a job exposure matrix based on national occupational hazard survey data. *Am J Ind Med.* 1991;20:163–174.
17. Ries LAG, Eisner MP, Kosary CL, Hankey BF, Miller BA, Clegg L, et al.. *SEER Cancer Statistics Review, 1973–1998.* Bethesda, MD: National Cancer Institute; 2001.
18. Edmonds LD, Layde PM, James LM, Flynt JW, Erickson JD, Oakley GP. Congenital malformations surveillance: two American systems. *Int J Epidemiol.* 1981;10:247–252.
19. Centers for Disease Control and Prevention. Available at: http://www.cdc.gov/nceh/cddh/BD/bdpghome.htm. Accessed January 2001.

20. Kramarow E, Lentzer H, Rooks R, Weeks J, Saydah S. *Health and Aging Chartbook. Health, United States, 1999*. Hyattsville, MD: National Center for Health Statistics; 1999.
21. United Nations. *1994 Demographic Yearbook*. New York, NY: United Nations; 1996.
22. World Health Organization. *World Statistics Annual 1994*. Geneva, Switzerland: World Health Organization; 1995.
23. International Agency for Research on Cancer. *Cancer Incidence in Five Continents*. Volume 6. Lyon, France: IARC; 1992.

5

Descriptive Epidemiology

LEARNING OBJECTIVES

By the end of this chapter the reader will be able to:

- Describe and provide examples of the three main elements of descriptive epidemiology: person, place, and time.
- Define the terms disease cluster and epidemic.
- Discuss the scientific and administrative uses of descriptive epidemiology.
- Describe the demographic characteristics of the U.S. population and its pattern of mortality by age.
- List the strengths and limitations of mortality data.
- Discuss the descriptive epidemiology of childhood lead poisoning, acquired immune deficiency syndrome (AIDS), and breast cancer.

Introduction

As described in Chapter 1, epidemiology is defined as the study of the distribution and determinants of disease frequency in human populations and the application of this study to control health problems.[1(p1),2(p55)] The portion of the definition pertaining to the distribution of disease is the domain of descriptive epidemiology, which involves the analysis of disease patterns according to the characteristics of *person*, *place*, and *time*. In other words, epidemiologists seek answers to the questions: Who is getting the disease? Where is it occurring? How is it changing over time? Variations in disease occurrence by these three characteristics provide useful information for understanding the health status of a population; for formulating hypotheses about the causes of disease; and for planning, implementing, and evaluating public health programs to control and prevent adverse health events. This chapter describes the components and uses of descriptive epidemiology and then provides examples of analyses of the patterns of death and of three important diseases in the United States.

Person

Personal characteristics that are usually available for descriptive epidemiology include age, sex, race and ethnic group, socioeconomic status, occupation, religion, and marital status. These attributes can be associated with major variations in disease occurrence. Age is probably the most important among them because it is associated with striking changes in disease rates. The frequency of most diseases increases with age. For example, the prevalence of elevated blood pressure in the period from 1988 to 1994 increased steadily with age from 8.6% of males aged 20 to 34 years to 64.2% of those aged 75 and older.[3] On the other hand, the incidence of some diseases declines with age. For example, whooping cough occurs predominantly in childhood, particularly among children younger than 5 years of age; cases among adolescents and adults are rare.[4(pp318–322)]

Why does disease occurrence vary dramatically with age? The answer is complicated because an individual's numerical age reflects both the aging process and that person's experiences. The latter includes the accumulation of harmful exposures as well as protective factors. For example, the prevalence of habits such as alcohol consumption increases with age (at least from the teenage years through middle age)[3] as does the prevalence of protective characteristics such as immunity to infectious diseases.

Sex is another personal characteristic associated with variations in disease occurrence. Certain diseases are more common among men, and others are more prevalent among women. A striking example of this type of variation is breast cancer, a disease for which less than 1% of cases occur among men and more than 99% occur among women.[5] The opposite is seen with AIDS, for which about 83% of cases have been among men.[6] Possible reasons for variations in disease rates between sexes include differences in: (1) hormone levels (for example, female hormones may protect women against heart disease); (2) habits such as the use of tobacco, alcohol, and drugs (which are more common among men); (3) sexual practices (for example, anal intercourse, a risk factor for AIDS transmission, is most commonly practiced among gay men); and (4) occupational exposures (men are more likely than women to hold jobs involving toxic exposures).

Race and ethnicity also have a profound influence on disease patterns. Fortunately, the measurement of these characteristics has improved over time. The U.S. Census currently distinguishes between more than 13 racial groups including whites, blacks, American Indians, Alaska Natives, Chinese, Filipinos, Japanese, Asian Indians, Koreans, Vietnamese, Native Hawaiians, Samoans, and Gaumanians.[7] The Census also identifies persons of Hispanic origin including Mexicans, Puerto Ricans, and Cubans.

The rates for many diseases in the United States are higher among minority groups, particularly blacks.[3] For example, diabetes is more common among blacks and Hispanics aged 70 years and older than among whites of the same age. In fact, the prevalence of diabetes is twice as high among minority women as among white women. In addition, non-Hispanic older blacks are 1.5 times more likely to report hypertension than non-Hispanic whites. These kinds of racial and ethnic differences in disease rates may stem from differences in socioeconomic status, health practices, psychosocial stress and resources, environmental exposures, discrimination, or access to health care. Because many of these factors are highly correlated, it is often difficult for epidemiologists to tease apart their contributions.

Socioeconomic status is also a prominent characteristic by which diseases vary. Commonly used measures of socioeconomic status include educational level, income, and occupation. The sinking of the Titanic is a historic example of health disparities between the poor and wealthy. Death rates among passengers of low socioeconomic status were twice as high as those among passengers of high socioeconomic status because the small supply of life jackets was preferentially given to wealthy passengers—particularly wealthy women and children.[8]

Today, large disparities for almost all measures of health exist between people with low and high incomes. For example, life expectancy is strongly related to family income; individuals with lower family income tend to die at younger ages than do those with higher family income.[9] During the period from 1979 to 1989, the average life expectancy among white adult men with a family income of at least $25,000 was 6.6 years longer than that among adult men with a family income of less than $10,000. The relationship between poverty and health is complex, because socioeconomic status is related to race, nutrition, risk factors such as smoking and alcohol use, environmental and occupational exposures, and access to and use of health care services.

Religious affiliation also influences disease rates. Like most of the personal characteristics described thus far, religion represents a mixture of factors including genetic, environmental, cultural, and behavioral factors. For example, Tay-Sachs disease, a degenerative disease of the brain and nervous system, is associated with a genetic mutation is that is present mainly among Jews of Eastern European decent.[10(pp347–350)] On the other hand, the likely reason for the 24% lower cancer rate among Mormons is their prohibition against two behaviors associated with cancer risk: cigarette smoking and alcohol consumption.[11]

It is not surprising that occupation influences disease patterns because potent and sustained exposures to harmful substances can occur on some jobs.[12(pp94–98)] One of the earliest associations between an occupation and disease was observed almost 200 years ago by Dr. Percival Pott, who noted that London chimney sweeps had a high rate of scrotal cancer. It was only many years later that the constituents of soot, called polycyclic aromatic hydrocarbons, were found to cause cancer in laboratory animals. Today, we know that the patterns of numerous diseases vary by occupation. For example, people with jobs in aluminum production, boot and shoe manufacturing, coal gasification, furniture making, iron and steel founding, rubber manufacturing, and nickel refining are known to have higher rates of cancer than the general population.

Finally, marital status is known to have an important effect on the patterns of disease and death. For example, suicide rates are higher among nonmarried individuals.[13] The highest rates occur among divorced and widowed persons, intermediate rates occur among singles, and the lowest rates occur among married persons. Data such as these suggest that the psychological and economic support associated with marriage exerts a protective effect against certain adverse health events.[14,15] Alternatively, it is possible that the characteristics that lead a person to marry may be responsible for this protection.[16]

Place

Place can be defined in terms of geopolitical units such as countries or states or in terms of natural geographic features such as mountains or rivers. The characteristics of place encompass numerous aspects of the environment including the physical environment (such as climate, water, and air), biological environment (such as flora and fauna), and social environment (such as cultural traditions). For example, malaria occurs in parts of the world where all these facets of the environment are conducive to the life cycle of the *Anopheles* mosquito, the vector that carries disease from one host to another.[17] Physical conditions that are necessary for the development and survival of the mosquito include a favorable temperature (20° to 30°C is optimal), adequate humidity, moderate rainfall, and the presence of standing or gently flowing water. Biological factors beneficial to the mosquito include plants that can collect small pools of water. Social factors that encourage transmission of the disease include the proximity of homes to mosquito breeding sites, housing construction that facilitates mosquito entry, and certain occupations that increase a person's exposure to mosquitos such as those involving outdoor work at night.

The scale of geographic comparisons can range from a global scale, in which rates are compared between continents and countries; to a regional one, in which states and cities are compared; to a local one, in which neighborhoods are examined. Regardless of the scale that is used, striking geographic patterns of infectious and noninfectious diseases are often observed. For example, almost all cases of malaria are limited to Africa south of the Sahara desert, central and southeast Asia, eastern Asia and Oceania, and Central and, South America (see Figure 5–1).

Rates of chronic diseases such as cancer also show tremendous worldwide variation (see Table 5–1). For example, rates of liver cancer among males are more than 112 times higher in Thailand and China than rates in the Netherlands.[18(pp9–54)] Epidemiologists hypothesize that higher rates of hepatitis infection in the Far East account for this particular difference.[19(pp155–157)]

An example of disease variation on a regional scale is the east-to-west decline across Canada and the United States in the prevalence of birth defects involving the spinal cord and brain (such as spina bifida and anencephaly). Data from the 1960s indicate that the prevalence in eastern Canada was at least twice as high as that of western Canada.[20(pp251–336)] Although we know that an adequate diet (particularly the consumption of the vitamin folic acid around the time of conception) reduces the risk of these birth defects, it is not known whether this or some other factor accounts for the east–west gradient.

An example of neighborhood variation in disease occurrence is the distribution of childhood lead poisoning within the city of Boston. During the 1980s, the prevalence of childhood lead poisoning was highest in 28 city

Areas where malaria transmission occurs
Areas with limited risk
No malaria

FIGURE 5–1. World Distribution of Malaria

Source: World Health Organization, 2001

TABLE 5-1 International Range of Cancer Incidence

Cancer Site	Country with high rate	Rate*	Country with low rate	Rate*	Ratio (high to low)
Males					
Liver	China	90.0	Netherlands	0.8	112.5
Stomach	Japan	93.3	India	2.1	44.4
Bladder	Italy	34.0	United States (Los Angeles)	1.8	18.9
Females					
Cervix	Peru	54.6	Israel	2.6	21.0
Lung	New Zealand	62.2	India	1.4	44.4
Ovary	Switzerland	17.0	Mali	1.0	17.0

* Rate per 100,000 population. The rates were age-adjusted to eliminate the differences in cause-specific death rates due to differences in the age composition of people dying of that cause. (See Chapter 3 for details on age-adjustment.)
Source: Data from Ries LAG. Rates. In: Harras A, Edwards BK, Blot WJ, Ries LAG, eds. *Cancer Rates and Risks.* NIH pub no 96-691. Bethesda, Md: National Cancer Institute 1996:24–27.

block areas. The residences in these areas contain lead-based paint, and the surrounding soil has high levels of lead contamination.

Migrant studies are one of the ways that epidemiologists investigate the effect of place on disease occurrence. These studies compare the rates of disease among natives of a home land to rates among immigrants (and their offspring) and among natives of the adopted country. For example, migrant studies have found that the rate of prostate cancer is low among Japanese in Japan, intermediate among Japanese immigrants to Hawaii, and high among Hawaiian whites.[21(pp185–187)] If the rate of disease among migrants approaches that of the host country, epidemiologists hypothesize that environmental factors may cause the disease. In the case of prostate cancer, those environmental factors may include dietary characteristics such as consumption of animal fat and vitamin A.

Time

Analysis of the changes in disease and death rates over calendar time provides epidemiologists with useful information for causal research and public health planning and evaluation. The scale of time that is examined depends on the disease and can range from decades or years to months, weeks, days, or hours. For example, the death rate from lung cancer has increased dramatically among women over the 30-year period from the 1960s through the 1990s.[5] Over the same period, there has been a dramatic decline in deaths from stomach cancer. Both of these are examples of long-term or secular trends.

Short-term trends are commonly examined for infectious diseases. For example, the 1976 outbreak of Legionnaires' disease at a Philadelphia convention occurred over a 1-month period.[22] Short-term trends are also relevant for noninfectious diseases that follow climatic changes such as heat waves, hurricanes, and pollution episodes. For example, the 4-day 1952 smog disaster in London was associated with an increase in cardiovascular and respiratory deaths, particularly among the elderly.[23] More recently, temporal elevations in air pollution levels in Philadelphia were associated with concomitant increases in death rates from chronic obstructive pulmonary disease, pneumonia, heart disease, and stroke.

Other types of temporal changes include periodic or regular fluctuations occurring on an annual, weekly, or even daily basis. Seasonal variations in disease frequency are the most common type of periodic fluctuations. For example, influenza peaks every winter season, and eastern equine encephalitis crests in summer and early fall in temperate regions of the world.[4(pp31-35)] Regarding weekly and diurnal variations, a study found that heart attacks occur most frequently on weekends and Mondays, and in the morning and afternoon.[24]

What can we infer from time trends? First, they may result from concomitant changes in exposure to causal agents and/or susceptibility to the disease. However, it is also possible that temporal changes in disease and death rates result from parallel fluctuations in diagnostic capabilities, disease definition or reporting methods, the accuracy of the enumeration of the denominator population, or age distribution of the population. For example, the increased prevalence of certain birth defects of the heart (such as ventricular septal defects) over the last decade stems, in part, from the use of sophisticated ultrasounds that can detect heretofore undiagnosed cases.[25] In addition, when examining mortality rates over time, epidemiologists must consider the influence of improvements in treatment that increase survival. How do we know which factor or factors are responsible for a particular time trend? Information gathering and detailed analysis of all possible explanations provide useful clues, but in many cases the answers are never learned.

Disease Clusters and Epidemics

Disease Clusters in Place and Time

A disease cluster is defined as an "aggregation of relatively uncommon events or disease in space and/or time in amounts that are believed or perceived to be greater than could be expected by chance."[2(pp30-31)] Thus, the hallmark of a cluster is the occurrence of cases of disease close together in space (spatial clustering), time (temporal clustering), or both space and time (spatio-temporal clustering).

A well-known historical disease cluster is known as "eleven blue men."[26(pp1–13)] Here, 11 derelicts were found ill or unconscious in a single neighborhood of New York City over the course of a single day. This finding would not have prompted much concern on the part of health authorities were it not for the unusual blue color of the men's skin. Given this peculiar symptom, the investigating epidemiologist easily identified the condition as methemoglobinemia, which results from the ingestion of sodium nitrite. This disease is so rare that the occurrence of 11 cases is far more than that expected by chance. A follow-up investigation found that a local restaurant where all the men had eaten had mistakenly put sodium nitrite instead of sodium chloride in its "salt" shakers.

More recently, a cluster of leukemia cases occurred in Woburn, Massachusetts, over an 11-year period.[27] Two of the eight wells supplying drinking water to the town were discovered to be contaminated with several chlorinated organic chemicals. Follow-up investigations confirmed that the cluster was real and found that the individuals with leukemia were more likely than others to live in homes that received water from the two contaminated wells.

Epidemiologists have varying opinions about the usefulness of investigating the causes of disease clusters because follow-up investigations often fail to produce fruitful results and they consume scarce resources.[28,29] Fruitful results are scarce because good information on exposure to the responsible agent is rarely available.[29] This is particularly true for diseases that have a long induction period where the likely cause (such as contaminated air or water) may have long since disappeared. Characteristics of clusters that are more likely to produce useful results are those involving diseases with a few unique and well-understood causes, a sufficient number of cases, and an environmentally persistent and measurable agent.

Epidemics

Analysis of disease incidence by person, place, and time is used to determine if an epidemic is occurring. An epidemic is defined as "the occurrence in a community or region of cases of an illness, specific health-related behavior, or other health-related events *clearly in excess of normal expectancy*. The community or region and time period in which the cases occur are specified precisely."[5(p54)] Thus, an epidemic occurs when the rate of disease increases to a level higher than what is usually seen in a particular population and time period. The number of cases that indicate the presence of an epidemic varies according to the disease, the population size, and previous experience with the disease. Thus, even the occurrence of one or two cases of a disease might be considered an epidemic. However, worldwide epidemics involving millions of people, termed pandemics, also occur. For example, four influenza pandemics have occurred in the past 100 years.[5(pp224–229)]

Although epidemics have traditionally been linked to infectious disease outbreaks (such as outbreaks of food poisoning and AIDS), epidemics of noninfectious diseases and conditions also occur. For example, MacMahon and Yen described the occurrence of an epidemic of neural tube birth defects (such as anencephaly and spina bifida) during the 1920s and 1930s in Boston, Massachusetts, and Providence, Rhode Island.[30] Delivery records revealed a baseline prevalence of these defects of about 2.0 per 1000 births (the normal expectancy). Subsequently, the prevalence increased until it peaked at 4.7 per 1000 births during the period from 1930 to 1935. Rates declined thereafter, and were lower than baseline by the end of the observation period (see Figure 5–2).

The most interesting aspect of this epidemic was that its occurrence went unrecognized until the late 1960s, when MacMahon and Yen conducted their study. The authors attribute this lapse to the insidious onset and decline of the epidemic and to the familiarity of these defects among hospital clinicians. Although they never learned the cause of the epidemic, MacMahon and Yen speculated that it might have been related to the consumption of moonshine liquor during the federal prohibition of alcoholic beverages (1920 to 1933). Now we know that the consumption of the vitamin folic acid prevents the occurrence of neural tube defects.[31]

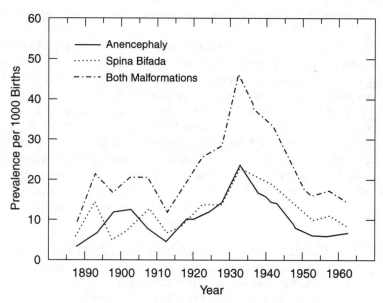

FIGURE 5–2. Frequency of Anencephaly and Spina Bifida in Two Hospitals Combined, 1885–1965

Source: Reprinted from MacMahon B, Yen S. Unrecognized epidemic of anencephaly and spina bifida. *Lancet.* 1971;1:32.

Main Uses of Descriptive Epidemiology

There are two main purposes for describing disease occurrence by person, place, and time—one is scientific and the other is administrative (see Table 5–2). Scientists examine the distribution of disease to search for clues about causes of disease and to generate specific hypotheses about these causal relationships. Public health administrators and planners examine these patterns to establish priorities, plan, and evaluate the effectiveness of clinical and public health programs.

Generating Hypotheses about Causal Relationships

Exactly what is a hypothesis? According to the *American Heritage Dictionary*, a hypothesis is "a tentative explanation for an observation, phenomenon, or scientific problem that can be tested by further investigation."[32(p866)] Thus, a hypothesis is usually a specific statement that attempts to explain certain observations. The process of generating hypotheses is a creative endeavor that combines these observations with biomedical information often from other fields such as genetics, biochemistry, physiology, and toxicology. For example, an epidemiologist might hypothesize that the high incidence of stomach cancer in Japan is due to the consumption of pickled foods because physiological data show that the nitrites in the pickled foods can combine with nitrogen-containing foods to form carcinogens in the stomach.[33(pp191–913)]

Although epidemiologists do not follow a rigid set of steps to generate a hypothesis, they often rely on several types of comparisons during the process. First, investigators often compare groups with very different disease rates and try to identify different characteristics that may account for the disparate rates. For example, the large differences in infant mortality rates according to race may be explained by documented racial differences in access to prenatal care.[3] Second, researchers often look for common characteristics that link the affected groups. For example, increased death rates from the cancer non-Hodgkin's lymphoma have been observed among diverse occupational groups including agricultural workers, rubber workers, chemists, and dry cleaners. Solvents are the single exposure

TABLE 5–2   Main Elements and Uses of Descriptive Epidemiology

Elements	Person (age, sex, race, religion, socioeconomic class)
	Place (country, state, city, neighborhood)
	Time (year, season, month, week, day, hour)
Uses	Assessing the health status of a population
	Generating hypotheses about causal factors
	Planning and evaluating public health programs

that all of these occupations have in common.[34(pp170–174)] Third, when examining changes in disease rates over time or from place to place, epidemiologists search for concomitant variation of a likely causal factor. For example, the large increase in lung cancer deaths among men over the last 60 years is attributed to the increased prevalence of cigarette smoking over the same time period.[35] The increase in lung cancer deaths among women trails behind that of men (it started in 1960), because women adopted cigarette smoking more recently than men. Fourth, it is helpful to look for analogies with other better known diseases. For example, at the beginning of the AIDS epidemic, researchers noted that many of its descriptive features resembled those of hepatitis B, a virally transmitted disease.[36(p103)] These features included "characteristics associated with a sexually active life style" such as a history of sexually transmitted diseases and large numbers of non steady sexual partners and percutaneous needle exposures.[36(p103)] Thus, these similarities led investigators to postulate a viral etiology of AIDS early in the epidemic.

Public Health Planning and Evaluation

Public health administrators and planners use descriptive epidemiology to establish priorities, allocate resources, and plan and evaluate the effectiveness of programs. On a national level, the U.S. Department of Health and Human Services has used descriptive data to provide baseline estimates and plan goals and objectives for *Healthy People 2010,* a comprehensive plan for "promoting health and preventing illness, disability, and premature death" in the U.S. population.[37] The plan has two overarching goals: to increase the quality and years of healthy life and to eliminate health disparities. These goals are supported by specific objectives in 28 focus areas including access to quality health services; cancer; diabetes; environmental health; family planning; health communication; HIV; maternal, infant, and child health; medical product safety; physical activity and fitness; sexually transmitted diseases; substance abuse; tobacco use; and food safety. The plan uses "leading health indicators" to illustrate individual behaviors, physical and social environmental factors, and health system issues that significantly affect the health of individuals and communities.

Example: Patterns of Mortality in the United States According to Age

In order to illustrate the main elements and uses of descriptive epidemiology, this section describes the pattern of mortality in the United States according to age.

Demographic Characteristics of the U.S. Population

First, it is necessary to present background demographic characteristics of the U.S. population.

SIZE The 2000 Census enumerated 281,421,906 individuals in the U.S. population.[7] This number represents a 13% increase since the 1990 Census and an 87% increase since the 1950 Census. Officials anticipate that population growth will continue slowly for the foreseeable future. Population growth stems both from a "natural increase" (where the number of births exceeds the number of deaths) and from immigration from other countries.

SEX RATIO According to the 2000 Census, the U.S. population consisted of 138,053,563 males and 143,368,343 females, resulting in an overall sex ratio of 96.3 males for every 100 females.[7] The sex ratio varies with age. There are more males than females (105 males for every 100 females) among individuals younger than 18 years of age, and fewer males than females (93.4 males for every 100 females) among those 18 years and older. There are only 70 men for every 100 women among individuals aged 65 years and older.

AGE STRUCTURE The median (or the midpoint) age of the U.S. population has increased steadily over time, rising from 26 years in 1970 to 35.3 years in 2000.[7] This increase reflects the "aging of the population." That is, the proportion of U.S. adults, particularly elderly adults, has grown over time. In 1970, adults aged 65 years and older formed 10.8% of the population; by 2000 they formed 12.4% (see Table 5–3). The median age is expected to con-

TABLE 5-3   Age Distribution of U.S. Resident Population, 1970 and 2000

Age (in years)	1970 Number (in thousands)	Percent	2000 Number (in thousands)	Percent
14 and younger	57,900	28.5	60,253	21.4
15–24	35,441	17.4	39,184	13.9
25–34	24,907	12.3	39,892	14.2
35–44	23,088	11.4	45,149	16.0
45–54	23,220	11.4	37,678	13.4
55–64	18,590	9.1	24,275	8.6
65–74	12,435	6.1	18,391	6.5
75–84	6,119	3.0	12,361	4.4
85 years and older	1,511	0.7	4,240	1.5

Source: Data from Kramarow E, Lentzer H, Rooks R, Weeks J, Saydah S. *Health and Aging Chartbook. Health, United States, 1999.* Hyattsville, MD: National Center for Health Statistics, 1999. U.S. Census Bureau. Census, 2000. Available at: http://www2.census.gov/census_2000/datasets/demographic_profile>. Accessed July 2001.

tinue to increase because the elderly population is growing at a faster rate than is the population as a whole.

RACE According to the 2000 Census, the U.S. population is predominantly white (75.1%) and not of Hispanic origin (87.5%)[7] (see Figure 5–3). However, many racial and ethnic groups are represented, with blacks making up the plurality of the other races and Mexicans predominating among people of Hispanic origin. The racial and ethnic diversity of the U.S. population is expected to increase in the coming years.

Natality

The number of live births occurring in the United States increased from nearly 3.8 million in the mid 1980s to almost 4.2 million in 1990, and then declined to about 3.9 million in 1997 when the crude birth rate was 14.5 per 1000 population for all races combined.[3]

Birth rates have been consistently higher among black women than white women (17.7 versus 13.9 per 1000 population in 1997). When 1997 rates are broken down further by age, blacks have higher birth rates than whites from ages 10 through 24 years, and whites have higher rates from ages 25 through 49 years (see Figure 5–4).

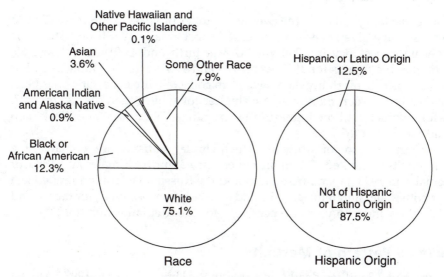

FIGURE 5–3. Distribution of Race and Hispanic Origin Among U.S. Resident Population, 2000

Source: Data from U.S. Census Bureau. *Census 2000.* Available at: http://www2.census.gov/census_2000/datasets/demographic_profile. Accessed July 2001.

*Live births per 1000 population

FIGURE 5–4. Live Births, Crude Birth Rates, and Birth Rates by Age and Race of Mother: United States, 1997

Source: Data from Kramarow E, Lentzer H, Rooks R, Weeks J, Saydah S. *Health and Aging Chartbook. Health, United States, 1999.* Hyattsville, MD: National Center for Health Statistics; 1999:110–113.

Life Expectancy

Life expectancy—that is, the average number of years of life remaining to a person at a given age—has increased substantially over time.[3] The average life expectancy in 1900 was 47.3 at birth and 11.9 years at age 65. Comparable figures for 1997 were 76.5 and 17.7 years (see Table 5–4). For as long as U.S. mortality data have been collected, life expectancy has been higher for women than men, and higher for whites than blacks. In 1997, white women had the highest life expectancy (79.9 years) and black men had the lowest (67.2 years).

Compared to countries for which similar statistics are available, the United States ranked 25th in life expectancy at birth for males and 19th for females in 1995. Japan ranked first and the Russian Federation ranked last for both males and females (76.4 and 82.9 years, respectively, for Japan, and 58.3 years and 71.6 years, respectively, for the Russian Federation).

Overall Pattern of Mortality

More than 2.3 million deaths occurred in the United States in 1997.[3] Almost 62% of these deaths could be accounted for by three causes: heart disease, cancer, and cerebrovascular disease (see Table 5–5). These three diseases were the leading causes among white males, white females, and black females. However unintentional injuries supplanted cerebrovascular disease as the third leading cause of death among black males. Leading sites for cancer deaths were the lung, prostate, and colon-rectum among men; and lung, breast, and colon-rectum among women[5] (see Table 5–6). Other important causes of death for both men and women were chronic lung diseases, unintentional injuries, infectious diseases (including pneumonia and influenza), diabetes, suicides, kidney diseases, and liver diseases.[3]

TABLE 5–4   Life Expectancy at Birth and at 65 Years of Age According to Race and Sex: United States, 1997

		Remaining life expectancy in years	
Race	*Sex*	*At birth*	*At 65 years*
All races	Both sexes	76.5	17.7
	Males	73.6	15.9
	Females	79.4	19.2
Whites	Both sexes	77.1	17.8
	Males	74.3	16.0
	Females	79.9	19.3
Blacks	Both sexes	71.1	16.1
	Males	67.2	14.2
	Females	74.7	17.6

Source: Data from Kramarow E, Lentzer H, Rooks R, Weeks J, Saydah S. *Health and Aging Chartbook. Health, United States, 1999.* Hyattsville, MD: National Center for Health Statistics; 1999:139.

TABLE 5–5   Leading Causes of Death: Number and Percentage of Deaths in the U.S. Population, 1997

Rank	*Cause of death*	*Number of deaths*	*Percentage of total deaths*
1	Heart diseases	726,974	31.4
2	Cancer	539,577	23.3
3	Cerebrovascular diseases	159,791	6.9
4	Chronic obstructive lung diseases	109,029	4.7
5	Unintentional injuries	95,644	4.1
6	Pneumonia and influenza	86,449	3.7
7	Diabetes	62,636	2.7
8	Suicide	30,535	1.3
9	Kidney diseases	25,331	1.1
10	Liver diseases	25,175	1.1

Source: Data from Kramarow E, Lentzer H, Rooks R, Weeks J, Saydah S. *Health and Aging Chartbook. Health, United States, 1999.* Hyattsville, MD: National Center for Health Statistics; 1999:151–154.

TABLE 5-6   Death Rates for the Five Leading Cancer Sites for Males and Females, United States, 1992–1998

Sex and cancer site	Death rates*
Males	
Lung and bronchus	69.3
Prostate	24.5
Colon and rectum	20.9
Pancreas	9.8
Non-Hodgkin's lymphoma	8.2
Females	
Lung and bronchus	34.0
Breast	24.7
Colon and rectum	14.3
Ovary	7.5
Pancreas	7.2

* Rates are per 100,000 and are age-adjusted to the 1970 U.S. standard.
Source: Data from Ries LAG, Eisner MP, Kosary CL, Hankey BF, Miller BA, Clegg L, et al, eds. *SEER Cancer Statistics Review, 1973–1998.* Supplemental Materials No.2: *Rates and Trends by Site and Sex for 1992–1998.* Bethesda, MD: National Cancer Institute; 2001.

Mortality Rates by Age

In the U.S. population, there is a *J*-shaped relationship between age and the rate of death[3] (see Figure 5–5). That is, mortality rates are relatively high during the first year of life. They decline until age 14, and then increase thereafter with each age group. Because age is such an important determinant of death, the remainder of this section describes the rates and important causes of death for each age group.

INFANTS (LESS THAN 1 YEAR OF AGE) The infant mortality rate is considered a sensitive indicator of the overall health of a population. In 1997, the leading causes of infant deaths were congenital anomalies, disorders relating to low birthweight and short gestation, sudden infant death syndrome, and respiratory distress syndrome. Although U.S. rates have declined over time (from 10.9 to 7.3 over the period from 1983 to 1996), there is a great disparity between racial and ethnic groups[3] (see Figure 5–6). For example, during this period, the rate among blacks was more than twice that of whites. Among countries with comparable data, the U.S. infant mortality rate ranked 25th after countries such as Finland (which had the lowest rate), Singapore, Sweden, Norway, Japan, Hong Kong, France, and Switzerland.

CHILDREN (1 TO 14 YEARS OF AGE) In 1997, major causes of death among children aged 1 to 14 were unintentional injuries, malignant neoplasms,

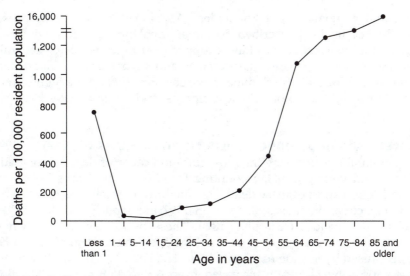

FIGURE 5–5. Death Rates for all Causes According to Age: United States, 1997

Source: Data from Kramarow E, Lentzer H, Rooks R, Weeks J, Saydah S. *Health and Aging Chartbook. Health, United States, 1999.* Hyattsville, MD: National Center for Health Statistics; 1999:160–163.

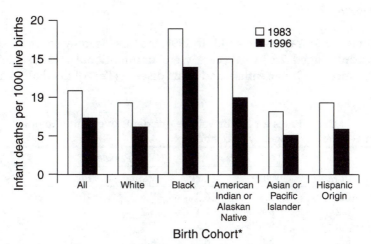

*A birth cohort consists of all individuals who were born in a given period of time (e.g., a year).

FIGURE 5–6. Infant Mortality Rate According to Mother's Race, 1983 and 1996 Birth Cohorts

Source: Data from Kramarow E, Lentzer H, Rooks R, Weeks J, Saydah S. *Health and Aging Chartbook. Health, United States, 1999.* Hyattsville, MD: National Center for Health Statistics; 1999:129.

congenital anomalies, and homicides.[3] Motor vehicle accidents caused about half of the deaths ascribed to unintentional injuries. Although deaths from motor vehicle accidents have dropped over time, they have generally been higher among males than females and higher among blacks than whites (see Table 5–7). Black males have consistently had the highest rates of death caused by motor vehicle accidents, and white females have had the lowest.

ADOLESCENTS AND YOUNG ADULTS (15 TO 24 YEARS OF AGE) In 1997, unintentional injuries were the most common cause of death among adolescents and young adults, accounting for 42% of the deaths in this age group.[3] Again, most of these deaths resulted from motor vehicle accidents.

Other common causes of death in 1997 included homicides (19% of deaths) and suicides (13% of deaths). These two causes of death have exhibited large increases over time in this age group. From 1950 to 1997, deaths caused by suicide rose from 4.5 to 11.4 per 100,000 population, and those caused by homicide increased from 6.3 to 16.8 per 100,000. Both whites and blacks have experienced increases in homicides, but the rates among blacks have been consistently higher than rates among whites (see Table 5–8). Black men had almost nine times the homicide rate of white men in this age group in 1997 (113.3 versus 13.2 per 100,000). Black females had higher rates than white females (13.3 versus 3.2 per 100,000), but homicide rates for females have always been much lower than those among males.

ADULTS (25 TO 64 YEARS OF AGE) In 1997, the three leading causes of death among adults aged 25 to 44 years were unintentional injuries (20% of deaths), cancer (16% of deaths), and heart disease (12% of deaths).[3] Among

TABLE 5–7 Death Rates for Motor Vehicle Accidents over Time Among Children 1–14 Years of Age, by Race and Sex

		Males		Females	
Year	All races	White	Black	White	Black
1970	10.5	12.5	16.3	7.5	10.2
1980	8.2	9.8	11.4	6.2	6.3
1985	7.0	8.3	9.7	5.4	5.1
1990	6.0	6.6	8.9	4.8	5.3
1995	5.3	5.9	7.8	4.3	5.1
1997	5.1	5.4	7.6	4.1	5.6

Source: Data from Kramarow E, Lentzer H, Rooks R, Weeks J, Saydah S. *Health and Aging Chartbook. Health, United States, 1999.* Hyattsville, MD: National Center for Health Statistics; 1999:185–188.

adults aged 45 to 64 years, cancer ranked first (35% of deaths), heart disease ranked second (27% of deaths), and unintentional injuries was a distant third (5% of deaths).

From 1950 through 1998, age-adjusted mortality rates for all types of cancer combined have increased by 3.5% among adult men and women.[5] Mortality rates have increased for many types of cancer, including esophagus, liver, lung and bronchus, melanoma of the skin, prostate, kidney, brain, non-Hodgkin's lymphoma, and multiple myeloma. On the other hand, they have decreased for other types of cancer including stomach, colon and rectum, cervix and uterine, breast, ovary, and leukemia.

Deaths caused by heart disease have also declined substantially over time among U.S. adult men and women. Men experience higher mortality rates from heart disease than women at all ages. For example, in 1997, male mortality rates from heart disease were 2.4 times higher than were rates among women aged 55 to 64 years (see Figure 5–7).

ELDERLY ADULTS (65 YEARS OF AGE AND OLDER) As one would expect, the elderly population experiences the highest mortality rates of all age groups.[3] In 1997, the leading causes of death in this age group were heart disease (35% of deaths), cancer (22%), and cerebrovascular disease (8%). Death rates have declined considerably over time among the "younger" elderly. For example, from 1970 through 1997, death rates for heart disease declined by 51.6% among men and women aged 65 to 74 years. In 1997, the overall death rate among the "younger" elderly was higher among men than among women; however, the rates were similar at the oldest ages. For example, men who were 65 to 69 years of age had 1.7 times the death rate of women of the same age, but the death rates were nearly identical for men and women aged 95 years and older.

TABLE 5–8 Death Rates for Homicides Among White and Black Males, 15–24 Years of Age

Year	White males	Black males
1950	3.7	58.9
1960	4.4	46.4
1970	7.9	102.5
1980	15.5	84.3
1985	11.0	65.9
1990	15.4	138.3
1995	16.5	132.0
1997	13.2	113.3

Source: Data from Kramarow E, Lentzer H, Rooks R, Weeks J, Saydah S. *Health and Aging Chartbook. Health, United States, 1999.* Hyattsville, MD: National Center for Health Statistics; 1999:189–191.

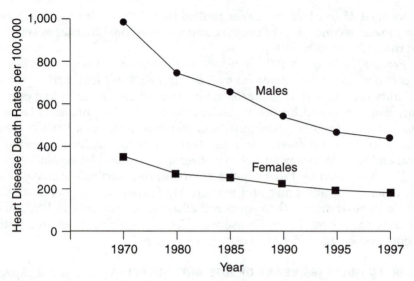

FIGURE 5-7. Heart Disease Death Rates over Time Among Men and Women, Aged 55–64 Years

Source: Data from Kramarow E, Lentzer H, Rooks R, Weeks J, Saydah S. *Health and Aging Chartbook. Health, United States, 1999.* Hyattsville, MD: National Center for Health Statistics; 1999:164–166.

Strengths and Limitations of Mortality Data

There are many advantages to using mortality data to learn about the health status of a population. First, because this information is completely reported for the entire country, it can be used to study fatal illnesses on a national, state, city, or neighborhood level. Second, the National Center for Health Statistics conducts extensive and ongoing analysis of deaths and produces readily available statistics for public health practitioners. Third, death rates provide information on the ultimate impact of a disease.

As previously described, numerous patterns are evident in the U.S. mortality data. For example,

- Life expectancy has increased over time, is higher for women than men, and is higher for whites than blacks.

- Death rates increase from adolescence onward.

- Leading causes of death vary among age groups (unintentional injuries predominate among the young, and chronic diseases predominate among adults and the elderly).

- Many cause-specific death rates—particularly those due to motor vehicle accidents, and homicides—are higher among blacks than among whites.

■ Many cause-specific death rates—particularly those due to heart disease and lung cancer—are higher among males than among females.

Although mortality patterns such as these provide useful information for etiologic research and public health planning and administration, mortality data also have important limitations. First, information about cause of death may be inaccurate because it is sometimes difficult for physicians to assign a single underlying cause of death—particularly when numerous conditions are present or when insufficient clinical, laboratory, and autopsy data are available. Second, mortality data are inadequate for examining nonfatal diseases. Thus, they give an incomplete picture of the health status of a population. This is particularly true for children and young adults whose mortality rates are low. Even among older and elderly adults, nonfatal conditions such as arthritis and visual and hearing impairments are of great concern because of their significant impact on daily living.

Examples: Three Important Causes of Morbidity in the United States

The remainder of this chapter focuses on three important causes of morbidity in the United States: childhood lead poisoning, AIDS, and breast cancer. Studying the patterns of these diseases in terms of person, place, and time can help us understand their causes and preventions.

Background and Descriptive Epidemiology of Childhood Lead Poisoning

Childhood lead poisoning is considered "one of the worst environmental threats to children in the United States."[38] Very high blood lead levels can lead to convulsions, coma, and even death; moderately elevated levels can adversely affect the brain, kidney, and blood-forming tissues. In fact, blood lead levels as low as 10 μg/dL have been associated with decreased IQ scores, growth deficits, and impaired vitamin D metabolism.[39]

According to one expert, lead poisoning threatens the health of our nation's children because "lead has subtly become an intrinsic part of our contemporary ways of life."[40(pp43–45)] A naturally occurring element in the earth's crust, lead's unique properties of softness, malleability, and imperviousness have made it "one of the most useful metals in the industrial world." Lead has been used in storage batteries, sewer pipes, roofing materials, solder for food cans and electronic equipment, containers for corrosive liquids, and gasoline. Perhaps its most infamous use has been to enhance the durability and brightness of paint. In fact, Dutch Boy paint advertisements from the 1930s encouraged consumers to purchase lead-based paint because "it lasts."[41]

The National Health and Nutrition Examination Surveys (NHANES) serve as the primary data source on the descriptive epidemiology of elevated blood lead levels among U.S. children.[42] Venous blood lead measurements were obtained in NHANES II (1976–1980), the Hispanic Health and Nutrition Examination Survey (HHANES) (1982–1984), NHANES III phases 1 (1988–1991) and 2 (1991–1994), and NHANES 1999. The following sections provide information on how children's blood lead levels have changed over time, what characteristics are associated with elevated levels, and what areas of the United States are most affected. Data on children aged 1 to 5 years are presented because children of this age have physiological and behavioral characteristics that place them at high risk of lead poisoning.[39] For example, young children absorb and ingest more lead and have a blood brain barrier that is less developed than older children and adults.

PERSON   In the late 1980s, children aged 1 to 2 years had the highest prevalence of elevated blood lead levels.[42] Average levels among boys were slightly higher than among girls. Non-Hispanic blacks had the highest average blood lead levels, followed by Mexican Americans and non-Hispanic whites. The prevalence of elevated blood lead levels was inversely related to the head of household's income and educational level (see Tables 5–9 and 5–10).

PLACE   Average blood lead levels were highest among children living in the Northeast region of the United States, intermediate among those living in the South and Midwest, and lowest among those living in the West. Children who lived in large urban areas (more than 1 million residents) had the highest average blood lead levels, children who resided in smaller urban areas (less than 1 million residents) had intermediate levels, and those who lived in rural areas had the lowest levels (see Table 5–10).

TIME   Average blood lead levels among children aged 1 to 5 years declined by 76% from 15.0 μg/dL in 1976–1980 (NHANES II) to 3.6 μg/dL in 1988–1991 (NHANES III) (see Figure 5–8). The drop in blood lead levels was less among non-Hispanic black children (72%), particularly those from low-income families who lived in large urban areas (60%), than it was among non-Hispanic white children (77%). Data from NHANES 1999 indicate that the drop in blood lead levels continued through the 1990s. By 1999, the average blood lead level among children aged 1 to 5 years was 2.0 μg/dL.[43]

DISCUSSION   The dramatic reduction in children's blood lead levels has been hailed as "one of the most remarkable public health achievements of the decade,"[38] and is likely the result of concerted governmental action over the last 20 years to reduce lead levels in many sources.[39] For example, the introduction of unleaded gasoline for automobiles in the 1970s greatly reduced airborne lead levels, and the phase-out of cans with lead-soldered seams decreased lead levels in food.

However, the continuing racial and economic disparities in the prevalence of childhood lead poisoning are disconcerting. As an editorial in the *Journal of the American Medical Association* stated: "The U.S. strategy must begin to focus more than ever on poor, nonwhite, and inner-city children. We must intensify our efforts to screen these children, identify the sources of lead exposure, and eliminate or reduce these exposures."[38]

The main sources of exposure among poor, inner-city children include old leaded paint and contaminated soil and dust in and around homes. Even though lead-based paint was banned for residential use in 1978, an estimated 57 million housing units contain lead-based paint because they

TABLE 5–9 Mean Blood Lead Levels (µg/dL) for Children Aged 1–5 Years by Sex, and Race/Ethnicity: United States, 1988–1991

	Race/Ethnicity		
Age and gender	*Non-Hispanic whites*	*Non-Hispanic blacks*	*Mexican Americans*
1–2 years			
Boys	3.5	6.3	4.2
Girls	3.6	5.8	4.8
3–5 years			
Boys	2.9	5.9	4.0
Girls	3.0	5.0	3.6

Source: Data from Brody DJ, Pirkle JL, Kramer RA, Flegal KM, Matte TD, Gunter EW, et al. Blood lead levels in the U.S. population: phase 1 of the third National Health and Nutrition Examination Surveys (NHANES III, 1988 to 1991). *JAMA.* 1994;272:280.

TABLE 5–10 Percentage of Children Aged 1–5 Years with Blood Lead Levels Above 10 µg/dL by Race/Ethnicity, Income Level, Urban Status: United States, 1988–1991

	All (%)	*Non-Hispanic white (%)*	*Non-Hispanic black (%)*	*Mexican American (%)*
Income level				
Low	16.3	9.8	28.4	8.8
Mid	5.4	4.8	8.9	5.6
High	4.0	4.3	5.8	0.0
Urban status				
Central city, ≥ 1 million	21.0	6.1	36.7	17.0
Central city, ≤ 1 million	16.4	8.1	22.5	9.5
Non-central city	5.8	5.2	11.2	7.0

Source: Reprinted from Brody DJ, Pirkle JL, Kramer RA, Flegal KM, Matte TD, Gunter EW, et al. Blood lead levels in the U.S. population: phase 1 of the third National Health and Nutrition Examination Surveys (NHANES III, 1988 to 1991). *JAMA.* 1994;272:282.

FIGURE 5–8. Blood Lead Levels for Children Aged 1–5 Years: United States, Second National Health and Nutrition Examination Survey (1976–1980, top) and Phase 1 of the Third National Health and Nutrition Examination Survey (1988–1991, bottom).

Source: Reprinted from Pirkle JL, Brody DJ, Gunter EW, Kramer RA, Paschal DC, Flegal KM, et al. The decline in blood lead levels in the United States: the National Health and Nutrition Examination Surveys (NHANES). *JAMA*.1994;272:285.

were built before the ban. Activities to clean up these sources and prevent future cases of lead poisoning must be left to the individual property owners.

Background and Descriptive Epidemiology of AIDS

The AIDS epidemic officially started in the United States in 1981 when several cases of *Pneumocystis carinii* pneumonia and Kaposi's sarcoma (a rare cancer of the blood vessels) were reported among previously healthy, young homosexual men living in New York and California.[44,45] These cases were notable because *Pneumocystis carinii* pneumonia had previously occurred only among immunocompromised individuals and Kaposi's sarcoma had occurred mainly among elderly men.

Today, AIDS is defined as a "specific group of diseases or conditions which are indicative of severe immunosuppression related to infection with the human immunodeficiency virus (HIV)."[6] AIDS is considered a chronic disease with a wide spectrum of clinical manifestations that start with a flu-like illness, followed first by a long asymptomatic phase and later by a progressively debilitating symptomatic phase.[46] The final stage is characterized by numerous complications such as HIV wasting syndrome and opportunistic infections like *Pneumocystis carinii* pneumonia. Data on the occurrence of AIDS in the United States come from the Division of HIV/AIDS Prevention at the Centers for Disease Control and Prevention.

INCIDENCE AND MORTALITY From 1981 through 1999, 733,374 cases of AIDS were reported in the United States.[6] Of these cases, 99% were diagnosed among adults and adolescents, and only 1% were diagnosed among children less than 13 years of age. In 1999, the overall incidence rate of AIDS among adult and adolescent men was 32.4 per 100,000; the incidence rate among adult and adolescent women was 9.3 per 100,000.

Although many treatments that delay disease progression and prolong survival have become available over the last decade, the cumulative mortality of AIDS remains high. Since 1981, 59% of adults and 58% of children diagnosed with AIDS have died. Although the annual number of deaths among persons with AIDS has declined markedly since 1995, AIDS remains an important cause of death among individuals aged 25 to 44 years.

TIME Figure 5–9 shows the number of adult cases diagnosed with AIDS from 1985 through 1999 using the 1993 case definition and adjusting for reporting delays. Note that the number of reported AIDS cases rose steadily from 1985 through 1992 and declined considerably from 1993 through 1999.[6] These

FIGURE 5–9. Estimated Incidence of AIDS and Deaths of Adults with AIDS, 1985–June 1999, United States

Source: Reprinted from Centers for Disease Control and Prevention. *HIV/AIDS surveillance—general epidemiology.* L173 slide series (through 1999). Available at: http://www.cdc.gov/hiv/graphics/surveillance.htm. Accessed September 2001.

trends were partly caused by the distorting effect of the 1993 expansion of the AIDS case definition. Individuals who formerly did not meet the case definition were reclassified as having AIDS, and so the number of new cases rose rapidly—particularly during 1991 and 1992. The recent decline in AIDS incidence is the result of new HIV treatments that delay disease progression.

PLACE Data on the global occurrence of AIDS come from the World Health Organization. Recent estimates of the AIDS epidemic present a grim picture. At the end of 1999, 34.3 million adults and children were estimated to be living with HIV/AIDS.[47] Most of these individuals live in two areas of the world: sub- Saharan Africa (71%), and South and Southeast Asia (16%). Only about 3% of people living with HIV/AIDS reside in North America, and most of these individuals live in the United States (see Figure 5–10).

In the United States, there is considerable geographic variation in the annual rate of AIDS.[6] In 1999, the lowest rates were in North Dakota (1.1 per 100,000 population), Montana (1.5 per 100,000), and Idaho (2.0 per 100,000). The highest rates were in Florida (36.2 per 100,000), New York (42.3 per 100,000), and the District of Columbia (161.5 per 100,000) (see Figures 5–11 and 5–12). Metropolitan areas with 500,000 or more people had higher rates (21.7 per 100,000) than did metropolitan areas with fewer people (10.2 per 100,000), and nonmetropolitan areas (6.2 per 100,000). The metropolitan areas with the highest rates were San Francisco (50.8 per 100,000), Fort Lauderdale (61.2 per 100,000), Miami (65.3 per 100,000), and New York City (72.7 per 100,000). The pattern of geographic variation in the United States is similar for males and females.

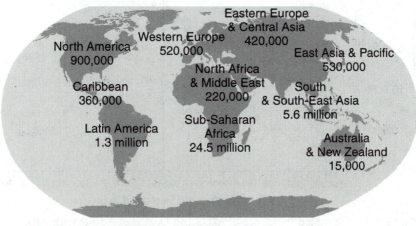

FIGURE 5–10. Global Distribution of HIV/AIDS

Source: Reprinted from Joint United Nations Programme on HIV/AIDS. *Report on the Global HIV/AIDS Epidemic, June 2000.* Geneva Switzerland: UNAIDS; 2000:6.

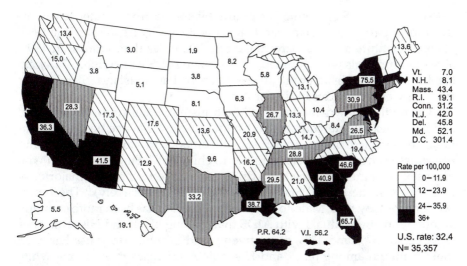

FIGURE 5–11. Male Adult/Adolescent AIDS Annual Rates per 100,000 Population for Cases Reported in 1999, United States

Source: Reprinted from Centers for Disease Control and Prevention. *HIV/AIDS Surveillance Report.* 1999;11(no 2):12.

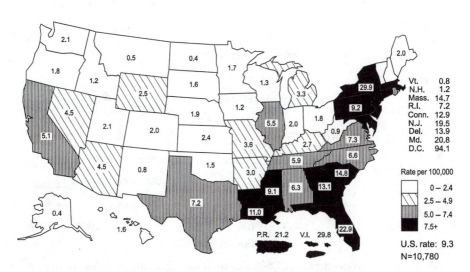

FIGURE 5–12. Female Adult/Adolescent AIDS Annual Rates per 100,000 Population for Cases Reported in 1999, United States

Source: Reprinted from Centers for Disease Control and Prevention. *HIV/AIDS Surveillance Report.* 1999;11(no 2):12.

PERSON The AIDS epidemic has gradually shifted from whites to minority groups, particularly blacks and Hispanics[6] (see Figure 5–13). Since 1996, blacks constitute a larger percentage of AIDS cases than whites. In 1999, 32% of individuals who were reported to have AIDS were white, 47% were black, 19% were Hispanic, 1% were Asian or Pacific Islander, and fewer than 1% were American Indian or Alaskan Native.

Currently known modes of viral transmission include homosexual and heterosexual intercourse, injection with nonsterile needles, transplantation of infected tissue, transfusion of blood and clotting factors, and transmission from an infected mother to child.[48(p89)] Since 1981, men who have sex with men and injecting drug users have formed the majority of male cases in the United States (56% and 22%, respectively).[6] These proportions vary by race. Male-to-male sexual contact has been more common among white individuals with AIDS than among black and Hispanic ones (75% versus 37% and 43%, respectively), and injecting drug use has been more common among black and Hispanic AIDS cases than among white ones (34% and 36% versus 9%, respectively).

A history of injecting drug use and heterosexual contact with an infected man (who was often an injecting drug user) has accounted for the majority of AIDS cases among women since 1981 (42% and 40%, respectively).[6] In contrast to male cases, the proportion of female cases associated with a particular exposure category was similar across racial groups.

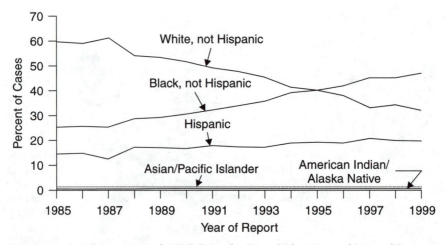

FIGURE 5–13. Proportion of AIDS Cases by Race/Ethnicity and Year of Report, 1985–1999, United States

Source: Reprinted from Centers for Disease Control and Prevention. *HIV/AIDS surveillance—general epidemiology.* L173 slide series through 1999). Available at: http://www.cdc.gov/hiv/graphics/surveillance.htm. Accessed September 2001.

Having a mother with or at risk for HIV infection has accounted for 91% of pediatric cases.[6] Thus, the vast majority of infants and children with AIDS acquire the disease from an infected mother either before, during, or after birth. Other modes of transmission among children include transfusions with infected blood and other products.

DISCUSSION AIDS surveillance data are used to track the spread of the epidemic and to plan and evaluate prevention and treatment programs.[6] For example, several areas of the United States have implemented needle-exchange programs among intravenous drug users (in which possibly infected "dirty" needles are exchanged for clean ones). A 1996 analysis found that injecting drug users who participated in New York City syringe-exchange programs were about 70% less likely to become infected with HIV than drug users who did not participate. As another example, educational programs have been conducted primarily in the gay male community to promote "safer-sex" practices such as the use of condoms and sexual abstinence.[50] However, because behavioral interventions may not be effective over the long term, the development of a preventive vaccine for AIDS has recently gained momentum.

Background and Descriptive Epidemiology of Breast Cancer Among Women

Breast cancer is an abnormal growth in a woman's mammary gland that is characterized by a tendency to invade the surrounding tissues and spread to new locations. The most common types of breast cancer arise in the lining of the ducts or in the lobules of the breast. Like other types of cancer, a malignancy of the breast is thought to develop through a multistep process known as carcinogenesis.[51] The first step in this process, called initiation, involves DNA damage and genetic changes. Initiation is followed by numerous promotion steps that help the cancerous cells grow and establish a blood supply. Growth continues until the cancer is detected by a screening test (such as a mammogram) or produces physical symptoms (such as a lump or nipple discharge). Often many years of inapparent disease elapse between initiation and the cancer diagnosis. For breast cancer, this period may be as long as 20 to 30 years.[52]

The best available epidemiologic data on breast cancer in the United States come from the National Cancer Institute's Surveillance Epidemiology and End Results (SEER) Program (described in Chapter 4).

INCIDENCE AND MORTALITY Approximately 192,200 cases of female breast cancer were reported in 1998, making it the most commonly diagnosed cancer among women in the United States.[5] During the period from 1996 to 1998, the estimated lifetime risk (the lifetime cumulative incidence) of breast cancer for women was 13.24%. From 1992 through 1997, 63% of all women diagnosed with breast cancer were diagnosed with localized disease (no sign of the cancer in the lymph nodes), 28% were diagnosed with regional disease (some evidence of lymph node involvement), and 6% were diagnosed with distant disease (evidence of cancer spread to organs such as the lungs and bone). The stage was unknown for the remaining 3% of women diagnosed with breast cancer.

From 1992 to 1997, the average 5-year relative survival rate among women diagnosed with breast cancer was 85.5%. (The relative survival rate is defined as the ratio of the observed survival rate for a group with cancer to the expected rate among a similar group without cancer.) As expected, women diagnosed with localized disease had much better survival (96.4%) than those diagnosed with regional (77.7%) and distant disease (21.1%).

Although the 5-year survival data are encouraging, they represent only the short-term consequences of the disease. The ultimate impact of breast cancer can be assessed solely by examining mortality rates. With an age-adjusted mortality rate of 22.7 per 100,000 women in 1998, breast cancer ranked second only to lung cancer among female cancer deaths.

TIME Age-adjusted incidence rate of breast cancer among all women increased from 82.6 per 100,000 women in 1973 to 118.1 per 100,000 women in 1998.[5] This increase was quite steep for most of the 1980s but has attenuated in recent years. These time trends for white and black women were similar (see Figure 5–14).

Since 1973, mortality rates have fallen by 18.1% among white women, and they have increased by 12.5% among black women.[5] These mortality trends vary by age at diagnosis. Among white women, mortality rates declined by 29.4% among those under the age of 50 years, but only by 8.2% for those aged 50 years and older. Among black women, mortality rates declined by 5.6% among those under the age of 50 years but increased by 25.7% among those aged 50 years and older.

PERSON Many individual characteristics such as age, race, socioeconomic level, and religion are associated with the risk of breast cancer.[53] Breast cancer incidence rates rise sharply with age. The increase is very steep from age 40 through 74 years and then levels off (see Figure 5–15). Incidence rates are highest among white women, intermediate among blacks and Hispanics, and lowest among Asian women. They are also higher among Jewish women and among women of high socioeconomic status. Various reproductive characteristics also influence a woman's risk of breast cancer.[54] For example, a younger age at menarche and older age at menopause are associated with a higher risk, and surgical removal of both ovaries is associated with a lower risk.

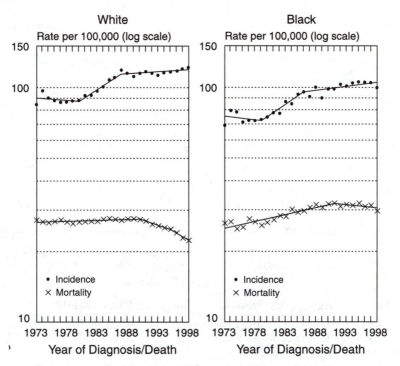

FIGURE 5–14. Breast Cancer Incidence and Mortality Over Time for White and Black Females

Source: Reprinted from Ries LAG, Eisner MP, Kosary CL, Hankey BF, Miller BA, Clegg L, et al., eds. *SEER Cancer Statistics Review, 1973–1998.* Figure IV-1. Bethesda, MD: National Cancer Institute; 2001.

PLACE Incidence rates are highest in North America and northern Europe, intermediate in southern Europe and South America, and lowest in Africa and Asia.[55] Breast cancer rates are four to five times higher in the United States than in Japan. However, the magnitude of the difference between the two countries is diminishing because rates in Japan have risen dramatically over the last few years.

When women migrate from one country to another, they generally adopt the incidence rate of their new country. The change can occur quickly or take several generations and appears to depend on the rate of acculturation. For example, a study of Japanese immigrants to the United States found that the immigrants had slightly higher breast cancer rates than women in Japan but that the immigrants' daughters had markedly increased rates.

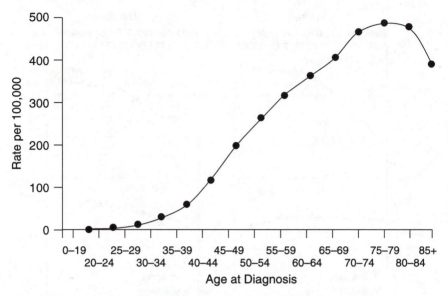

FIGURE 5-15. Age-specific Breast Cancer Incidence Rates, 1994–1998

Source: Data from Ries LAG, Eisner MP, Kosary CL, Hankey BF, Miller BA, Clegg L, et al., eds. *SEER Cancer Statistics Review, 1973–1998.* Table IV-2. Bethesda, MD: National Cancer Institute; 2001.

Death rates from breast cancer also vary dramatically within the United States (see Figure 5–16). They are highest in the Northeast, intermediate in the West and Midwest, and lowest in the South.[56] Highest rates in the Northeast are found in parts of New York, New Jersey, Massachusetts, Connecticut, and Rhode Island.[57] The highest rate west of the Mississippi River is in San Francisco.

DISCUSSION Because the epidemiologic data are so consistent, many of the characteristics described above are considered "established" risk factors for breast cancer[55] (see Table 5–11). Most of these characteristics also fit into the well-accepted hypothesis that ovarian hormones such as estrogen and progesterone play a crucial role in breast cancer development.[58] For example, the low rates among women in Japan and other Asian countries can be accounted for by low serum levels of these hormones. Furthermore, the association with family history and Jewish religion may be partly explained by two recently discovered gene alterations (BRCA1 and BRCA2) that predispose a woman to breast and ovarian cancer. Alterations of one of the genes (BRCA1) have been found in families in which several members have breast or ovarian cancer[59] and among Jews of Eastern European descent.[60]

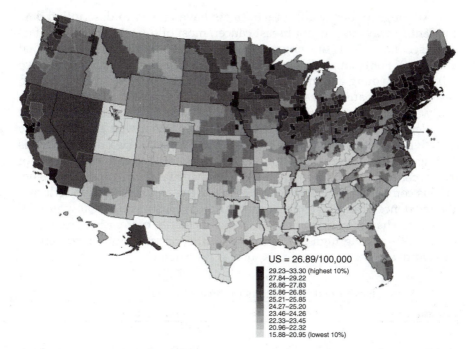

US = 26.89/100,000

29.23–33.30 (highest 10%)
27.84–29.22
26.86–27.83
25.86–26.85
25.21–25.85
24.27–25.20
23.46–24.26
22.33–23.45
20.96–22.32
15.88–20.95 (lowest 10%)

FIGURE 5–16. Breast Cancer Deaths per 100,000 White Women by State Economic Area

Source: Reprinted from: Devesa SS, Grauman DG, Blot WJ, Pennello G, Hoover RN, Fraumeni JF Jr. *Atlas of Cancer Mortality in the United States, 1950–1994.* NIH pub. no. (NIH) 99-4564. Washington, DC: U.S. Government Printing Office; 1999. Available at: http://www.dceg.cancer. gov/atlas/download/gif-gs/breswf7g.gif. Accessed March 2002.

Unfortunately, the established risk factors cannot account for all cases of breast cancer. Many women with breast cancer (from 45% to 75%) do not have any of the high-risk characteristics.[61]

Clearly more research is needed to determine additional risk factors for breast cancer. Factors associated with breast cancer in some studies but for which uncertainty still exists include breastfeeding, long-term use of oral contraceptives, estrogen replacement therapy for menopausal symptoms, and alcohol consumption.[55] In addition, hypotheses have been postulated involving exposure to electromagnetic fields[62] and environmental estrogens.[63] The environmental estrogens, termed xenoestrogens, are a diverse group of chemicals including pesticides, plasticizers, and detergents that have been released into the environment in great quantities.[64] Hypotheses about electromagnetic fields and xenoestrogen as risk factors for breast cancer are biologically plausible, because exposure to these items is thought to influence a woman's estrogen levels.

Although public health practitioners have looked to descriptive data to identify ways to prevent breast cancer, most of the established risk factors (see Table 5–11) are not modifiable by behavioral or environmental changes.[55] For example, it is unlikely that a woman would choose to have a baby at a young age in order to reduce her risk of breast cancer later in life. Postmenopausal obesity is the only established risk factor that appears fairly amenable to modification.

Nevertheless, several studies are currently under way to evaluate the effectiveness of preventive measures. The Women's Health Initiative is testing the hypothesis that a low-fat diet in adulthood reduces the risk of breast cancer.[51] In addition, the STAR (Study of Tamoxifen and Raloxifene) Trial is comparing the effectiveness of raloxifene and tamoxifen in reducing the incidence of invasive breast cancer among postmenopausal women.[65] Tamoxifen has been shown to reduce the incidence of invasive breast cancer by 49% among high-risk women,[66] but concern about its side effects has led to studies of other drugs such as raloxifene.

TABLE 5–11   Established Risk Factors for Breast Cancer

Characteristic	High-risk group
Age	Old
Country of birth	North America, Northern Europe
Place of residence in United States	Urban areas, Northeast
Mother and/or sister with breast cancer	Yes
History of cancer in one breast	Yes
History of benign proliferative breast disease	Yes
Nodular densities on the mammogram	Yes
Atypical cells in nipple aspirate fluid	Yes
Moderate to high doses of radiation to chest	Yes
Socioeconomic status	High income
Race	
Breast cancer at $\geq$ 45 years of age	White
Breast cancer at < 40 years of age	Black
Religion	Jewish
Age at first full-term birth	$\geq$ 30 years at first birth
Age at menarche and menopause	$\leq$ 11 years at menarche and $\geq$ 55 years at menopause
Obesity	
Breast cancer at $\geq$50 years of age	Obese
Breast cancer at < 50 years of age	Thin
Surgical removal of ovaries before age 40	No

Source: Adapted from Kelsey JL. Breast cancer epidemiology. *Epidemiol Rev.* 1993;15:256–263.

Although breast cancer cannot yet be prevented, survival may be improved through early diagnosis via breast self-examination and mammography. Current guidelines from the American Cancer Society recommend that the monthly practice of breast self-examination begin at age 20 and that screening mammography begin by age 40.[67] They also recommend that women in their 40s receive a mammogram every 1 to 2 years, and those 50 years and older receive one annually. Descriptive data on screening mammography are used to monitor compliance with these recommendations. Use of mammography among women over 40 years of age increased by 112% from 1987 through 1994.[3] However, poor and elderly women had lower mammography rates than their wealthier and younger counterparts, and so more outreach is needed for these groups.

Summary

Descriptive epidemiology involves the analysis of disease patterns by person, place, and time. Personal characteristics include age, sex, race and ethnicity, and socioeconomic status. Place, which is usually defined in geopolitical units such as countries, encompasses the physical environment (such as water and air), biological environment (such as flora and fauna), and social environment (such as cultural traditions). Time trends are examined for short- and long-term changes (ranging from days to decades), as well as cyclical fluctuations.

The principal reasons for describing disease rates by person, place, and time are: (1) to assess the health status of a population, (2) to generate hypotheses about causal factors for disease, and (3) to plan and evaluate public health programs. Descriptive analyses can also be used to identify a disease cluster, defined as the occurrence of cases close together in space and time, and a disease epidemic, defined as a number of cases that is clearly in excess of normal expectancy.

The analysis of U.S. mortality rates by age reveals numerous patterns, including higher death rates due to unintentional injuries among the young than among older individuals, higher death rates due to motor vehicle accidents and homicides among blacks than among whites, and lower death rates from heart disease and lung cancer among females than among males. Although mortality data have many advantages, including complete reporting and easy access, they also have several disadvantages, including inaccurate information on cause of death and insufficient data on serious nonfatal diseases. Thus, epidemiologists rely on other data sources to learn about descriptive patterns of important fatal and nonfatal illnesses such as childhood lead poisoning, AIDS, and breast cancer. For example, the NHANES, the primary data source on the descriptive epidemiology of childhood lead poisoning in the United States, reveals continuing racial and economic disparities in children's blood lead levels, despite significant decreases in all groups over time. Similarly, descriptive statistics on HIV and AIDS from the Centers for Disease Control and Prevention and the World Health Organization show a lower prevalence in the United States than in other parts of the world, especially sub-Saharan Africa. In addition, breast cancer data from the National Cancer Institute's Surveillance, Epidemiology and End Results Program indicate that breast cancer is the most commonly diagnosed cancer among U.S. women and that rates are highest among white women, women of high socioeconomic status, and women residing in the Northeast.

References

1. MacMahon B, Trichopoulos D. *Epidemiology: Principles and Methods.* 2nd ed. Boston; MA: Little, Brown and Co; 1996.
2. Last JM, ed. *A Dictionary of Epidemiology.* 3rd ed. New York, NY: Oxford University Press; 1995.
3. Kramarow E, Lentzer H, Rooks R, Weeks J, Saydah S. *Health and Aging Chartbook. Health, United States, 1999.* Hyattsville, MD: National Center for Health Statistics; 1999.
4. Benenson AS, ed. *Control of Communicable Diseases in Man.* Washington, DC: American Public Health Association; 1990.
5. Ries LAG, Eisner MP, Kosary CL, Hankey BF, Miller BA, Clegg L, et al., eds. *SEER Cancer Statistics Review, 1973–1998.* Bethesda, MD: National Cancer Institute; 2001.
6. Centers for Disease Control and Prevention. *HIV/AIDS Surveillance Report.* 1999;11:1–44.
7. U.S. Census Bureau. Available at: http://www2.census.gov/census_2000/datasets/demographic_profile. Accessed July 2001.
8. Wade WC. *The Titanic: End of a Dream.* New York, NY: Rawson Wade; 1979.
9. Pamuk E, Makuc D, Heck K, Reuben C, Lochner K. *Socioeconomic Status and Health Chartbook. Health, United States, 1998.* Hyattsville, MD: National Center for Health Statistics; 1998.
10. Davis RL, Robertson DM, eds. *Textbook of Neuropathology.* 2nd ed. Baltimore, MD: Williams and Wilkins; 1991.
11. Lyon JL, Gardner K, Gress RE. Cancer incidence among Mormons and non-Mormons in Utah (United States), 1971–85. *Cancer Causes Control.* 1994;5:149–156.
12. Blair A. Occupation. In: Harras A, Edwards BK, Blot WJ, Ries LAG, eds. *Cancer Rates and Risks.* NIH pub no 96-691. Bethesda, MD: National Cancer Institute; 1996.
13. Monk M. Epidemiology of suicide. *Epidemiol Rev.* 1987;89:51–69.
14. McIntosh JH, Berman K, Holliday FM, Byth K, Chapman R, Piper DW. Some factors associated with mortality in perforated peptic ulcer: a case-control study. *J Gastroenterol Hepatol.* 1996;11:82–87.
15. Ebrahim S, Wannamethee G, McCallum A, Walker M, Shaper AG. Marital status, change in marital status, and mortality in middle-aged British men. *Am J Epidemiol.* 1995;142:834–842.

16. Goldman N, Korenman S, Weinstein R. Marital status and health among the elderly. *Soc Sci Med.* 1995;40:1717–1730.
17. Clyde DF. Recent trends in the epidemiology and control of malaria. *Epidemiol Rev.* 1987;9:219–243.
18. Ries LAG. Rates. In: Harras A, Edwards BK, Blot WJ, Ries LAG, eds. *Cancer Rates and Risks* NIH pub no 96-691. Bethesda, MD: National Cancer Institute; 1996:24–27.
19. DiBisceglie A, Tabor E. Liver. In: Harras A, Edwards BK, Blot WJ, Ries LAG, eds. *Cancer Rates and Risks* NIH pub no 96-691. Bethesda, MD: National Cancer Institute; 1996.
20. Little J, Elwood JM. Epidemiology of neural tube defects. In: Kiely M, ed. *Reproductive and Perinatal Epidemiology.* Boca Raton, FL: CRC Press; 1991.
21. Hayes RB. Prostate. In: Harras A, Edwards BK, Blot WJ, Ries LAG, eds. *Cancer Rates and Risks.* NIH pub no 96-691. Bethesda, MD: National Cancer Institute; 1996.
22. Fraser DW, Tsai TR, Orenstein W, Parkin WE, Beecham HJ, Sharrar RG, et al and the Field Investigation Team. Legionnaires' disease: description of an epidemic of pneumonia. *N Engl J Med.* 1977;297:1189–1197.
23. Schwartz J. What are people dying of on high air pollution days? *Environ Res.* 1994;64:26–35.
24. Van der Palen J, Doggen CJ, Beaglehorn R. Variation in the time and day of onset of myocardial infarction and sudden death. *N Zealand Med J.* 1995;108: 332–334.
25. Martin GR, Perry LW, Ferencz C. Increased prevalence of ventricular septal defects: epidemic or improved diagnosis. *Pediatrics.* 1989; 83:200–203.
26. Roueche B. *Eleven Blue Men and Other Narratives of Medical Detection.* New York, NY: Berkeley Publishing Co; 1953.
27. Lagakos S, Wessen B, Zelen M. An analysis of contaminated well water and health effects in Woburn, Massachusetts. *J Am Stat Assoc.* 1986;81:583–595.
28. Rothman KJ. A sobering start for the cluster busters' conference. *Am J Epidemiol.* 1990;132:S6–S13.
29. Neutra RR. Counterpoint from a cluster buster. *Am J Epidemiol.* 1990;132:1–8.
30. MacMahon B, Yen S. Unrecognized epidemic of anencephaly and spina bifida. *Lancet.* 1971;1:31–33.
31. Werler MM, Shapiro S, Mitchell AA. Peri-conceptional folic acid exposure and risk of occurrent neural tube defects. *JAMA.* 1993;269:1257–1261.
32. Pickett JP, exec. ed. *The American Heritage Dictionary of the English Language.* 4th ed. Boston, MA: Houghton Mifflin Co; 2000.
33. Kneller R. Stomach. In: *Cancer Rates and Risks.* Harras A, Edwards BK, Blot WJ, Ries LAG, eds.. NIH pub no 96-691. Bethesda, MD; National Cancer Institute; 1996.
34. Zahm S. Non-Hodgkin's lymphoma. In: Harras A, Edwards BK, Blot WJ, Ries LAG, eds. *Cancer Rates and Risks.* NIH pub no 96-691. Bethesda, MD: National Cancer Institute; 1996.
35. Escobedo LG, Peddicord JP. Smoking prevalence in US birth cohorts: the influence of gender and education. *Am J Public Health.* 1996;86:231–236.

36. Alter MJ, Francis DP. Hepatitis B virus transmission between homosexual men: a model of the acquired immune deficiency syndrome (AIDS). In: Ma P, Armstrong D, eds. *The Acquired Immune Deficiency Syndrome and Infections of Homosexual Men.* Yorke Medical Books; 1984.

37. US Department of Health and Human Services. Available at: http://www.health.gov/healthypeople/document. Accessed January 2000.

38. Goldman LR, Carra J. Childhood lead poisoning in 1994 [editorial]. *JAMA.* 1994;272:315–316.

39. Centers for Disease Control and Prevention. Preventing Lead Poisoning in Young Children: A Statement by the Centers for Disease Control. Atlanta GA: Public Health Service; 1991.

40. Lin-Fu J. Historical perspective on health effects of lead. In: *Dietary and Environmental Lead: Human Health Effects.* Elsevier Science Publishers BV; 1985.

41. Rabin R. Warnings unheeded: a history of child lead poisoning. *Am J Public Health.* 1989;79:1668–1674.

42. Brody DJ, Pirkle JL, Kramer RA, Flegal KM, Matte TD, Gunter EW, et al. Blood lead levels in the US population: phase 1 of the third National Health and Nutrition Examination Surveys (NHANES III, 1988 to 1991). *JAMA.* 1994;272: 277–283.

43. Lofgren JP, Macias MHS, Russakow S, et al. Blood lead levels in young children—United States and selected states, 1996–1999. *MMWR.* 2000;49: 1133–1137.

44. Gottlieb MS, Schanker HM, Fan PT, Saxon A, Weisman JD, Pozalski I. *Pneumocystis* pneumonia—Los Angeles. *MMWR.* 1981;30:250–252.

45. Friedman-Kien A, Laubenstein L, Marmor M, et al. Kaposi's sarcoma and *Pneumocystis* pneumonia among homosexual men—New York City and California. *MMWR.* 1981;30:305–308.

46. Steger KA. Epidemiology, natural history, and staging. In: Libman H, Witzburg RA, eds. *HIV Infection: A Clinical Manual.* 2nd ed. Boston, MA: Little, Brown and Co; 1993.

47. Joint United Nations Programme on HIV/AIDS (UNAIDS). *Report on the Global HIV/AIDS Epidemic, June 2000.* Geneva, Switzerland: UNAIDS; 2000.

48. Kaslow RA, Francis DP. Epidemiology: general considerations. In: Kaslow RA, Francis DP, eds. *The Epidemiology of AIDS: Expression, Occurrence, and Control of Human Immunodeficiency Virus Type 1 Infection.* New York, NY: Oxford University Press; 1989.

49. Des Jarlais DC, Marmor M, Paone D, Titus S, Shi Q, Perlis T, Jose B. HIV incidence among injecting drug users in New York City syringe-exchange programmes. *Lancet;* 1996;348:987–991.

50. Miller RL. Assisting gay men to maintain safer sex: an evaluation of an AIDS service organization's safer sex maintenance program. *AIDS Educ Prev.* 1995;7: 48–63.

51. Greenwald P, Kelloff G, Burch-Whitman C, Kramer BS. Chemoprevention. *CA Cancer J Clin.* 1995;45:31–49.

52. Schottenfeld D, Haas JF. Carcinogens in the workplace. *CA Cancer J Clin.* May-June 1979; 29:144.

53. Kelsey JL, Horn-Ross PL. Breast cancer: magnitude of the problem and descriptive epidemiology. *Epidemiol Rev.* 1993;15:7–16.

54. Kelsey JL, Gammon MD, John EM. Reproductive factors and breast cancer. *Epidemiol Rev.* 1993;15:36–47.

55. Kelsey JL. Breast cancer epidemiology. *Epidemiol Rev.* 1993;15:256–263.

56. Sturgeon SR, Schairer C, Gail M, McAdams M, Brinton LA, Hoover RN. Geographic variation in mortality from breast cancer among white women in the US *J Natl Cancer Inst.* 1995;87:1846–1853.

57. Devesa SS, Grauman DG, Blot WJ, Pennello G, Hoover RN, Fraumeni JF Jr. *Atlas of Cancer Mortality in the United States, 1950–1994.* NIH pub no (NIH) 99-4564 Washington, DC: US Government Printing Office; 1999.

58. Pike MC, Spicer DV, Dahmoush L, Press MF. Estrogens, progestogens, normal breast cell proliferation and breast cancer risk. *Epidemiol Rev.* 1993;15:17–35.

59. Struewing JP, Brody LC, Erdos MR, Kase RG, Giambarresi TR, Smith SA, et al. Detection of eight BRCA1 mutations in 10 breast/ovarian cancer families, including 1 family with male breast cancer. *Am J Hum Genet.* 1995;57:1–7.

60. Struewing JP, Abeliovich D, Peretz T, Avishai N, Kaback MM, Collins FS, et al. The carrier frequency of the BRCA1 185delAG mutation is approximately 1 percent in Ashkenazi Jewish individuals. *Nat Genet.* 1995;11:198–200.

61. Garfinkel L. Perspectives on cancer prevention [editorial]. *CA Cancer J Clin.* 1995;45:5–7.

62. Stevens RG. Electric power use and breast cancer: a hypothesis. *Am J Epidemiol.* 1978;125:556–561.

63. Davis DL, Bradlow HL, Wolff M, Woodruff T, Hoel DG, Anton-Culver H. Medical hypothesis: xenoestrogens as preventable causes of breast cancer. *Environ Health Perspect.* 1993;101:372–377.

64. Colborn T, vom Saal FS, Soto AM. Developmental effects of endocrine-disrupting chemicals in wildlife and humans. *Environ Health Perspect.* 1993;101:378–384.

65. Jubelirer SJ, Crowell EB. The STAR (Study of Tamoxifen and Raloxifene) trial in West Virginia. *W Va Med J.* 2000;96:602–604.

66. Fisher B, Constantino JP, Wickerham DL, Redmond CK, Kavanah M, Cronin WM, et al. Tamoxifen for prevention of breast cancer: report of the National Surgical Adjuvant Breast and Bowel Project P-1 Study. *J Natl Cancer Inst.* 1998; 90:1371–1388.

67. American Cancer Society. *Cancer Facts and Figures –2001.* Atlanta, GA: American Cancer Society; 2001.

EXERCISES

1. The following data give some of the descriptive epidemiology of ectopic pregnancy in the United States. An ectopic pregnancy is a pregnancy that occurs outside the uterus, primarily in the fallopian tubes. It may lead to tubal rupture, internal bleeding, and even death.

Number and Prevalence of Ectopic Pregnancy by Year—United States, 1970–1992

Year	Number	Prevalence (per 1000 reported pregnancies)
1970	17,800	4.5
1975	30,500	7.6
1980	52,200	10.5
1985	78,400	15.2
1989	88,400	16.0
1992	108,800	19.7

Prevalence of Ectopic Pregnancy by Race and Age—United States, 1970–1989

Race	Age group (years)	Prevalence (per 1000 reported pregnancies)
White	15–24	6.1
	25–34	13.7
	35–44	19.0
	All ages, 15–44	10.3
Black	15–24	8.2
	25–34	22.6
	35–44	30.1
	All ages, 15–44	14.7
All races	15–24	6.6
	25–34	15.4
	35–44	21.5
	All ages, 15–44	11.3

Source: Data from Golder TE, Lawson HW, Xia, Z et al. Surveillance for ectopic pregnancy—United States, 1970–1989. *MMWR.* 1993;42:73–85. Current trends in ectopic pregnancy—United States, 1990–1992. *MMWR.* 1995; 44:46–48.

A. Based on these data, briefly describe each of the following using words and numbers:
   i.   The change in prevalence from 1970 to 1992
   ii. The difference in prevalence between blacks and whites
   iii. The difference in prevalence by age
B. Do these data suggest that there is an epidemic of ectopic pregnancy in the United States?
C. Data such as these are used to generate hypotheses about the causes of disease. Using any information in the tables, briefly describe a hypothesis that might explain one of these descriptive features.
D. Data such as these are also used by public health administrators and planners to establish priorities, allocate resources, and plan and evaluate the effectiveness of treatment and prevention programs. Briefly describe how these data might be used to allocate resources for the prevention and treatment of ectopic pregnancy.

6

Overview of Epidemiologic Study Designs

LEARNING OBJECTIVES

By the end of this chapter, the reader will be able to:

- Distinguish between experimental and observational studies.
- Describe the key characteristics of experimental, cohort, case–control, cross-sectional, and ecologic studies regarding subject selection, data collection, and analysis.
- Identify the design of a particular study.
- Discuss the factors that determine when a particular design is indicated.

Introduction

As described in Chapter 1, epidemiology is the study of the distribution and determinants of disease frequency in human populations and the application of this study to control health problems.[1(p1),2(p55)] The term *study* includes both *surveillance,* whose purpose is to monitor aspects of disease occurrence and spread that are pertinent to effective control,[3(p507)] and *epidemiologic research,* whose goal is to harvest valid and precise information about the causes, preventions, and treatments for disease. The term *disease* refers to a broad array of health-related states and events including diseases, injuries, disabilities, and death.

Epidemiologic research encompasses several types of study designs, including experimental studies and observational studies such as cohort and case–control studies. Each type of epidemiologic study design simply represents a different way of harvesting information. The selection of one design over another depends on the particular research question, concerns about validity and efficiency, and practical and ethical considerations. For example, experimental studies, also known as trials, investigate the role of some factor or agent in the prevention or treatment of a disease. In this type of study, the investigator assigns individuals to two or more groups that either receive or do not receive the preventive or therapeutic agent. Because experimental studies closely resemble controlled laboratory investigations, they are thought to produce the most scientifically rigorous data of all the designs.

However, because experimental studies are often infeasible because of difficulties enrolling participants, high costs, and thorny ethical issues, most epidemiologic research is conducted using observational studies. Observational studies are considered "natural" experiments because the investigator lets nature take its course. Observational studies take advantage of the fact that people are exposed to noxious and/or healthy substances through their personal habits, occupation, place of residence, and so on. The studies provide information on exposures that occur in natural settings, and they are not limited to preventions and treatments. Furthermore, they do not suffer from the ethical and feasibility issues of experimental studies. For example, although it is unethical to conduct an experimental study of the impact of drinking alcohol on the developing fetus by assigning newly pregnant women to either a drinking or nondrinking group, it is perfectly ethical to conduct an observational study by comparing women who choose to drink during pregnancy with those who decide not to do so.

The two principal types of observational studies are cohort and case–control studies. A classical cohort study examines one or more health effects of exposure to a single agent. Subjects are defined according to their exposure status and followed over time to determine the incidence of health outcomes. In contrast, a classical case–control study examines a single disease in relation to exposure to one or more agents. Cases who have the disease of interest and controls who are a sample of the population that produced the cases are defined and enrolled. The purpose of the control group is to provide information on the exposure distribution in the population that gave rise to the cases. Investigators obtain and compare exposure histories of cases as well as controls.

Additional observational study designs include cross-sectional studies and ecologic studies. A cross-sectional study examines the relationship between a disease and an exposure among individuals in a defined population at a point in time. Thus, it takes a snapshot of a population and measures the exposure prevalence in relation to the disease prevalence. An ecologic study evaluates an association using the population rather than the individual as the unit of analysis. The rates of disease are examined in relation to factors described on the population level. Both the cross-sectional and ecologic designs have important limitations that make them less scientifically rigorous than cohort and case-control studies. These limitations are discussed later in this chapter.

An overview of these study designs is provided in Table 6–1. The goal of all these studies is to determine the relationship between an exposure and a disease with validity and precision using a minimum of resources. *Validity* is defined as the lack of bias and confounding. *Bias* is an error committed by the investigator in the design or conduct of a study that leads to a false association between the exposure and disease. *Confounding*, on the other hand, is not the fault of the investigator but rather reflects the fact that epidemiologic research is conducted among free-living humans with unevenly distributed characteristics. As a result, epidemiological studies that try to determine the relationship between an exposure and disease are susceptible to the disturbing influences of extraneous factors known as confounders. *Precision* is the lack of random error, which leads to a false association between the exposure and disease just by "chance," an uncontrollable force that seems to have no assignable cause.[4(p309)] Bias, confounding, and random error are covered in greater detail in Chapters 10 through 12.

Several factors help epidemiologists determine the most appropriate study design for evaluating a particular association, including the hypothesis being tested, state of knowledge, the frequency of the exposure and the disease, and the expected strength of the association between the two. This chapter provides: (1) an overview of five epidemiologic study designs—experimental, cohort, case–control, cross-sectional, and

TABLE 6–1   Main Types of Epidemiologic Studies

Type of study	Characteristics
Experimental	Studies preventions and treatments for diseases; investigator actively manipulates which groups receive the agent under study.
Observational	Studies causes, preventions, and treatments for diseases; investigator passively observes as nature takes its course.
Cohort	Typically examines multiple health effects of an exposure; subjects are defined according to their exposure levels and followed for disease occurrence.
Case–control	Typically examines multiple exposures in relation to a disease; subjects are defined as cases and controls, and exposure histories are compared.
Cross-sectional	Examines relationship between exposure and disease prevalence in a defined population at a single point in time.
Ecological	Examines relationship between exposure and disease with population-level rather than individual-level data.

ecological designs—and (2) a description of the settings in which the three main study designs—experimental, cohort, and case–control—are most appropriate. Chapters 7 through 9 describe these three study designs in more detail.

Overview of Experimental Studies

Definitions and Classification

An experimental study, also known as a trial, investigates the role of some agent in the prevention or treatment of a disease. In this type of study, the investigator assigns individuals to two or more groups that either receive or do not receive the preventive or therapeutic agent. The group that is allocated the agent under study is generally called the treatment group, and the group that is not allocated the agent under study is called the comparison group. Depending on the purpose of the trial, the comparison group may receive no treatment at all, an inactive treatment such as a placebo, or another active treatment.

The active manipulation of the agent by the investigator is the hallmark that distinguishes experimental studies from observational ones. In the latter, the investigator acts as a passive observer merely letting nature take its course. Because experimental studies more closely resemble controlled laboratory investigations, most epidemiologists believe that experimental studies produce more scientifically rigorous results than do observational studies.

Experimental studies are commonly classified by their objective—that is, by whether they investigate a measure that prevents disease occurrence or a measure that treats an existing condition. The former is known as a preventive or prophylactic trial, and the latter is known as a therapeutic or clinical trial. In preventive trials, agents such as vitamins or behavioral modifications such as smoking cessation are studied to determine if they are effective in preventing or delaying the onset of disease among healthy individuals. In therapeutic trials, treatments such as surgery, radiation, and drugs are tested among individuals who already have a disease.

Selection of Study Population

During the recruitment phase of an experimental study, the study population—which is also called the experimental population—is enrolled on the basis of eligibility criteria that reflect the purpose of the trial, as well as scientific, safety, and practical considerations. For example, healthy or high-risk individuals are enrolled in prevention trials, while individuals with specific diseases are enrolled in therapeutic trials. Additional inclusion and exclusion criteria are used to restrict the study population by factors such as gender and age.

The study population must include an adequate number of individuals in order to determine if there is a true difference between the treatment and comparison groups. An investigator determines how many subjects to include by using formulas that take into account the anticipated difference between the groups, the background rate of the outcome, and the probability of making certain statistical errors.[5(pp142–146)] In general, smaller anticipated differences between the treatment and comparison groups require larger sample sizes.

Consent Process and Treatment Assignment

All eligible and willing individuals must give consent to participate in an experimental study. The process of gaining their agreement is known as *informed consent*. During this process, the investigator describes the nature and objectives of the study, the tasks required of the participants, and the benefits and risks of participating. The process also includes obtaining the participant's oral or written consent.

Individuals are then assigned to receive one of the two or more treatments being compared. Randomization, "an act of assigning or ordering that is the result of a random process,"[6(p220)] is the preferred method for assigning the treatments because it is less prone to bias than other methods and because it produces groups with very similar characteristics, if the study size is sufficient. Random assignment methods include flipping a coin, using a random number table (commonly found in statistics textbooks), and using a computerized random number generator.

Treatment Administration

In the next phase of a trial, the treatments are administered according to a specific protocol. For example, in a therapeutic trial participants may be asked to take either an active drug or an inactive drug known as a placebo. The purpose of placebos is to match as closely as possible the experience of the comparison group with that of the treatment group. The principle underlying the use of placebos harkens back to laboratory animal experiments where, except for the test chemical, all important aspects of the experimental conditions are identical for all groups. Placebos permit study participants and investigators to be masked—that is, to be unaware of the participant's treatment assignment. Masking of subjects and investigators helps prevent biased ascertainment of the outcome, particularly when end points involve subjective assessments.

Maintenance and Assessment of Compliance

All experimental studies require the active involvement and cooperation of participants. Although participants are apprised of the study requirements when they enroll, many fail to follow the protocol exactly as required as the trial proceeds. The failure to observe the requirements of the protocol is known as noncompliance, and this may occur in the treatment group, the comparison group, or both. Reasons for not complying include toxic reactions to the treatment, waning interest, and desire to seek other therapies. Noncompliance is problematic because it results in a smaller difference between the treatment and comparison groups than truly exists, thereby diluting the real impact of a treatment.

Because good compliance is an important determinant of the validity of an experimental study, many design features are used to enhance a participant's ability to comply with the protocol requirements.[7] These include designing an experimental regimen that is simple and easy to follow, enrolling motivated and knowledgeable participants, presenting a realistic picture of the required tasks during the consent process, maintaining frequent contact with participants during the study, and conducting a run-in period before enrollment and randomization. The purpose of the run-in period is to ascertain which potential participants are able to comply with the study regimen. During this period, participants are placed on the test or comparison treatment to assess their tolerance and acceptance and to obtain information on compliance.[6(p143)] Following the run-in period, only compliant individuals are enrolled in the trial.

Ascertaining the Outcomes

During the follow-up stage of an experimental study, the treatment and comparison groups are monitored for the outcomes under study. If the study's goal is to prevent the occurrence of disease, the outcomes may include the precursors of disease or the first occurrence of disease (that is, incidence). If the study is investigating a new treatment among individuals who already have a disease, the outcomes may include disease recurrence, symptom improvement, length of survival, or side effects. The length of follow-up depends on the particular outcome under study. It can range from a few months to a few decades.

Usually, all reported outcomes under study are confirmed in order to guarantee their accuracy. Confirmation is typically done by masked investigators who gather corroborating information from objective sources such as medical records and laboratory tests. High and comparable follow-up rates are needed to ensure the quality of the outcome data. Follow-up is adversely affected when participants withdraw from the study (these individuals are called dropouts) or cannot be located or contacted by the investigator (these individuals are termed lost to follow-up). Reasons for dropouts and losses include relocation, waning interest, and adverse reactions to the treatment.

Analysis

The classic analytic approach for an experimental study is known as an intent-to-treat or treatment assignment analysis. In this analysis, all individuals who were randomly allocated to a treatment are analyzed, regardless of whether they completed the regimen or received the treatment.[8] An intent-to-treat analysis gives information on the effectiveness of a treatment under everyday practice conditions. The alternative to an intent-to-treat analysis is known as an efficacy analysis, which determines the treatment effects under ideal conditions, such as when participants take the full treatment exactly as directed.

Overview of Cohort Studies

Definitions

A cohort is defined as a group of people with a common characteristic or experience. In a cohort study, healthy subjects are defined according to their exposure status and followed over time to determine the incidence of symptoms, disease, or death. The common characteristic for grouping subjects is their exposure level. Usually two groups are compared, an "exposed" and "unexposed" group. The unexposed group is called the referent group or comparison group.

Cohort study is the term that is typically used to describe an epidemiologic investigation that follows groups with common characteristics. Other expressions that are used include *follow-up, incidence,* and *longitudinal study.* There are several additional terms for describing cohort studies that depend on the characteristics of population from which the cohort is derived, whether the exposure changes over time, and whether there are losses to follow-up. The term *fixed cohort* is used when the cohort is formed on the basis of an irrevocable event such as undergoing a medical procedure. Thus, an individual's exposure in a fixed cohort does not change over time. The term *closed cohort* is used to describe a fixed cohort with no losses to follow up. In contrast, a cohort study conducted in an *open population* is defined by exposures that can change over time such as cigarette smoking. Cohort studies in open populations may also experience losses to follow-up.

Timing of Cohort Studies

Three terms are used to describe the timing of events in a cohort study: prospective, retrospective, and ambidirectional. In a *prospective cohort study,* participants are grouped on the basis of past or current exposure and are followed into the future in order to observe the outcomes of interest. When the study commences, the outcomes have not yet developed and the investigator must wait for them to occur. In a *retrospective cohort study,* both the exposures and outcomes have already occurred when the study begins. Thus, this type of investigation studies only prior outcomes and not future ones. An *ambidirectional cohort study* has both prospective and retrospective components. The decision to conduct a retrospective, prospective, or ambidirectional study depends on the research question, practical constraints such as time and money, and the availability of suitable study populations and records.

Selection of the Exposed Population

The choice of the exposed group in a cohort study depends on the hypothesis being tested, the exposure frequency, and feasibility considerations such as the availability of records and ease of follow-up. Special cohorts are used to study the health effects of rare exposures such as uncommon workplace chemicals, unusual diets, and uncommon lifestyles. Special cohorts are often selected from occupational groups (such as rubber workers) or religious groups (such as Mormons) where the exposures are known to occur. General cohorts are typically assembled for common exposures such as cigarette smoking and alcohol consumption. These cohorts are often selected from professional groups such as nurses or from well-defined geographic areas in order to facilitate follow-up and accurate ascertainment of the outcomes under study.

Selection of Comparison Group

There are three sources for the comparison group in a cohort study: an internal comparison group, the general population, and a comparison cohort. An internal comparison group consists of unexposed members of the same cohort. An internal comparison group should be used whenever possible, because its characteristics will be most similar to the exposed group. The general population is used for comparison when it is not possible to find a comparable internal comparison group. The general population comparison is based on preexisting population data on disease incidence and mortality. A comparison cohort consists of members of another cohort. It is the least desirable option because the comparison cohort, while not exposed to the exposure under study, is often exposed to other potentially harmful substances and so the results can be difficult to interpret.

Sources of Information

Cohort study investigators typically rely on many sources for information on exposures, outcomes, and other key variables. These include medical and employment records, interviews, direct physical examinations, laboratory tests, biological specimens, and environmental monitoring. Some of these sources are preexisting, and others are designed specifically for the study. Because each type of source has advantages and disadvantages, investigators often use several sources to piece together all of the necessary information.

Health care records are used to describe a participant's exposure history in studies of possible adverse health effects stemming from medical procedures. The advantages of these records include low expense and a high level of accuracy and detail regarding a disease and its treatment. Their main disadvantage is that information on many other key characteristics, apart from basic demographic characteristics, is often missing.

Employment records are used to identify individuals for studies of occupational exposures. Typical employment record data includes job title, department of work, years of employment, and basic demographic characteristics. Like medical records, they usually lack details on exposures and other important variables.

Because existing records such as health care and employment records often have limitations, many studies are based on data collected specifically for the investigation. These include interviews, physical examinations, and laboratory tests. Interviews and self-administered questionnaires are particularly useful for obtaining information on lifestyle characteristics (such as use of cigarettes or alcohol), which are not consistently found in records.

Whatever the source of information, it is important to use comparable procedures for obtaining information on the exposed and unexposed groups. Biased results may occur if different sources and procedures are used. Thus, all resources used for one group must be used for the other. In addition, it is a good idea to mask investigators to the exposure status of a subject so that they make unbiased decisions when assessing the outcomes. Standard outcome definitions are also recommended to guarantee both accuracy and comparability.

Approaches to Follow-Up

Loss to follow-up occurs either when the participant no longer wishes to take part or when he or she cannot be located. Because high rates of follow-up are critical to the success of a cohort study, investigators have developed many methods to maximize retention and trace study participants.[9] For prospective cohort studies, strategies include collection of information (such as full name, Social Security number, and date of birth) that helps locate participants as the study progresses. In addition, regular contact is recommended for participants in prospective studies. These contacts might involve requests for up-to-date outcome information or newsletters describing the study's progress and findings.[9] The best strategy to use when participants do not initially respond is to send additional mailings.

When participants are truly lost to follow-up, investigators employ a number of strategies.[9] These include sending letters to the last known address with "Address Correction Requested"; checking telephone directories, directory assistance, newly available Internet resources such as the "White Pages," vital statistics records, driver's license rosters, and voter registration records; and contacting relatives, friends, and physicians identified at baseline.

Analysis

The primary objective of the analysis of cohort study data is to compare the occurrence of symptoms, disease, and death in the exposed and unexposed groups. If it is not possible to find a completely unexposed group to serve as the comparison, then the least exposed group is used. The occurrence of the outcome is usually measured using cumulative incidence or incidence rates, and the relationship between the exposure and outcome is quantified using absolute or relative difference between the risks or rates, as described in Chapter 3.

Overview of Case–Control Studies

The case–control study has traditionally been viewed as an inferior alternative to the cohort study. In the traditional view, subjects are selected on the basis of whether they have or do not have the disease. Those who have the disease are termed *cases*, and those who do not have the disease are termed *controls*. The exposure histories of cases and controls are then obtained and compared. Thus, the central feature of the traditional view is the comparison of the cases' and controls' exposure histories. This differs from the logic of experimental and cohort study designs, in which the key comparison is disease incidence between the exposed and unexposed (or least exposed) groups.

Over the last two decades, the traditional view that a case–control study is a backwards cohort study has been supplanted by a modern view that asserts that it is merely an efficient way to learn about the relationship between an exposure and disease.[10] More specifically, a case–control study is a method of sampling a population in which researchers identify and enroll cases of disease and a sample of the source population that gave rise to the cases. The sample of the source population is known as the control group. Its purpose is to provide information on the exposure distribution in the population that produced the cases, so that the rates of disease in exposed and nonexposed groups can be compared. Thus, the key comparison in the modern view is the same as that of a cohort study.

Selection of Cases

The first step in the selection of cases for a case–control study is the formulation of a disease or case definition. A case definition is usually based on a combination of signs and symptoms, physical and pathological examinations, and results of diagnostic tests. It is best to use all available evidence to define with as much accuracy as possible the true cases of disease.

Once investigators have created a case definition, they can begin case identification and enrollment. Typical sources for identifying cases are hospital or clinic patient rosters, death certificates, special surveys, and reporting systems such as cancer or birth defects registries. Investigators consider both accuracy and efficiency in selecting a particular source for case identification. The goal is to identify as many true cases of disease as quickly and cheaply as possible.

Another important issue in selecting cases is whether they should be incident or prevalent. Researchers who study the causes of disease prefer incident cases because they are usually interested in the factors that lead to developing a disease rather than factors that affect its duration. However, sometimes epidemiologists have no choice but to rely on prevalent cases (for example, when studying the causes of insidious diseases whose exact onset is difficult to pinpoint). Studies using prevalent cases must be interpreted cautiously, because it is impossible to determine if the exposure is related to the inception of the disease, its duration, or a combination of the two.

Selection of Controls

Controls are a sample of the population that produced the cases. The guiding principle for the valid selection of controls is that they come from the same base population as the cases. If this condition is met, then a member of the control group who gets the disease under study *would* end up as a case in the study. This concept is known as the *would criterion*, and its fulfillment is crucial to the validity of a case–control study. Another important principle is that controls must be sampled independently of exposure status. In other words, exposed and unexposed controls should have the same probability of selection.

Epidemiologists use several sources for identifying controls in case–control studies. They may sample: (1) individuals from the general population, (2) individuals attending a hospital or clinic, (3) friends or relatives identified by the cases, or (4) individuals who have died. Population controls are typically selected when cases are identified from a well-defined population such as residents of a geographic area. These controls are usually identified using voter registration lists, driver's license rosters, telephone directories, and random digit dialing (a method for identifying telephone subscribers living in a defined geographic area).

Population controls have one principal advantage that makes them preferable to other types of controls. Because of the manner in which population controls are identified, investigators are usually assured that the controls come from the same population as the cases. Thus, investigators are usually confident that population controls are comparable to the cases with respect to demographic and other important variables. However, population controls have several disadvantages. First, they are time-consuming and expensive to identify. Second, these individuals do not have the same level of interest in participating as do cases and controls identified from other sources. Third, because they are generally healthy, their recall may be less accurate than that of cases who are likely reviewing their history in search of a "reason" for their illness.

Epidemiologists usually select hospital and clinic controls when they identify cases from these health care facilities. Thus, these controls have diseases or have experienced events (such as a car accident) for which they have sought medical care. The most difficult aspect of using these types of controls is determining which diseases or events are suitable for inclusion. In this regard, investigators should follow two general principles. First, the illnesses in the control group should, on the basis of current knowledge, be unrelated to the exposure under study. For example, a case–control study of cigarette smoking and emphysema should not use lung cancer patients as controls, because lung cancer is known to be caused by smoking cigarettes. Second, the control's illness should have the same referral pattern to the health care facility as the case's illness. For example, a case–control study of acute appendicitis should use patients with other acute conditions as controls. Following this principle will help ensure that the cases and controls come from the same source population.

There are several advantages to the use of hospital and clinic controls. Because they are easy to identify and have good participation rates, hospital and clinic controls are less expensive to identify than population controls. In addition, because they come from the same source population they will have comparable characteristics to the cases. Finally, their recall of prior exposures will be similar to the cases' recall, because they are also ill. The main disadvantage of this type of control is the difficulty in determining appropriate illnesses for inclusion.

In rare circumstances, deceased and "special" controls are enrolled. Deceased controls are occasionally used when some or all of the cases are deceased by the time data collection begins. Researchers usually identify these controls by reviewing death records of individuals who lived in the same geographic area and died during the same time period as the cases. The main rationale for selecting dead controls is to ensure comparable data collection procedures between the two groups. For example, if researchers collect data by interview, they would conduct proxy interviews with subjects' spouses, children, relatives, or friends for both the dead cases and dead controls.

However, many epidemiologists discourage the use of dead controls because these controls may not be a representative sample of the source population that produced the cases, which—by definition—consists of living people. Furthermore, the investigator must consider the study hypothesis before deciding to use dead controls, because they are more likely than living controls to have used tobacco, alcohol, or drugs.[11] Consequently, dead controls may not be appropriate if the study hypothesis involves one of these exposures.

In unusual circumstances, a friend, spouse, or relative (usually a sibling) is nominated by a case to serve as his or her control. These "special" controls are used because they are likely to share the cases' socioeconomic status, race, age, educational level, and genetic characteristics, if they are related to the cases. However, cases may be unwilling or unable to nominate people to serve as their controls. In addition, biased results are possible if the study hypothesis involves a shared activity among the cases and controls.

Methods for Sampling Controls

Epidemiologists use three main strategies for sampling controls in a case–control study. Investigators can select controls from the "non-cases" or "survivors" at the end of the case diagnosis and accrual period. This method of selection, which is known as *survivor sampling*, is the predominant method for selecting controls in traditional case–control studies. In *case-based* or *case-cohort* sampling, investigators select controls from the population at risk at the beginning of the case diagnosis and accrual period. In *risk set sampling*, controls are selected from the population at risk as the cases are diagnosed.

When case-based and risk set sampling methods are used, the control group may include future cases of disease. Although this may seem incorrect, modern epidemiologic theory supports it. Recall that both diseased and nondiseased individuals contribute to the denominators of the risks and rates in cohort studies. Thus, it is reasonable for the control group to include future cases of disease because it is merely an efficient way to obtain the denominator data for the risks and rates.

Sources of Exposure Information

Case–control studies are used to investigate the risk of disease in relation to a wide variety of exposures, including those related to lifestyle, occupation, environment, genes, diet, reproduction, and the use of medications.[12] Most exposures that are studied are complex, and so investigators must attempt to obtain sufficiently detailed information on the nature, sources, frequency, and duration of these exposures. Sources available for obtaining exposure data include in-person and telephone interviews; self-administered questionnaires; preexisting medical, pharmacy, registry, employment, insurance, birth, death, and environmental records; and biological specimens.[12] When selecting a particular source, investigators consider its availability, its accuracy, and the logistics and cost of data collection. Accuracy is a particular concern in case–control studies because exposure data are retrospective. In fact, the relevant exposures may have occurred many years before data collection, making it difficult to gather correct information.

Analysis

As described above, controls are a sample of the population that produced the cases. However, in most instances the sampling fraction is not known, so the investigator cannot fill in the total population in the margin of a two-by-two table or obtain the rates and risks of disease. Instead, the researcher obtains a number called an *odds*, which functions as a rate or risk. An odds is defined as the probability that an event will occur divided by the probability that it will not occur. In a case–control study, epidemiologists typically calculate the odds of being a case among the exposed (a/b) compared to the odds of being a case among the nonexposed (c/d). The ratio of these two odds is expressed as follows:

$$\frac{a/b}{c/d} \text{ or } \frac{ad}{bc}$$

This ratio, known as the disease odds ratio, provides an estimate of the relative risk just as the incidence rate ratio and cumulative incidence ratio do. Risk or rate differences are not usually obtainable in a case–control study. However, it is possible to obtain the attributable proportion among the exposed. Analytic issues for case–control studies are described in more detail in Chapter 9.

Case–Crossover Study

The case–crossover study is a relatively new variant of the case–control study that was developed for settings in which the risk of the outcome is increased for only a brief time following the exposure.[13] The period of increased risk following the exposure is termed the hazard period.[14] In the case–crossover study, cases serve as their own controls, and the exposure frequency during the hazard period is compared to that from a control period. Because cases serve as their own controls, this design has several advantages including the elimination of confounding by characteristics such as gender and race and the elimination of a type of bias that results from selecting unrepresentative controls. In addition, because variability is reduced, this design requires fewer subjects than the traditional case–control study.

When Is It Desirable to Use a Particular Study Design?

The goal of every epidemiologic study is to gather correct and sharply defined data on the relationship between an exposure and a health-related state or event in a population. The three main study designs represent different ways of gathering this information. Given the strengths and weaknesses of each design, there are circumstances for which a particular type of study is clearly indicated. These situations are described in the following paragraphs.

Experimental Studies

Investigators conduct an experimental study when they wish to learn about a prevention or treatment for a disease. In addition, they conduct this type of study when they need data with a high degree of validity that is simply not possible in an observational study. The high degree of validity in an experimental study stems mainly from investigators' ability to randomize subjects to either the treatment group or the comparison group and thereby control for distortions produced by confounding variables. A high level of validity may be needed for studying a prevention or treatment that is expected to have a small effect—usually defined as a difference of 20% or less between groups. A difference of this size is difficult to detect using an observational study because of uncontrolled bias and confounding. When the difference between groups is small, even a small degree of bias or confounding can create or mask an effect.

Although most scientists agree that well-conducted experimental studies produce more scientifically rigorous data than do observational studies, several thorny issues make it difficult to conduct experimental studies. These issues include noncompliance, the need to maintain high follow-up rates, high costs, physicians' and patients' reluctance to participate, and numerous ethical issues. Investigators must address all of these issues when considering this design. In particular, it is ethical to conduct experimental studies only when there is a state of equipoise within the expert medical community regarding the treatment. Equipoise is a "state of mind characterized by legitimate uncertainty or indecision as to choice or course of action."[6(p88)] In other words, there must be genuine confidence that a treatment may be worthwhile in order to administer it to some individuals and genuine reservations about the treatment in order to withhold it from others.

Observational Studies

Observational studies can be used to study the effects of a wider range of exposures than experimental studies, including preventions, treatments, and possible causes of disease. For example, observational studies provide information to explain the causes of disease incidence and the determinants of disease progression, to predict the future health care needs of a population, and to control disease by studying ways to prevent disease and prolong life with disease. The main limitation of observational studies is investigators' inability to have complete control over disturbing influences or extraneous factors. As Susser states: "Observational studies have a place in the epidemiological armament no less necessary and valid than controlled trials; they take second place in the hierarchy of rigor but not in practicability and generalizability. . . . Even when trials are possible, observational studies may yield more of the truth than randomized trials."[15]

Once an investigator has decided to conduct an observational study, the next decision is usually whether to select a cohort or case–control design. Because a cohort study can provide information on a large number of possible health effects, this type of study is preferable when little is known about the health consequences of an exposure. A cohort study is also efficient for investigating a rare exposure, which is usually defined as a frequency of less than 20%.

Case–control studies are preferable when little is known about the etiology of a disease because they can provide information on a large number of possible risk factors. Case–control studies take less time and cost less money than cohort studies, primarily because the control group is a sample of the source population. Case–control studies are also more efficient than cohort studies for studying rare diseases because fewer subjects are needed, and for studying diseases with long induction and latent periods because long-term prospective follow-up is avoided. (A long induction and latent period means that there is a long time between the causal action of an exposure and the eventual diagnosis of disease.[16]) Because of their relatively smaller sample size, case–control studies are preferred when the exposure data are difficult or expensive to obtain. Finally, they are desirable when the population under study is dynamic because it is difficult to keep track of a population that is constantly changing. Tracing is required for a typical cohort study but not a typical case–control study.

Case-control studies have a few important disadvantages. First, because of the retrospective nature of the data collection, there is a greater chance of bias. Some epidemiologists have argued that case–control studies are not well suited for detecting weak associations—those with odds ratios less than 1.5—because of the likelihood of bias.[17] Second, because data collection is retrospective, it may be difficult to establish the correct temporal relationship between the exposure and disease.

If an investigator has decided to conduct a cohort study, he or she must make one more choice: should it be a retrospective or prospective cohort study? This decision depends on the particular research question, the practical constraints of time and money, and the availability of suitable study populations and records. For example, a retrospective design must be used to study historical exposures. In making this decision, the investigator must also take into account the complementary advantages and disadvantages of retrospective and prospective cohort studies. For example, retrospective cohort studies are more efficient than prospective ones for studying diseases with long induction and latent periods. However, minimal information is usually available on the exposure, outcome, confounders, and contacts for follow-up because retrospective cohort studies typically rely on existing records that were not designed for research purposes. In addition, the use of retrospective data makes it more difficult to establish the correct temporal relationship between the exposure and disease.

In prospective cohort studies, investigators can usually obtain more detailed information on exposures and confounders because they have more control of the data collection process and can gather information directly from the participants. Follow-up may be easier because the investigator can obtain tracing information from participants and can maintain periodic contact with subjects. Prospective cohort studies are considered less vulnerable to bias than retrospective studies, because the outcomes have not occurred when the cohort is assembled and the exposures are assessed. In addition, it is easier for investigators to establish a clear temporal relationship between exposure and outcome. A decision tree depicting the choices between the three main study designs is shown in Figure 6–1.

Other Types of Studies

In addition to the three main study designs described above, two other types of studies are commonly conducted in epidemiologic research: cross-sectional and ecologic studies (see Table 6–2). Although both are popular, these designs have important limitations that are not present in the other observational designs.

Cross–Sectional Studies

A cross-sectional study "examines the relationship between diseases (or other health-related characteristics) and other variables of interest as they exist in a defined population at one particular time."[2(p40)] Unlike populations studied in cohort and case–control studies, cross-sectional study

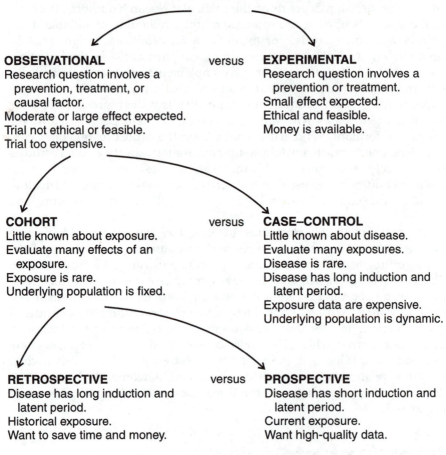

Goal: To Harvest Valid and Precise Information on Association
Between Exposure and Disease Using a Minimum of Resources

OBSERVATIONAL versus **EXPERIMENTAL**

Research question involves a prevention, treatment, or causal factor.
Moderate or large effect expected.
Trial not ethical or feasible.
Trial too expensive.

Research question involves a prevention or treatment.
Small effect expected.
Ethical and feasible.
Money is available.

COHORT versus **CASE–CONTROL**

Little known about exposure.
Evaluate many effects of an exposure.
Exposure is rare.
Underlying population is fixed.

Little known about disease.
Evaluate many exposures.
Disease is rare.
Disease has long induction and latent period.
Exposure data are expensive.
Underlying population is dynamic.

RETROSPECTIVE versus **PROSPECTIVE**

Disease has long induction and latent period.
Historical exposure.
Want to save time and money.

Disease has short induction and latent period.
Current exposure.
Want high-quality data.

FIGURE 6–1. Decision Tree for Choosing Among Study Designs

populations are commonly selected without regard to exposure or disease status. Cross-sectional studies take a snapshot of a population at a single point in time and so measure the exposure prevalence in relation to the disease prevalence. In other words, current disease status is examined in relation to current exposure level.

Cross-sectional studies are carried out for public health planning and for etiologic research. Most governmental surveys conducted by the National Center for Health Statistics are cross-sectional in nature (see Chapter 4 for more details). For example, the National Survey of Family Growth is a periodic population-based survey focusing on factors that

TABLE 6–2   Key Features of Cross-Sectional and Ecologic Studies

Cross-sectional studies

- Examine association at a single point in time, and so measure exposure prevalence in relation to disease prevalence.

- Cannot infer temporal sequence between exposure and disease if exposure is a changeable characteristic.

- Other limitations may include preponderance of prevalent cases of long duration and healthy worker survivor effect.

- Advantages include generalizability and low cost.

Ecologic studies

- Examine rates of disease in relation to a population-level factor.

- Population-level factors include summaries of individual population members, environmental measures, and global measures.

- Study groups are usually identified by place, time, or a combination of the two.

- Limitations include the ecological fallacy and lack of information on important variables.

- Advantages include low cost, wide range of exposure levels, and the ability to examine contextual effects on health.

affect maternal and child health. Its most recent cycle was based on a national probability sample of almost 11,000 civilian, noninstitutionalized women aged 15 to 44 years. In-person interviews gathered information on a woman's ability to become pregnant; pregnancy history; use of contraceptives, family planning, and infertility services; and breastfeeding practices.

Cross-sectional studies are fairly common in occupational settings using data from preemployment physical examinations and company health insurance plans.[18(p144)] For example, investigators conducted a cross-sectional study to determine the relationship between low back pain and sedentary work among crane operators, straddle-carrier drivers, and office workers.[19] All three groups had sedentary jobs that required prolonged sitting. Company records were used to identify approximately 300 currently employed male workers aged 25 through 60 years who had been employed for at least 1 year in their current job. Investigators assessed the "postural load" by observing workers' postures (such as straight upright position, forward or lateral flexion) and movements (such as sitting, standing, and walking). The investigators found that the prevalence of current and recent low back pain was more common among crane operators and straddle-carrier drivers than office workers. The crane operators and straddle-carrier drivers had two to three times the risk of low back pain than did the office workers. The authors postulated that these differences resulted from crane operators' and straddle-carrier drivers' more frequent adoption of "non-neutral" trunk positions involving back flexion and rotation while on the job.[19]

Unfortunately, when epidemiologists measure the exposure prevalence in relation to disease prevalence in cross-sectional studies, they are not able to infer the temporal sequence between the exposure and disease. They cannot tell which came first—the exposure or the disease. This occurs when the exposure under study is a changeable characteristic such as a place of residence or a habit such as cigarette smoking. Consider, for example, a hypothetical cross-sectional study of cigarette smoking and the risk of tubal infertility conducted among patients seeking treatment at an infertility clinic. The current smoking status of women who have a diagnosis of tubal infertility is compared with that of fertile women whose husbands are the source of the infertility. If the frequency of cigarette smoking is three times greater among the infertile women, one could conclude that there is a moderately strong association between smoking and tubal infertility. However, it is difficult to know if smoking caused the infertility, because the women may have begun smoking after they began having difficulties achieving a pregnancy. This is quite possible, given that precise onset of infertility is difficult to determine and that medical treatment for infertility usually does not begin until a couple has been trying to conceive for at least 1 year. This is an important limitation of cross-sectional studies, because epidemiologists must establish the correct temporal sequence between an exposure and a disease in order to support the hypothesis that an exposure causes a disease (see Chapter 15 for more details).

Another disadvantage of cross-sectional studies is that such studies identify a high proportion of prevalent cases of long duration. People who die soon after diagnosis or who recover quickly are less likely to be identified as diseased. This can bias the results if the duration of disease is associated with the exposure under study.

Still another bias may occur when cross-sectional studies are conducted in occupational settings. Because these studies include only current and not former workers, the results may be influenced by the selective departure of sick individuals from the workforce. Those who remain employed tend to be healthier than those who leave employment. This phenomenon, known as the "healthy worker survivor effect," generally attenuates an adverse effect of an exposure. For example, the strength of the association observed in the study of low back pain among sedentary workers may have been biased by the self-selection out of employment of workers with low back pain.

Cross-sectional studies also have several advantages. First, when they are based on a sample of the general population, their results are highly generalizable. This is particularly true of the cross-sectional surveys conducted by the National Center for Health Statistics. Second, they can be carried out in a relatively short period of time, thereby reducing their cost. Furthermore, the temporal inference problem can be avoided if an inalterable characteristic, such as a genetic trait, is the focus of the investigation. It can also be avoided if the exposure measure reflects not only present but also past exposure. For example, an x-ray fluorescence (XRF) measurement of an individual's bone lead level reflects that person's cumulative exposure over many years.[20] Thus, a cross-sectional study of infertility and bone lead levels using XRF measurements would not suffer from the same temporal inference problem as the study of infertility and cigarette smoking described above.

Ecologic Studies

A classical ecologic study examines the rates of disease in relation to a factor described on a population level. Thus, "the units of analysis are populations or groups of people rather than individuals."[2(p52)] The population-level factor may be an aggregate measure that summarizes the individual members of the population (for example, the proportion of individuals above the age of 65 years), an environmental measure that describes the geographic location where the population resides or works (for example, the air pollution level), or a global measure that has no analog on the individual level (such as the population density or existence of a specific law or health care system).[21(p460)] Thus, the two key features that distinguish a traditional ecologic study from other types of epidemiologic studies are: (1) the population unit of analysis and (2) an exposure status that is the property of the population.

Ecologic studies usually identify groups by place, time, or a combination of the two.[21(p463)] For example, researchers conducted an ecologic study with groups identified by place to determine the association between air pollution and mortality rates.[22] The study authors obtained 1978–1981 air pollution levels from monitoring stations throughout the United States and 1980 mortality rates for 305 Standard Metropolitan Statistical Areas (SMSAs). SMSAs are geographic areas that typically include a city and its surrounding areas.[2(pp160–161)] The investigators examined correlations between the air pollution variables (such as total suspended particulates and sulfates) and mortality. They observed a positive association between annual mean sulfate concentration and total mortality. That is, SMSAs with high sulfate concentrations tended to have high mortality rates (for example, Scranton, Pennsylvania), while those with low sulfate concentrations tended to have low mortality rates (for example, Salt Lake City, Utah) (see Figure 6–2).

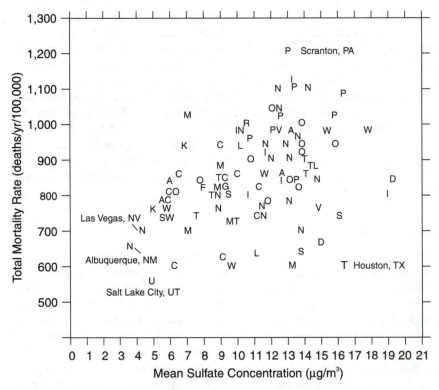

FIGURE 6–2. Plot of Total Mortality Rate versus Annual Mean Sulfate Concentration in an Ecologic Study

Source: Reprinted from Ozkaynak H, Thurston GD. Association between 1980 US mortality rates and alternative measures of airborne particle concentration. *Risk Analysis.* 1987;7:454.

Ecologic studies that identify groups by time often compare disease rates over time in geographically defined populations.[21(p464)] For example, investigators conducted an ecologic study to compare HIV seroprevalence changes over time among injecting drug users in cities with and without needle-exchange programs.[23] The investigators hypothesized that introduction of needle-exchange programs (programs that allow drug users to obtain clean needles and syringes free of charge) would decrease HIV transmission and lead to lower seroprevalence rates. The authors obtained information on HIV seroprevalence among injecting drug users during the 1980s and 1990s from published studies and from unpublished reports from the Centers for Disease Control and Prevention. They obtained information on the implementation of the needle-exchange programs from published reports and experts. They found that the average HIV seroprevalence *increased* by 5.9% per year in 52 cities without needle-exchange programs, and it *decreased* by 5.8% per year in 29 cities with needle-exchange programs. Thus, the average annual change in seroprevalence was 11.7% lower in cities with needle-exchange programs.

A special type of time-trend ecologic study tries to separate the effects of three time-related variables: age, calendar time, and year of birth.[21(p465)] For example, a recent ecologic study examined homicide mortality data from the United States during the period 1935 through 1994 in order to understand better these three time-related variables.[24] The authors found that death rates caused by homicide doubled over this period, and that most of the increase occurred from 1960 through 1974. Peak ages for homicide deaths ranged from 20 to 39 years. No associations with year of birth were seen among women; however, there was a large increase in the risk of homicide mortality among men born around 1965. Men in this "birth cohort" accounted for the increase in homicide mortality from 1985 through 1994. The authors postulated that the increased prevalence of alcohol and drug abuse and the availability of lethal weapons may account for the association with year of birth among males.

Some investigations cannot be classified as traditional ecologic studies because they have both ecologic and individual-level components. Consider, for example, a "partially" ecologic study that was recently conducted in Norway to determine if chlorinated drinking water was associated with the occurrence of birth defects.[25] Chlorinated water contains numerous chemicals called disinfection byproducts that may be harmful to developing embryos. Because the study used group-level data on the exposure and individual-level data on the birth defects and confounding variables, it is considered partially ecologic. The study population consisted of children born in Norway from 1993 through 1995 who lived in an area with information on water chlorination (n = 141,077 children). Investigators examined the prevalence of birth defects in relation to the proportion of the population served by chlorinated water. They examined four groups of municipalities: those with 0% chlorinated water, 0.1% to 49.9% chlorinated water, 50 to 99.9% chlorinated water, and 100% chlorinated water. Individual-level characteristics that were controlled included maternal age and parity and place of birth, as obtained from the children's birth records. The study suggested there was a 15% increased risk of birth defects overall and a 99% increased risk of urinary tract defects among women whose water was chlorinated. However, the authors acknowledged that the study did not directly measure the concentrations of the disinfection byproducts on the individual level.

The lack of individual-level information leads to a limitation of ecologic studies known as the "ecological fallacy" or "ecological bias." The ecological fallacy means that "an association observed between variables on an aggregate level does not necessarily represent the association that exists at the individual level."[2(p51)] In other words, one cannot necessarily infer the same relationship from the group level to the individual level. In the Norway study, we do not know if the women who drank chlorinated water were the same women who gave birth to babies with defects. This is particularly true for the two middle exposure groups (municipalities with 0.1 to 49.9% and 50 to 99.9% of the population with chlorinated water), because women with chlorinated and unchlorinated water were grouped together. On a practical level, the ecological bias means that the investigator cannot fill in the cells of a two-by-two table from the data available in a traditional ecologic study.

Additional limitations of ecologic studies include investigators' inability to detect subtle or complicated relationships (such as a J-shaped or other curvilinear relationships) because of the crude nature of the data, and the lack of information on characteristics that might distort the association. For example, although the ecologic study of changes in HIV seroprevalence over time suggests that needle-exchange programs reduce HIV transmission, other factors may have accounted for this change, including the simultaneous implementation of other types of HIV prevention strategies.

In spite of these limitations, ecologic studies remain a popular study design among epidemiologists for several reasons.[21(p462)] They can be done quickly and inexpensively because they often rely on preexisting data. Their analysis and presentation are relatively simple and easy to understand. They have the ability to achieve a wider range of exposure levels than could be expected from a typical individual-level study. And, last but not least, epidemiologists have a genuine interest in ecologic effects. For example, ecologic studies can be used "to understand how context affects the health of persons and groups through selection, distribution, interaction, adaption, and other responses." As Susser states, "Measures of individual attributes cannot account for these processes; pairings, families, peer groups, schools, communities, cultures, and laws are all contexts that alter outcomes in ways not explicable by studies that focus solely on individuals."[26] This observation is particularly true for studies of the transmission of infectious disease. For example, investigators conducted an ecological analysis to determine the risk factors for dengue fever (a viral infection transmitted by the *Aedes aegypti* mosquito) in 70 Mexican villages.[27] They measured exposure by the average proportion of *Aedes* larvae among households in each village in relation to the proportion of affected individuals in the village. The study found a strong relationship between dengue antibody levels and the village-level larval concentrations. This association was not seen when an individual-level study was carried out, because it did not take into account transmission dynamics at the population level.

Summary

Epidemiolgists use both experimental and observational study designs to answer research questions. Each type of design represents a different way of harvesting the necessary information. The selection of one design over another depends on the research question and takes into account validity, efficiency, and ethical concerns.

For ethical reasons, experimental studies can only be used to investigate preventions and treatments for diseases. The hallmark of an experimental study is the investigator's active manipulation of the agent under study. Here, the investigator assigns subjects (usually at random) to two or more groups that either receive or do not receive the preventive or therapeutic agent. Investigators select this study design when they need data with a high degree of validity that is simply not possible in an observational study. However, experimental studies are expensive and often infeasible and unethical, and so most epidemiolgic research consists of observational studies.

Observational studies can be used to investigate a broader range of exposures including causes, preventions, and treatments for diseases. The two most important types of observational studies are the cohort study and the case–control study. Epidemiologists use a cohort study when little is known about an exposure, because this type of study allows investigators to examine many health effects in relation to an exposure. In a cohort study, subjects are defined according to their exposure levels and are followed for disease occurrence. In contrast, investigators use a case–control study when little is known about a disease, because this type of study allows researchers to examine many exposures in relation to a disease. In a case–control study, cases with the disease and controls are defined and their exposure histories are collected and compared.

Cross-sectional and ecologic studies are two other popular types of observational studies. Cross-sectional studies examine exposure prevalence in relation to disease prevalence in a defined population at a single point in time. Ecologic studies examine disease rates in relation to a population-level factor. Both types of design have important limitations absent from the other observational studies. An unclear temporal relationship between exposure and disease arises in cross-sectional studies of changeable exposures. Problems making cross-level inferences from the group to the individual (known as the ecological fallacy) occur in ecologic studies.

References

1. MacMahon B, Trichopoulos D. *Epidemiology Principles and Methods.* 2nd ed. Boston, MA: Little, Brown and Company; 1996.
2. Last JM. *A Dictionary of Epidemiology.* 3rd ed. New York, NY: Oxford University Press; 1995.

3. Benenson AS. *Control of Communicable Diseases in Man.* 15th ed. Washington, DC: American Public Health Association; 1990.

4. Pickett JP, exec. ed. *The American Heritage Dictionary of the English language.* 4th ed. Boston, MA: Houghton Mifflin; 2000.

5. Colton T. *Statistics in Medicine.* Boston, MA: Little, Brown and Company; 1974.

6. Meinert CL. *Clinical Trials Dictionary, Terminology and Usage Recommendations.* Baltimore, MD: The Johns Hopkins Center for Clinical Trials; 1996.

7. Friedman LM, Furberg CD, DeMets DL. *Fundamentals of Clinical Trials.* 2nd ed. Littleton, MA: PSG Publishing Co; 1985.

8. Newell DJ. Intention-to-treat analysis: implications for quantitative and qualitative research. *Int J Epidemiol.* 1992;21:837–841.

9. Hunt JR, White E. Retaining and tracking cohort study members. *Epidemiol Rev.* 1998;20:57–70.

10. Miettinen OS. The "case–control" study: valid selection of study subjects. *J Chron Dis.* 1985;38:543–548.

11. McLaughlin JK, Blot WJ, Mehl ES, Mandel JS. Problems in the use of dead controls in case–control studies. I. General results. *Am J Epidemiol.* 1985;121: 131–139.

12. Correa A, Stewart WF, Yeh H-C, Santos-Burgoa C. Exposure measurement in case–control studies: reported methods and recommendations. *Epidemiol Rev.* 1994;16:18–32.

13. Maclure M. The case-crossover design: a method for studying transient effects on the risk of acute events. *Am J Epidemiol.* 1991;133:144–153.

14. Mittleman MA, Maclure M, Robins JM. Control sampling strategies for case-crossover studies: an assessment of relative efficiency. *Am J Epidemiol.* 1995;142: 91–98.

15. Susser M. Editorial: The tribulations of trials—interventions in communities. *Am J Public Health.* 1995;85:156–158.

16. Rothman KJ. Induction and latent periods. *Am J Epidemiol.* 1981;114:253–259.

17. Austin H, Hill HA, Flanders WD, Greenberg RS. Limitations in the application of case–control methodology. *Epidemiol Rev.* 1994;16:65–76.

18. Monson RR. *Occupational Epidemiology.* 2nd ed. Boca Raton, FL: CRC Press; 1990.

19. Burdorf A, Naaktgeboren B, de Groot H. Occupational risk factors for low back pain among sedentary workers. *J Occup Med.* 1993;35:1213–1220.

20. Hu H. Bone lead as a new biologic marker of lead dose: recent findings and implications for public health. *Environ Health Perspect.* 1998;106:961–967.

21. Morgenstern H. Ecologic studies. In: Rothman KJ, Greenland S, eds. *Modern Epidemiology.* Philadelphia, PA: Lippincott-Raven Publishers; 1998.

22. Ozkaynak H, Thurston GD. Association between 1980 US mortality rates and alternative measures of airborne particle concentration. *Risk Anal.* 1987;7: 459–480.

23. Hurley SF, Jolley DJ, Kaldor JM. Effectiveness of needle-exchange programmes for prevention of HIV infection. *Lancet.* 1997;349:1797–1800.

24. Shahpar C, Li G. Homicide mortality in the United States, 1935–1994: age, period and cohort effects. *Am J Epidemiol.* 1999;150:1213–1222.

25. Magnus P, Jaakkola JJK, Skrondal A, Alexander J, Becher G, Krogh T, Dybing E. Water chlorination and birth defects. *Epidemiology.* 1999;10:513–517.
26. Susser M. The logic in ecological: I. The logic of analysis. *Am J Public Health.* 1994;84:825–829.
27. Koopman JS, Longini IM. The ecological effects of individual exposures and nonlinear disease dynamics in populations. *Am J Public Health.* 1994;84: 836–842.

EXERCISES

1. State the main difference between the following study designs:
   A. Observational and experimental studies
   B. Retrospective cohort and prospective cohort studies
   C. Cohort and case–control studies

2. Briefly describe a cross-sectional study and indicate its main limitation.

3. Briefly describe an ecologic study and indicate its main limitation.

4. State which observational study design is best (that is, most efficient and logical) in each of the following scenarios:
   A. Identifying the causes of a rare disease CASE CONTROL
   B. Identifying the long-term effects of a rare exposure Retrospective
   C. Studying the health effects of an exposure for which information is difficult and expensive to obtain CASE CONTROL
   D. Identifying the causes of a new disease about which little is known
   E. Identifying the short-term health effects of a new exposure about which little is known Prospective
   F. Identifying the causes of a disease with a long latent period CASE control

5. Which type of study is being described in each of the following scenarios?
   A. A study that examines the death rates from cervical cancer in each of the 50 U.S. states in relation to the average percentage of women in each state undergoing annual PAP smear screening. ecological
   B. A study that compares the prevalence of back pain among current members of the plumbers and pipefitters union with that of current members of the bakers and confectionary union. cross section
   C. A study that evaluates the relationship between breast cancer and a woman's history of breastfeeding. The investigator selects women with breast cancer and an age-matched sample of women who live in the same neighborhoods as the women with breast case control

cancer. Study subjects are interviewed to determine if they breast-fed any of their children.

D. A study that evaluates two treatments for breast cancer. Women with stage 1 breast cancer are randomized to receive either lumpectomy alone or lumpectomy with breast radiation. Women are followed for 5 years to determine if there are any differences in breast cancer recurrence and survival. *expiramentle*

E. A study of the relationship between exposure to chest irradiation and subsequent risk of breast cancer that was begun in 2001. In this study, women who received radiation therapy for postpartum mastitis (an inflammation of the breast that occurs after giving birth) in the 1940s were compared to women who received a nonradiation therapy for postpartum mastitis in the 1940s. The women were followed for 40 years to determine the incidence rates of breast cancer in each group.

Retrospective cohort

7

Experimental Studies

LEARNING OBJECTIVES

By the end of this chapter, the reader will be able to:

- Distinguish between the types of experimental studies, including individual versus community trials, preventive versus therapeutic trials, parallel versus crossover trials, and simple versus factorial trials.
- State the established sequence for conducting trials of new drugs.
- Describe the key features of conducting experimental studies, including the enrollment and consent process, randomization, use of placebos and masking, maintenance and assessment of compliance, follow-up and ascertaining the outcomes, and data analysis.
- Discuss the special ethical issues of experimental studies, including equipoise and use of placebo controls.

Introduction

An experimental study, commonly known as a trial, involves the use of designed experiments to investigate the role of some agent in the causation, prevention, or treatment of a disease. In this type of study, the investigator assigns individuals to two or more groups that either receive or do not receive a preventive or therapeutic treatment. The active manipulation of the treatment by the investigator is the hallmark that distinguishes experimental studies from observational ones.

Because experimental studies more closely resemble controlled laboratory investigations, most epidemiologists believe that, if well conducted, they produce more scientifically rigorous results than do observational studies. In a laboratory experiment, the investigator regulates all important aspects of the experimental conditions, permitting the experimental subjects to differ only for the purpose of testing the hypothesis. For example, a laboratory experiment testing the toxicity of a chemical is conducted on genetically similar animals (such as mice, rats).[1] Animals are assigned (usually by chance) to either the test or control group. Using identical routes of administration (for example, by mouth or injection), the chemical under investigation is given to the test group while an inert chemical such as a salt solution is dispensed to the control group. All experimental animals are kept in the same physical environment, are fed the same diet, and follow the same daily schedule. Thus, the only difference between the two groups is the dissimilar chemical (test versus inert), deliberately introduced by the investigator.

Although experimental studies conducted among free-living humans can never achieve the same degree of control as laboratory animal experiments, many aspects of human experimental research emulate the principles of laboratory research. This chapter describes the design, conduct, and analysis of experimental studies among humans. First, an overview of experimental studies is presented, followed by a detailed discussion of each aspect of an experimental study. The chapter concludes with a discussion of the numerous special considerations in experimental studies that make them scientifically rigorous but difficult to perform.

Overview of Experimental Studies

Investigators must formulate a hypothesis before launching an epidemiologic study. Hypothesis generation is a creative endeavor in which an investigator proposes a specific idea to explain a set of observations. Next, the epidemiologist must decide which type of study design will efficiently provide valid information to either support or refute the hypothesis. The appropriate study design is determined by considering the state of knowledge, the frequency of the exposure and disease, and the expected strength of the association between the two. In addition, several practical and ethical problems must be solved when experimental studies are conducted.

Once the study has been designed, a research proposal is written and funding is solicited. At this time, the investigators usually request approval for the study from the ethics committee of the participating institutions. The ethics committee, also called the institutional review board, reviews all studies to ensure that the research is ethical and legitimate.[2(p89)] The review is particularly important in experimental studies because a state of equipoise must exist for the study to be ethical. Equipoise is characterized by genuine uncertainty about the risks and benefits of the test treatment. That is, there must be sufficient certainty that the test treatment might be beneficial in order to administer it to some individuals while, at the same time, sufficient doubt about its benefits in order to withhold it from others.

Next, during the recruitment phase, investigators enroll individuals in the study on the basis of specific eligibility criteria. The eligibility criteria consist of inclusion and exclusion criteria that stem from both scientific and practical concerns. For example, the CAPRIE (Clopidogrel versus Aspirin in Patients at Risk of Ischemic Events) experimental study compared the effectiveness of clopidogrel in reducing the risk of heart attacks and strokes with that of aspirin among patients with atherosclerotic vascular disease.[3] Inclusion criteria consisted of an established diagnosis of recent stroke, heart attack, or peripheral arterial disease. Exclusion criteria included contraindications to the study drugs because of potential side effects, and geographic factors that made participation unrealistic. The eligibility criteria influence the generalizability of the study—that is, the larger population to whom the study results are applicable.

Subsequently, eligible individuals must give formal consent to participate, usually by signing a consent form that has been approved by the ethics committee. Investigators then use either random or nonrandom methods to assign individuals to receive one of the two or more treatments being compared. Random assignment, usually termed randomization, is preferred because its unpredictable nature makes it less prone to bias. The group that is allocated to the agent under study is generally called the treatment group, and the other group is called the comparison or control group. The comparison group may receive no treatment at all, an inactive treatment such as a placebo, or another active treatment. Often the active treatment given to the comparison group is the current standard of care. For example, the CAPRIE study compared a new drug (clopidogrel) to the standard treatment (aspirin). Because the aspirin treatment, while effective, had serious potential side effects such as gastrointestinal bleeding, there was great interest in finding another effective treatment with fewer adverse effects.[3]

In the next phase of a trial, the treatments are administered according to a specific protocol. For example, the CAPRIE study patients were asked to take tablets of clopidogrel or aspirin every day with their morning meal for at least 1 year.[3]

During the follow-up stage, the treatment and comparison groups are monitored for the outcomes under study. If the goal of the study is to prevent the occurrence of disease, the outcome may include the precursors of disease or the first occurrence of disease (that is, incidence). On the other hand, if the study is testing a new treatment among individuals who already have a disease, outcomes may include disease recurrence, symptom improvement, length of survival, or side effects. In the CAPRIE therapeutic study, outcome measures included the recurrence of stroke and heart attacks, primary brain hemorrhage, and leg amputation.[3]

The length of time that subjects are followed depends on the outcomes being studied. Only a few months may be needed in a short-term study of drug side effects, but a decade may be necessary for examining slowly developing diseases such as cancer. During follow-up, investigators maintain contact with participants through periodic visits, phone calls, or letters. Losses to follow-up and dropouts must be kept to a minimum during this phase to ensure a successful trial. For example, in the CAPRIE study, follow-up visits with physicians took place several times a year for up to 3 years, and so the number of losses to follow-up and dropouts was quite low.[3]

All reported outcomes of interest are confirmed in order to guarantee their accuracy. Confirmation is usually done by masked investigators who gather corroborating information from objective sources such as medical records. Masking, which means that the investigator is unaware of the participant's treatment assignment, reduces the chance of making a biased assessment of the outcome and so improves the rigor of the study.

During the follow-up stage, investigators assess participants' level of compliance with the treatment regimen. That is, they determine if participants are following exactly the study protocol. In the CAPRIE study, follow-up visits included questions about the use of study medications and any other drugs.[3] Fortunately, fewer than 1% of the patients were completely noncompliant (that is, they never took the study drugs as directed). Noncompliance is problematic, because it makes it more difficult for investigators to determine if an experimental treatment is effective.

The classical approach to the analysis of an experimental study is known as an intent-to-treat analysis. Here, all individuals allocated to a treatment are analyzed as representing that treatment, regardless of whether they completed or even received the treatment. Investigators take this approach to preserve the baseline comparability of the groups and to provide information on the effectiveness of a treatment under real-life conditions.

Types of Experimental Studies

Experimental studies can be classified in several ways, depending on their design and purpose. The major types of categorization are described in the following sections and are summarized in Table 7–1.

Individual versus Community Trials

Trials are often distinguished according to the method by which the treatment is assigned. Most commonly conducted are individual trials, in which the treatment is allocated to individual persons. For example, a recent individual trial among adults infected with human immunodeficiency virus (HIV) compared the effectiveness of treatment with a single drug (zidovudine or didanosine alone) versus treatment with two drugs (zidovudine and didanosine, or zidovudine and zalcitabine) in

TABLE 7–1 Types of Experimental Studies

Type	Defining characteristic
Individual	Treatment is allocated to individuals.
Community	Treatment is allocated to entire community.
Preventive	Prophylactic agent is given to healthy or high-risk individuals to prevent disease occurrence.
Therapeutic	Treatment is given to diseased individuals to reduce the risk of recurrence, improve survival, or improve quality of life.
Parallel	Each group receives one treatment. Treatments are administered concurrently.
Crossover	Each group receives all treatments one after another. The treatment order differs for each group. Washout period may intervene between treatments.
Simple	Each group gets one treatment.
Factorial	Each group gets two or more treatments.

slowing disease progression and improving survival.[4] In this study, 2467 HIV-infected individuals were each randomly assigned to one of four daily regimens, with roughly 600 patients in each group. Each patient was treated for an average of 18 weeks and followed for an average of 143 weeks. Outcome measures including decline in immune function, progression to acquired immune deficiency syndrome (AIDS), and death were measured in each patient and later aggregated by treatment group.

In community trials, which are less common, the treatment is allocated to an entire community. A well-known community trial was the Newburgh–Kingston Caries Fluorine Study, which was conducted to determine if increasing fluoride levels in drinking water would reduce the incidence of dental caries among resident children.[5] Children who lived in the community of Newburgh, New York, served as the treatment group. Beginning in 1944, fluoride was added to the town's drinking water supply to raise its concentration from about 0.1 to 1 part per million (ppm). The children of Kingston, New York, a similarly sized community about 35 miles away, served as the comparison group. The fluoride level (0.1 ppm) of its water supply was left unchanged. Periodic dental examinations were conducted among school-aged children residing in each community for several years. Investigators assessed the efficacy of the fluoride treatment by comparing the prevalence of decayed, missing, or filled teeth among children in Newburgh to that of children in Kingston.

More recently, a community trial was conducted in Tanzania to test the hypothesis that improving medical and educational services for treating sexually transmitted diseases would reduce the incidence of HIV infection.[6] The study randomly assigned 12 pairs of health centers and their catchment populations either to receive the community intervention activities or to serve as a comparison. Key activities of the community-level intervention included training health center staff members in the treatment of sexually transmitted diseases, educating villagers about sexually transmitted diseases, regularly supplying medications to the health centers, and making available a diagnostic laboratory. The intervention activities were targeted toward the entire community served by the health center rather than toward specific individuals. The investigators conducted surveys in the intervention and comparison communities before and after the intervention to determine if there were any changes in incidence rates of HIV infection.

Preventive versus Therapeutic Trials

Another way to classify experimental studies is according to their purpose—that is, whether they investigate a measure that prevents disease occurrence (known as a preventive or prophylactic trial) or a measure that treats an existing condition (known as a therapeutic trial). Trials that prevent or delay the onset of disease among healthy individuals are called primary prevention trials, and those that prevent or delay progression among diseased individuals are termed secondary prevention trials.[2(pp.206,244)]

In some preventive trials, the alleged causal factor is reduced or removed. For example, the Boston Lead Free Kids Study tested the hypothesis that removing lead-contaminated soil from around children's homes would reduce their blood lead levels and their risk of lead poisoning.[7] In this instance, the suspected causal factor—lead-contaminated soil—was removed from yards and replaced with clean soil and ground cover.

In other preventive trials, agents such as vitamins (such as folic acid and vitamins A, C, and E), minerals (such as selenium and calcium), naturally occurring compounds (such as carotenoids and flavenoids), and drugs (such as cholesterol-lowering and antihypertensive drugs) are studied to determine if they are effective in reducing disease occurrence or recurrence.[8] Prevention trials may also involve behavior modifications such as dietary improvements (for example, low-cholesterol diet),[9] smoking cessation,[10] physical exercise,[11] and safer-sex educational programs.[12] The Women's Health Initiative, an ongoing randomized trial of about 65,000 postmenopausal women, combines several preventive measures as it examines the effects of eating a low-fat diet (with 20% of calories from fat), hormone replacement therapy, and calcium and vitamin D supplementation on the prevention of cancer, cardiovascular disease, and osteoporotic fractures.[13]

Some preventive trials are conducted among the general population and others among high-risk individuals. For example, the Women's Health Initiative is being conducted among healthy postmenopausal women whose baseline risk of disease is no higher than that of similarly aged women in the general population. On the other hand, the Breast Cancer Prevention (BCP) Trial determined the ability of tamoxifen to reduce breast cancer incidence and mortality among high-risk healthy women.[14] Here, risk was determined by current age, age at menarche and first live birth, family history of breast cancer, number of benign breast biopsies, and mammographic abnormalities. The BCP Trial focused on high-risk women rather than those from the general population, in part, because the benefits of taking tamoxifen presumably outweigh its risks only among high-risk women. Tamoxifen has been associated with an increased risk of endometrial cancer in several experimental and observational studies.[15]

Prevention trials usually take many years to conduct and require tens of thousands of participants because they often focus on reducing the incidence of diseases that typically occur at a yearly cumulative incidence of 1% or less.[16] For example, the BCP Trial enrolled about 13,000 women and followed them for more than 5 years.[14]

Whereas prevention trials are conducted among individuals without disease, therapeutic trials involve testing treatments such as surgery, radiation, and drugs among individuals who already have a disease. Therapeutic trials are commonly called clinical trials because they are conducted in a clinical setting among diseased patients and use a clinical outcome measure such as recurrence or side effects.[2(p42)] In therapeutic trials, a new therapy is usually compared to the standard treatment. The new therapy may consist of a new drug, a novel combination of existing drugs, a new therapy, or a technology improvement of an old therapy. These treatments are meant to reduce the recurrence of disease, improve survival, and improve the quality of life. Because therapeutic trials attempt to reduce the occurrence of relatively common outcomes (such as disease recurrence or death), they usually only take 1 or 2 years to conduct and generally involve only a few hundred patients.[16]

For example, a therapeutic trial was conducted among women with advanced ovarian cancer to determine if the plant-derived drug paclitaxel improved survival.[17] Women in the experimental group were treated with the new combination of paclitaxel and cisplatin, and those in the comparison group were treated with cisplatin and cyclophosphamide, the standard choice for more than a decade. The investigators enrolled 386 eligible women and followed them for 48 months. The investigators found that the new drug combination improved the length of progression-free and overall survival. Women who received the new drug combination lived an average of 5 more months without the disease worsening and 14 more months overall than did those who received the standard therapy.

New Drug Trials

There is a well-established sequence for carrying out therapeutic trials involving new drugs.[2(pp193–194)] A phase 1 drug trial is conducted to provide preliminary information on drug safety using a relatively small number of normal healthy volunteers. The exception is for cancer chemotherapeutic agents, which are conducted in patients who usually have advanced disease. This trial provides metabolic and pharmacologic profiles of the drug, including determination of the maximally tolerated dose. Next, a phase 2 trial is conducted on a larger number of diseased individuals to obtain preliminary information on efficacy and additional information on safety including side effects. Sometimes the Food and Drug Administration (the federal agency with the authority to approve drugs and devices for clinical use) approves drugs following phase 2 testing, but usually a phase 3 trial is needed to show an advantage of an experimental therapy over a standard one using an objective outcome such as improved survival.[18] Phase 3 trials also gather information on a drug's indications of use, recommended doses, and side effects—all necessary for administering appropriately the drug in clinical practice.[2(p193)] When a phase 3 trial is complete, the drug manufacturer can request to market the drug for the indication covered by the trial. After approval of the new drug application, a phase 4 trial and postmarketing surveillance may be conducted to determine long-term safety and efficacy of the drug. A phase 4 trial may be needed because rare and slowly developing adverse events may not become evident during the typical 3-year phase 3 trial.

Investigators do not always adhere to this rigid sequence for new drug trials, particularly for life-threatening diseases.[2(p194)] For example, two or more phases of a drug trial may be conducted concurrently. In addition, for serious diseases with few treatment options, "it has become commonplace for new drugs showing promise in early studies to be made widely available to patients who might benefit from them at the same time as the randomized trials designed to measure any such benefit are undertaken."[19] For example, more AIDS patients have received new drugs such as didanosine through "expanded-release" or "parallel-track" programs than through clinical trials.

Parallel versus Crossover Trials

Trials can also be described according to the method of treatment administration (see Table 7–1). In the simplest design, known as parallel treatment, individuals in each group simultaneously receive one study treatment. For example, in the drug efficacy study among women with advanced ovarian cancer, women in the experimental group received the new drug combination and women in the comparison group received the standard drug regimen over the same calendar period. Thus, the treatment and comparison groups consisted of entirely different women, and the treatments were administered during the same general time frame (see Figure 7–1).

PARALLEL DESIGN

Group 1——— Treatment A ——▶ Follow-up and outcome assessment

Group 2——— Treatment B ——▶ Follow-up and outcome assessment

CROSSOVER DESIGN

Group 1—— Treatment A —▶ Washout —▶Treatment B—▶ Follow-up and outcome assessment

Group 2—— Treatment B —▶ Washout —▶Treatment A—▶ Follow-up and outcome assessment

Time ——————————————————————————▶

FIGURE 7-1. Parallel and Crossover Treatment Study Designs

In a crossover trial design, two or more study treatments are administered one after another to each group. Thus, all trial participants receive all of the treatments—only the order of the treatments differs. In this type of trial, a person may serve as his or her own control. For example, if the drug efficacy trial among ovarian cancer patients were a crossover design, women in the experimental group would first receive the new drug combination and then the standard regimen while those in the comparison group would first receive the standard regimen and then the new drug combination. The groups usually switch treatments at the same time, and there is often a washout period between the end of one treatment and the start of another to give the body time to metabolize and excrete the initial treatment.

Simple versus Factorial Designs

Trials can also be categorized according to the number of treatments being tested (see Table 7–1). In a simple treatment design, each group receives a treatment consisting of one component (for example, a single drug). In contrast, two or more treatments are combined in a factorial treatment design. For example, the Women's Health Study is using a two-by-two-by-two factorial design to test these three hypotheses among 40,000 female health professionals aged 40 and over: (1) low-dose aspirin reduces the risk of cardiovascular disease, (2) the antioxidant vitamin E reduces the risk of cancer, and (3) beta-carotene reduces the risk of cancer.[20] As shown in Figure 7–2, investigators conducted three rounds of randomization (for each of the three treatments) in order to assign all possible combinations of the treatments to eight groups: (1) active aspirin, beta-carotene, and vitamin E; (2) active aspirin, beta-carotene placebo, active vitamin E; (3) active aspirin, active beta-carotene, and vitamin E placebo; (4) aspirin placebo, active beta-carotene, and active vitamin E; (5) active aspirin, beta-carotene

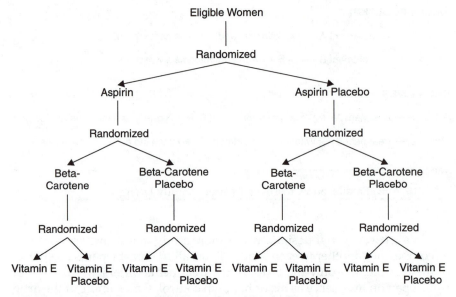

FIGURE 7–2. Two-by-two-by-two Factorial Study Design

Source: Data from Buring JE, Hennekens CH. Randomized trials of primary prevention of cardiovascular disease in women: an investigator's view. *Ann Epidemiol.* 1994;4:111–114.

placebo, and vitamin E placebo; (6) aspirin placebo, active beta-carotene, and vitamin E placebo; (7) aspirin placebo, beta-carotene placebo, and active vitamin E; and (8) aspirin placebo, beta-carotene placebo, and vitamin E placebos. The factorial design allows an investigator to test the separate and combined effects of several agents.

Study Population

The study population, also called the experimental population, consists of the people who are considered for enrollment in a trial. Thus, it consists of potential participants. The study population depends on the purpose of the trial and may include healthy, high-risk, or diseased individuals. The study population's characteristics are further defined by specific eligibility criteria. For example, a trial of the efficacy of the antiretroviral drug zidovudine in reducing the risk of maternal-infant HIV transmission enrolled women with the following characteristics: HIV-infected; pregnant and between 14 and 34 weeks' gestation; CD4 T-lymphocyte counts greater than 200 cells per cubic millimeter; normal levels of other blood, liver, and urine parameters; and no medical reason for needing antiretroviral therapy.[21] Women were excluded if they had abnormal ultrasound findings such as fetal anomalies or if they received any HIV therapy during the pregnancy. Only women who met all of these criteria were enrolled and randomly assigned to receive either zidovudine or placebo during pregnancy and labor.

Eligibility criteria such as these are based upon scientific, safety, and practical considerations. For example, only HIV-infected, pregnant women were included in the maternal-infant HIV transmission trial because, if the drug were found effective, it was intended to be used by this population.[21] In addition, women were excluded if the fetus had an anomaly that could increase the concentration of zidovudine or its metabolite and endanger its health. Finally, women with a medical reason for needing antiretroviral drugs were excluded because it would be unethical to assign such women to the placebo comparison group.

Although all individuals who meet the eligibility criteria can theoretically participate in a trial, practical constraints usually limit actual enrollment to individuals who investigators are able to recruit. Thus, participants of therapeutic trials are usually patients at the hospitals and clinics with which the investigators are affiliated. Trials that enroll healthy individuals may also recruit patients at these institutions, or participants may be identified through other sources such as newspapers and television. For example, the study of high-impact exercise on bone strength recruited healthy premenopausal women through local newspaper advertisements.[11]

Depending on the number of participants needed for the trial, one or many institutions may take part. A single-center trial is conducted at a single clinical site, whereas a multicenter trial includes two or more sites. Each clinical site enrolls individuals, administers the treatments, and collects data. For example, the maternal-fetal HIV transmission prevention trial was conducted at almost 50 institutions in the United States and France.[21] The large number of institutions was needed to accrue a sufficient number of subjects in a reasonable time frame.

Studies have shown that the characteristics of people who volunteer for trials are different from those who do not. In one study of cardiac arrhythmia, participants were more likely than nonparticipants to be male, young, and concerned about their health and to have no medical insurance (free health insurance was the reason for enrollment).[22]

Why do people volunteer for experimental studies? Many enroll because they want the best possible medical care, including new treatments that are otherwise unavailable. Still others participate for altruistic reasons such as a desire to help others with the disease or to leave something for posterity. It is important to keep in mind that the characteristics of trial volunteers may affect the generalizability of the results.

Sample Size

For investigators to determine if there is a true difference in effectiveness between the treatment and comparison groups, it is crucial that they enroll an adequate number of individuals in the experimental study. The term *statistical power* refers to "the ability of a study to demonstrate an association if one exists."[23(p128)] Unfortunately, numerous trials have erroneously reported null results (that is, no difference between the treatment and comparison groups) simply because their sample size was too small and statistical power was too low to detect clinically important differences.[24]

How do investigators decide how many subjects to include in a trial? Usually they determine the needed sample size using formulas that take into account the following factors: (1) the anticipated difference between the treatment and comparison groups, (2) the background rate of the outcome, and (3) the probability of making statistical errors known as *alpha* and *beta* errors.[25(pp142–146)]

Many therapeutic and most preventive trials require a very large number of participants in order to have sufficient statistical power to detect a meaningful effect. For most therapeutic trials, the large numbers are necessary primarily because the trial is being conducted to determine if a test treatment offers a small improvement over an existing treatment. In general, the smaller the anticipated difference between the treatment and comparison groups, the larger the necessary sample size. For the preventive trials, the large sample size is needed because the subjects are healthy at the start and the disease end points usually have a low incidence. Some researchers believe that meta-analysis, a statistical procedure that pools data from many small trials, is a viable alternative to conducting large trials.[26]

Consent Process

All eligible individuals must voluntarily agree to participate in a trial. The process of gaining their agreement, known as informed consent, must be reviewed and approved by the ethics committee (also called institutional review board) of the participating institutions. During the consent process, the investigator must describe, in simple language, the nature and objectives of the study; the treatments being investigated; tasks, procedures, and tests required of participants; method of treatment assignment; data to be collected; and, most important, likely benefits and risks of participating.[2(p54)] Investigators must assure participants that personal information obtained during the course of the study will be kept confidential, and that participants may withdraw from the study at any time without jeopardizing their medical care. The consent process includes giving oral or written consent according to a protocol that has been approved by the ethics committee.

Treatment Assignment

After they give their consent, eligible individuals are assigned to either the treatment or comparison group. Nonrandom and random assignment are two general methods for assigning treatments to participants. The non-random method most commonly used is alternation assignment, which is a systematic assignment method that is based on the order of enrollment. For example, the first enrolled person is assigned to the treatment group, the second is assigned to the comparison group, the third is assigned to the treatment group, and so on.

Although nonrandom assignment methods are simple and easy to follow, they are predictable and so may lead to situations that allow biased assignment. For example, if two subjects are enrolled at exactly the same time in the alternation assignment scheme, the investigators may have the discretion to assign one individual to the treatment group and the other to the comparison group. If the investigators make this assignment on the basis of a prognostic characteristic such as severity of illness (for example, they put the healthier person into the comparison group), and if they do this often enough, the study groups would be imbalanced and the results could be biased.

Random assignment is superior to nonrandom methods because it is less prone to this type of bias. Random treatment assignment, known as randomization, is defined as "an act of assigning or ordering that is the result of a random process."[2(p220)] Although the overall probability of being assigned to a particular group is known (for example, 50% are assigned to each group), there is no way to predict the order of future assignments from that of past ones. The lack of predictability is the key to minimizing bias.

Random methods include flipping a coin, using a random number table (commonly found in statistics textbooks), or a computer random number generator. Large trials often have a central office that handles the randomization so that the investigators who determine eligibility, enroll individuals, and administer the treatments are unaware of the assignment order ahead of time. In smaller trials without a central randomization office, treatment assignments are usually sealed in numbered opaque envelopes to safeguard the process.

Randomization has two main goals. First, as already described, it ensures that treatment assignment occurs in an unbiased fashion. Second, if the sample size is sufficiently large, it will usually control for known and unknown confounding variables by producing treatment and comparison groups with very similar baseline characteristics. (As is discussed further in Chapter 11, confounding is a nuisance that can distort results because risk factors are unevenly distributed across compared groups.) For example, in the very large CAPRIE study, approximately 19,000 patients with atherosclerotic vascular disease were randomly assigned to receive clopidogrel ($n = 9599$) or aspirin ($n = 9586$).[3] The baseline characteristics of the two groups were quite similar (for example, exactly the same proportion of males was in each group) (see Table 7–2). On the other hand, the maternal-infant HIV transmission study randomized a much smaller

TABLE 7–2   Baseline Characteristics of Patients in the CAPRIE Study

Characteristic	Clopidogrel group (n = 9599)	Aspirin group (n = 9586)
Male (%)	72	72
White (%)	95	95
Current cigarette smoker (%)	29	30
Patients with a history of:		
Hypertension (%)	52	51
Stable angina (%)	22	22
High cholesterol levels (%)	41	41

Source: Data from CAPRIE Steering Committee. A randomized, blinded trial of clopidogrel versus aspirin in patients at risk of ischemic events (CAPRIE). *Lancet.* 1996;348:1329–1339.

group of women (n = 477) to either the zidovudine or placebo group.[21] Randomization was less successful in achieving baseline comparability (for example, there was a 10% difference in the proportion of whites in each group) because the sample size was much smaller (see Table 7–3).

Investigators often use two additional procedures—blocking and stratification—with randomization in order to secure balanced groups. *Blocking* is used "to ensure balance in the mix of the treatment groups with regard to time of enrollment" and helps "eliminate the risk of differential secular trends in the makeup of treatment groups."[2(pp.28–29)] When blocking is used, randomization is conducted in groups or blocks of a certain size. For example, in a trial with a projected enrollment of 100 individuals (that is, 50 participants will ultimately be assigned to each of two groups), blocks of, say, 10 patients may be randomized at a time to ensure that equal numbers of patients are assigned to the two groups throughout the enrollment process.

Stratification accompanies randomization in order to ensure that key confounding variables are equally distributed between the treatment and comparison groups. In this method, individuals are first stratified or separated according to the confounding characteristic. Then, they are randomly assigned to either the treatment or comparison group within each stratum. For example, women in the maternal-fetal HIV transmission trial were stratified according to the stage of pregnancy at enrollment (one group was from 14 to 26 weeks pregnant, and the other was greater than 26 weeks pregnant). Then, women in each stratum were randomly assigned to receive either zidovudine or placebo (see Figure 7–3).[21] This was done because the investigators thought that zidovudine would be more effective if it were started earlier in pregnancy, and so they wanted to ensure that the two groups were nearly identical on this important characteristic. As shown in Table 7–3, the median age and the distribution of gestational age at entry were similar in the two groups.

TABLE 7–3 Baseline Characteristics of Patients in the Maternal-Infant HIV Transmission Trail

Characteristic	Zidovudine group (n = 239)	Placebo group (n = 238)
Median age at entry (years)	25	25
White (%)	48	38
Gestational age at entry		
Median (weeks)	26	27
14–26 weeks (%)	52	50
> 26 weeks (%)	48	50
Mean CD4 count at entry	560	538

Source: Data from Connor EM, Sperling RS, Gelber R, et al. Reduction of maternal-infant transmission of human immunodeficiency virus type 1 with zidovudine treatment. *N Engl J Med.* 1994;331:1173–1180.

Use of the Placebo and Masking

A placebo is defined as a "pharmacologically inactive substance given as a substitute for an active substance, especially when the person taking or receiving it is not informed whether it is an active or inactive substance."[2(p 195)] A placebo pill usually consists of a sugar-coated, inert substance. Its purpose is to match as closely as possible the experience of the comparison group with that of the treatment group. The principle underlying the use of placebos harkens back to laboratory animal experiments where, except for the test chemical, all important aspects of the

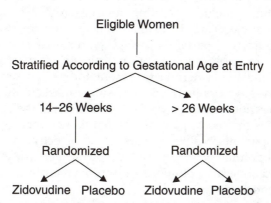

FIGURE 7–3. Depiction of Stratified Randomization in the Maternal-Infant HIV Transmission Study

Source: Data from Connor EM, Sperling RS, Gelber R, et al. Reduction of maternal-infant transmission of human immunodeficiency virus type 1 with zidovudine treatment. *N Engl J Med.* 1994;331:1173–1180.

experimental conditions are identical for the treatment and comparison groups. Thus, when placebo pills are used in drug trials among humans, they are purposely manufactured to be as similar as possible to the active drug in shape, size, texture, color, and taste.

When trials involve procedures rather than pills, sham procedures are administered to match as closely as possible the experience of the treatment and comparison groups. A sham procedure is defined as "a bogus procedure designed to resemble a legitimate one."[2(p248)] For example, in a study of the effectiveness of localized hyperthermia (heat) treatment for benign prostate enlargement, patients in the treatment group were given the hyperthermia treatment using a transrectal system that heated the prostate to 43°C, and patients in the sham comparison group underwent the same procedure except that the prostatic temperature was maintained at the usual body temperature of 37°C.[27]

Both placebos and sham procedures permit study participants, health care providers, and study investigators to be masked. That is, these parties do not know if a participant is in the treatment or comparison group. Several terms are commonly used to describe which individuals associated with an experimental study are masked. In a single-masked study, the participants but not the investigators are masked. In a double-masked study, both the participants and investigators administering the treatment are masked. In a triple-masked study, the participants, the investigators administering the treatment, and the investigators monitoring the effects of the treatment are masked. The latter investigators are usually members of a treatment effects monitoring committee that is charged with the regular review of collected data for evidence of adverse or beneficial treatment effects while the trial is being conducted and for recommending changes in a study treatment including ending the trial early.[2(p284)]

Masking of subjects and investigators helps prevent biased ascertainment of the outcome, particularly end points that involve subjective assessment. For example, patients but not physicians were masked in the study of localized hyperthermia treatment for benign prostate enlargement.[27] The investigators justified their single-masked study as follows: "This study does not include physician evaluations of the clinical status of the patient but is limited to parameters that were either measured . . . or obtained from patients."[27(p1048)] For example, objective measurements of urine flow and volume were obtained by physicians using uroflowmetry equipment, and subjective opinions of improvement were obtained from patient questionnaires.

In some studies, it is not possible to mask participants or investigators because of the nature of the treatments. For example, both participants and investigators administering the treatment were aware of a participants' group assignment in a therapeutic trial of breast cancer that compared the effectiveness of total mastectomy, lumpectomy, and lumpectomy combined with irradiation.[28] However, because the main outcomes under study—overall survival, disease-free survival, and recurrence—were objectively determined, the lack of masking should not have affected the results.

Many researchers have observed that participants who receive the placebos or sham procedures improve over the course of the experimental study. The beneficial effect produced by an inactive control treatment is known as the "placebo effect," and is thought to arise from the power of suggestion. That is, participants assigned to the placebo group improve just because they are told that they will. The related terms "halo" and "Hawthorne effects" are also used when the improvement stems from the attention received by participating in a study. This effect is analogous to the Heisenberg uncertainty principle in physics, which states that "the act of observing a phenomenon changes the phenomenon itself."[29(p59)] In epidemiologic terms, it means that participants, either consciously or unconsciously, change their behavior just because they are being studied. For example, patients in the study of localized hyperthermia treatment for prostate enlargement were asked 3 months after receiving the treatment or sham procedure if they thought that their condition had improved.[27] Fifty percent of the sham group and 63% of the treatment group reported that they were cured or markedly improved. However, based on objective data such as urine flow rates, investigators observed meaningful improvements only in the treatment group. Thus, it appears that the power of suggestion associated with the placebo effect led to a subjective but not objective improvement among the men in the sham group.

Maintenance and Assessment of Compliance

All experimental studies require the active involvement and cooperation of participants. In fact, taking part in a trial can be quite intrusive in a person's daily life. For example, required tasks in three recent therapeutic and preventive trials have included taking pills on a daily basis, exercising three times a week, quitting smoking, and making important dietary changes[4,9,11] (see Table 7–4).

Although participants are apprised of the study requirements when they enroll, many fail to follow the protocol exactly as required as the trial proceeds. The failure to observe the requirements of the protocol is known as *noncompliance*. There are many reasons for noncompliance including toxic reactions to the treatment, waning interest, inability to meet the demands of the study, desire to seek other therapies, disease progression, and death.

Noncompliance may occur among members of the treatment group, the comparison group, or both groups. For example, women in the

TABLE 7–4 Required Tasks and Reasons for Noncompliance in Three Experimental Studies

Title/purpose of trial	Tasks required of participants	Reasons for noncompliance
AIDS Clinical Trials Group Study 175. Compared effectiveness of monotherapy versus combination therapy for HIV infection.	Group 1: zidovudine three times a day. Group 2: zidovudine and zalcitabine three times a day. Group 3: zidovudine three times a day and didanosine two times a day. Group 4: didanosine two times a day.	Toxic reactions to the treatment, desire to seek other therapies, demands of the study (such as the number of required pills).
High-impact Exercise Study. Determined the effect of high-impact exercises on bone mineral density, muscle performance, and cardiorespiratory fitness.	Exercising group: Participate in high-impact exercise sessions three times a week for 18 months. Comparison group: Maintain current physical activity level.	Musculoskeletal injuries, lack of interest.
MRFIT Study. Examined the effect of reducing multiple risk factors on coronary heart disease mortality rates among high-risk men.	Special intervention group: receive counseling for smoking cessation, dietary advice to lower blood cholesterol levels, and stepped-care treatment for hypertension. Usual care comparison group: Use standard sources of health care.	Sizable reductions in blood pressure, serum cholesterol, and cigarette smoking occurred in the usual care group, perhaps because they became more health-conscious.

Source: Data from Hammer SM, et al. A trial comparing nucleoside monotherapy with combination therapy in HIV-infected adults with CD4 cell counts from 200 to 500 per cubic millimeter. *N Engl J Med.* 1996;335:1081–1090. Heinonen A, et al. Randomised controlled trial of effect of high-impact exercise on selected risk factors for osteoporotic fractures. *Lancet.* 1996;348:1343–1347. Multiple Risk Factor Intervention Trial Research Group. Multiple Risk Factor Intervention Trial: Risk factor changes and mortality rates. *JAMA.* 1982;248:1465–1477.

exercising treatment group of a high-impact exercise study were noncompliant when they did not participate in the exercise program as directed[11] (see Table 7–4). On the other hand, women in the nonexercising comparison group were noncompliant when they began exercising during the study period. According to the study investigators, both groups had a high level of compliance. Exercising individuals completed, on average, 83% of their exercise program (2.5 out of 3 sessions per week), and the physical activity level of the comparison group remained unchanged over the course of the study.[11]

However, not all studies have high levels of compliance. Perhaps the most well-known example of noncompliance in an experimental study was the Multiple Risk Factor Intervention Trial (MRFIT), a randomized primary prevention trial of the impact of smoking, blood cholesterol, and blood pressure reduction on coronary heart disease mortality in 12,866 high-risk men aged 35 to 57 years.[9] MRFIT included two groups of participants: (1) the special intervention group received dietary advice for lowering blood cholesterol levels, smoking cessation counseling, and stepped-care treatment for hypertension; (2) the usual care group received their typical sources of health care within the community. Noncompliance occurred when men in the usual care group quit smoking and lowered their blood pressure and cholesterol levels. The authors speculated that the comparison group changed their smoking and dietary habits like the rest of the U.S. population during the 1970s and 1980s.

Noncompliance is the bane of an investigator's life because it leads to two vexing problems. First, it results in a smaller difference between the treatment and comparison groups than truly exists. For example, the MRFIT study found that the special intervention group had only a 7.1% lower rate of coronary heart disease mortality than the usual care group. Second, noncompliance reduces the statistical power of the study, making it more difficult to detect an effect when it exists. Thus, when a study finds little or no difference between the treatment and comparison groups (null results), noncompliance should be considered a possible explanation.

Because good compliance is an important determinant of the validity of an experimental study, many study features are designed to enhance a participant's ability to comply with the protocol requirements.[30] First, investigators design experimental regimens that are simple and easy to follow. For example, it is much easier to comply with a regimen that requires taking one pill at the same time each day than one that requires taking numerous pills at different times. When a difficult treatment schedule cannot be avoided, compliance aides such as blister pill packs resembling monthly calendars and pill boxes with programmed alarms are used.

Second, investigators enroll motivated and knowledgeable participants who lead fairly organized lives. For example, investigators decided to enroll physicians in a randomized, double-masked, placebo-controlled primary prevention trial of cardiovascular disease and cancer, in part, because they believed that the physicians were more likely to comply with the daily regimen of taking aspirin and/or beta-carotene and would be easier to trace.[20]

Third, investigators present a realistic picture of the tasks required by the trial during the informed consent process. In this way, participants know exactly what they are getting themselves into.

Fourth, investigators obtain a detailed medical history from potential subjects so that they can exclude those with conditions that would preclude or make compliance difficult. For example, the CAPRIE trial excluded potential participants who had medical contraindications to the study drugs (for example, a history of aspirin sensitivity).[3]

Fifth, investigators mask study subjects in placebo-controlled studies because those in the comparison group might be less motivated to comply if they knew that they were receiving the placebo.

Sixth, researchers maintain frequent contact with participants (either in person or by mail) during the study. For example, in the CAPRIE study, follow-up visits involving a physical examination, laboratory tests, and questionnaire administration took place every month for the first 4 months and then every 4 months thereafter.[3]

Finally, investigators conduct a run-in or lead-in period before enrollment and randomization to ascertain which potential participants are able to comply with the study regimen. During this period (which may last several weeks or months), potential participants are placed on the test or control treatment "to assess their tolerance to or acceptance of a treatment, and to obtain information on treatment compliance."[2(p143)] When the run-in is over, investigators enroll only the compliant individuals. For example, in the Physician's Health Study, 33,223 eligible and willing subjects were enrolled in a run-in phase during which all participants were given active aspirin and beta-carotene placebo for 18 weeks.[31] After the run-in, investigators sent participants a questionnaire asking about their compliance, side effects, and willingness to continue with the trial. Only 22,071 physicians who could tolerate the medications and were good compliers, defined as taking two-thirds of the pills, were invited to continue in the trial.

Even when compliance-enhancement measures are used, investigators must still assess the extent of noncompliance. This can be done in several ways. First, investigators can question participants about the extent of their noncompliance. For example, in the high-impact exercise study, the investigators interviewed women in the nonexercising comparison group every 4 months to assess any changes in physical activity level. Second, if the trial requires taking pills, investigators can ask participants to return any unused pills. Investigators in the CAPRIE study used this method and found that only 86 patients (out of more than 19,000) never took any of the study drugs.[3] Third, investigators in medication trials can collect biological samples, such as blood or urine, to analyze for the presence of the treatment or its metabolite. For example, in an experimental study of the effectiveness of a calcium, vitamin, and selenium cocktail in reducing the growth of colorectal polyps, investigators analyzed stool calcium levels to assess patients' compliance.[32]

Ascertaining the Outcomes

During the follow-up period, investigators monitor the treatment and comparison groups for the outcomes under study. In preventive trials, the outcomes of interest are generally precursors of disease or the first occurrence of disease; in therapeutic trials, the outcomes typically include symptom improvement, length of survival, or disease recurrence. For example, outcome measures in the preventive study of high-impact exercise included bone mineral density (a measure of bone strength and important determinant of bone fracture risk), muscle performance, and cardiorespiratory fitness.[11] Outcome measures in the CAPRIE therapeutic study of patients with atherosclerotic vascular disease included the recurrence of fatal and nonfatal strokes, heart attacks, and brain hemorrhages.[3]

Usually one of these end points is designated as the primary outcome—that is, the main condition that the trial has been designed to evaluate, and the outcome used for the sample size calculations. The remaining end points, termed secondary outcomes, are considered less important. For example, the primary outcome in the CAPRIE study was the composite outcome cluster of first occurrence of stroke, heart attack, or vascular death.[3] Investigators determined that a sample of at least 18,000 patients was needed based on the expected frequency (14 to 25%) of the outcome cluster during the 3-year follow-up period.

In some trials, a surrogate outcome measure such as a laboratory test result that correlates with a clinical outcome is used instead of a clinical event.[26] For example, investigators might measure cholesterol levels, which are correlated with the occurrence of heart attacks. The purpose of surrogate measures is to reduce the length of follow-up, sample size, and cost of the study. For example, in experimental studies of AIDS treatments, CD4 lymphocyte levels have been used as surrogate measures of a treatment's effectiveness. Although most researchers agree that surrogate markers are useful for identifying promising treatments during the early phases of research, some warn that they may lead to false conclusions. For example, numerous experimental studies of AIDS treatments found that changes in CD4 counts were imperfectly correlated with the occurrence of opportunistic infections and survival.[33]

How long must investigators follow subjects to ascertain the outcomes under study? Only a few months may be needed for a short-term study of drug side effects, but a decade may be necessary for examining slowly developing outcomes such as cancer incidence. During the follow-up period, investigators obtain outcome information from participants through periodic medical visits, phone interviews, or mail questionnaires. For example, in the CAPRIE study, follow-up visits with physicians took place for up to 3 years.[3]

Accurate information on the outcomes is crucial to the success of a trial. Investigators work to ensure high-quality outcome data by developing strategies to achieve *high follow-up rates* and by incorporating a process known as *validation* in the study design.

Follow-up is adversely affected when participants either withdraw from the study (these are called dropouts) or cannot be located or contacted by the investigator (these individuals are termed lost to follow-up). Reasons for dropouts and losses include relocation, waning interest, and adverse reactions to the treatment. Dropouts and losses to follow-up pose a problem for researchers, because they lead to missing outcome data and, ultimately, a smaller study. In the CAPRIE study, no study subjects withdrew and only 0.2% of patients were lost to follow-up.[3] On the other hand, about 14% of participants in the high-impact exercise study dropped out because of musculoskeletal problems, injuries, pregnancy, relocation, and loss of interest.[11] Thus, the already small sample size of 98 women was reduced to 84.

The problem of missing data is further aggravated if the follow-up rates of the treatment group differ from those of the comparison group and if attrition is related to the outcome. This combination of events can lead to incorrect results. For example, many more women in the exercise group than the comparison group dropped out of the high-impact exercise study.[11] If the bone strength of women who dropped out differed from those who remained, the study results could be biased. Methods for minimizing dropouts and losses include designing a simple protocol, enrolling motivated individuals who lead organized lives, and maintaining frequent contact. In addition, follow-up is often facilitated by obtaining the name of a friend or relative of the study participant at enrollment. Ideally, this person does not live with the participant yet will always know the participant's whereabouts.

The process known as validation helps to ensure accurate outcome data. Validation means that investigators verify or corroborate the occurrence of the outcome using several sources. For example, researchers often review medical records to confirm the occurrence of events reported by patients. Whenever possible, corroborating evidence should be objective in nature, such as laboratory test results and physical findings. It is good practice for the investigators who perform the validation to be masked. For example, in the CAPRIE study, masked members of a central validation committee were responsible for determining the accuracy all of the non-fatal outcomes and reported causes of death.[3] The evidence for each reported outcome was reviewed independently by two committee members, and any disagreements were resolved by the entire committee.

Data Analysis

As described in Chapter 3, the results of an experimental study may be arranged in a two-by-two table and the measures of association calculated. For example, let us examine the results of the experimental study of maternal-infant HIV transmission (see Table 7–5).[21] The cumulative incidence of HIV infection was 13/180 or 7.2% among infants whose mothers received zidovudine, and 40/183 or 21.9% among infants whose mothers received placebos. Thus, the relative risk, as estimated by the cumulative incidence ratio, was 0.33. This means that infants whose mothers took zidovudine had one third the risk of becoming HIV infected than did the infants whose mothers took placebos. Stated differently, there was a 67% relative reduction in the risk of HIV transmission among the zidovudine group (null relative risk of $1.00 - 0.33 = 0.67$ or 67%). The attributable risk or absolute difference in the cumulative incidence of infection was −14.1% (the difference between 7.2% and 21.9%). In other words, 14 HIV infections among every 100 infants whose mothers were given placebos would have been prevented if these mothers had received zidovudine.

Although the mathematical calculations of experimental study data are straightforward, a few conceptual issues regarding the analysis of experimental studies deserve mention. The first relates to composition of the analytic groups. In the classical analytic approach, known as an intent-to-treat or treatment assignment analysis, all individuals who are randomly allocated to a treatment are analyzed, regardless of whether they complete or even receive the treatment.[34] An intent-to-treat analysis would compare everyone who was randomly assigned to treatment 1 with everyone who was assigned to treatment 2 (see Figure 7–4). Thus, this analysis would compare the outcomes of those who completed combined with those who did not complete treatment 1 (groups A and B) with the out-

TABLE 7–5 Reduction of Maternal-Infant Transmission of HIV with Zidovudine Treatment

Treatment	Infant HIV infected		Total
	Yes	No	
Yes (Zidovudine)	13	167	180
No (Placebo)	40	143	183

Source: Data from Connor EM, et al. Reduction in maternal-infant transmission of human immunodeficiency virus type 1 with zidovudine treatment. *N Engl J Med.* 1994;331:1173–1180.

FIGURE 7–4. Analysis Groups in a Randomized Experimental Study

comes of those who completed combined with those who did not complete treatment 2 (groups C and D).

What is the purpose of an intent-to-treat analysis? First, it preserves the benefits of randomization. That is, it preserves baseline comparability of the groups for known and unknown confounders. Second, it maintains the statistical power of the original study population. Third, because good and poor compliers differ from one another on important prognostic factors, it helps ensure that the study results are unbiased.[30] For example, the Coronary Drug Project studied the impact of several lipid-lowering drugs, including clofibrate, among men with a history of myocardial infarction.[35] Investigators found that only 15.0% of the "good" compliers versus 24.6% of the "poor" compliers in the clofibrate group died during the follow-up period. Surprisingly, a similar pattern was seen among the "good" and "poor" compliers who were taking the placebo.

Still another reason for conducting an intent-to-treat analysis is that it gives information on the effectiveness of a treatment under everyday practice conditions. It answers the question, "How well does the treatment work among those who are offered it?" If a test treatment is found to be effective, it will be used in clinical settings where people may not comply exactly with the prescribed regimen because of toxicity, lack of interest, and so forth. Thus, an analysis that excludes noncompliers gives an overly optimistic view of how well the treatment will work in real life.

The alternative to an intent-to-treat analysis is known as an efficacy analysis. This type of analysis determines the treatment effects under ideal conditions. It answers the question, "How well does the treatment work among those who take the full treatment as directed?"[34] In Figure 7–4, an efficacy analysis would compare the outcomes of those who completed treatment 1 and those who completed treatment 2 (groups A and C), and would ignore the outcomes of participants who failed to complete treatment 1 or treatment 2 (groups B and D). Proponents of this approach argue that it is merely answering a different question than the intent-to-treat analysis. However, others find it problematic because the compared groups (for example, groups A and C) may not be similar.

Sometimes investigators conduct both types of analysis in a given study. For example, the CAPRIE study investigators first conducted an intent-to-treat analysis that was based on all randomized patients regardless of their compliance with the study protocol. In addition, they also conducted an "on-treatment" analysis that included only outcomes that occurred while patients were on the study medication or within 28 days of early discontinuation of the medication.[3] In the intent-to-treat analysis, investigators found 939 events during 17,636 person-years at risk in the clopidogrel group and 1021 events during 17,519 person-years at risk in the aspirin group, resulting in a relative risk of 0.913. The on-treatment analysis, based on somewhat different numbers, found a similar result—a relative risk of 0.906.

A second issue that arises in the analysis of experimental studies pertains to determining the effectiveness of the treatment among different subgroups. For example, the maternal-infant HIV transmission study conducted analyses to evaluate the effectiveness of zidovudine in reducing transmission among women of different races, ages, stages of pregnancy, and delivery characteristics.[21] Some investigators pejoratively call such subgroup analyses "data dredging" or "exploratory," because they are usually done on an ad hoc basis (that is, without the benefit of a hypothesis stated at the start of the study).[26] Others believe that it is acceptable to analyze subgroups if they are defined ahead of time and intended. Still others believe that, because data do not magically change on the basis of investigators' prior plans, subgroup analyses provide valuable and valid information—regardless of an investigator's original hypothesis. Nevertheless, subgroup analyses are usually based on fewer subjects than analyses using the entire sample; thus, although results of subgroup analysis may be accurate, they are unlikely to be as precise as those from the whole study population.

Generalizability

Generalization is a judgment in which the investigator relates the conclusions of a trial "beyond the setting of the trial and the particular people studied in the trial . . . to the broader setting of general medical care and to a more heterogeneous set of patients."[2(p107)] The group of people to whom the study results may be applied or generalized is termed the reference population. The original eligibility criteria that determine the composition of the study population, in turn, determine the appropriate reference population. Investigators' ability to generalize the results of a study to a broader context is affected by the study participants' physiological, behavioral, and cultural characteristics. For example, the maternal-infant HIV transmission study included only women with mildly symptomatic HIV disease. For this reason, the investigators stated, "It is not clear whether the result of this trial can be extrapolated to . . . women with more advanced disease" because of physiological differences between these groups.[21]

Because the racial and gender compositions of a study population are such important determinants of generalizability, the National Institutes of Health (NIH), a federal agency that provides funding for many experimental studies, has encouraged the inclusion of women and members of minority groups in order to increase the applicability of trials.[36] Moreover, the NIH requires that every proposed trial include sufficient numbers of women and minorities to enable comparison of treatment responses separately between the gender and racial/ethnic groups.

Special Issues in Experimental Studies

A number of practical issues make it difficult to conduct an experimental study. First, experimental studies are very expensive. For example, the Cancer Cooperative Program of Randomized Trials cost about $75 million per year.[36] Second, many physicians and patients are reluctant to participate in experimental research. Physicians are hesitant to participate because they believe that such trials will hamper their ability to maintain a personalized relationship with their patients.[37] The necessity of standardized approaches to patient workup and monitoring and the additional work and oversight involved in trials also contribute to physicians' reluctance. In addition, because experimentation still has a negative connotation in our society, patients are often unwilling to serve as "guinea pigs" for the advancement of science.

In addition to these practical issues, epidemiologists must consider numerous ethical issues when designing and conducting experimental studies. Most researchers believe that it is ethical to conduct experimental studies—particularly randomized, placebo controlled trials—only when there is a state of equipoise or equilibrium regarding the treatment within the expert medical community. Equipoise is a "state of mind characterized by legitimate uncertainty or indecision as to choice or course of action."[2(p88)] In other words, there must be genuine confidence that a treatment may be worthwhile in order to administer it to some individuals and genuine reservations about the treatment in order to withhold it from others. Furthermore, physicians who already have developed opinions about the effectiveness of a treatment (even though the treatment has not been tested adequately) are reluctant to enroll their patients in a trial if there is a chance that their patients will not get the preferred treatment.

Equipoise is not a static state, and a shift in equipoise sometimes occurs during the course of a trial. The shift often occurs when a clear benefit or adverse effect is observed for the test treatment in an interim data analysis from the ongoing trial. Such an analysis is usually conducted by a treatment effects monitoring committee, a semiindependent group with varied backgrounds (such as clinicians, medical ethicists, and biostatisticians) who examine the accumulating data for detecting early evidence of harm or benefit that may require early termination. Early terminations have occurred in major trials of both therapeutic and preventive treatments including the maternal-infant HIV transmission study.[21,38] When the effectiveness of zidovudine in reducing maternal-fetal HIV transmission was observed in the first interim data analysis, study investigators stopped enrolling additional patients and all women were offered the zidovudine treatment.[21]

Another ethical concern about experimental studies involves the use of placebo controls. Rothman and Michels argue forcefully that randomized clinical trials are unethical when they administer placebos to the comparison group if effective treatments are available.[39] For example, Fabre conducted a trial in 1990 that randomly assigned patients with major depression to either a new medication (buspirone) or a placebo.[40] This study took place at a time when numerous effective treatments were available for severe depression.[41(pp47-76)] When two participants attempted to commit suicide during the course of the study, they were removed from the study and placed on one of the standard medications.[40]

Why do investigators use placebos in these settings? Usually they offer scientific reasons such as the need to control for the placebo and Hawthorne effects. However, no scientific principle mandates investigators to compare an experimental treatment to a placebo rather than to another effective treatment, and scientific principles should never supersede the well-being of study participants.[39]

Summary

Well-conducted experimental studies are thought to produce more scientifically rigorous results than do observational studies. This is because of several distinctive features of experimental studies including the random assignment of participants to treatment and comparison groups to eliminate baseline differences between the groups and to reduce the likelihood of biased allocation, and the use of placebo controls to permit masked ascertainment of the outcomes. On the other hand, several practical issues make it difficult for epidemiologists to conduct experimental studies, including participants' noncompliance with the treatment regimen, the need to maintain high follow-up rates over extended periods of time, high cost, and physicians' and patients' reluctance to participate. In addition, experimental studies pose numerous ethical issues. For example, a state of equipoise regarding the treatment must exist within the medical community. That is, there must be genuine confidence that a treatment may be worthwhile in order to administer it to some individuals and genuine reservations about the treatment in order to withhold it from others.

References

1. Hodgson E, Guthrie, FE eds. *Introduction to Biochemical Toxicology.* New York, NY: Elsevier Science Publishing Co; 1980.
2. Meinert CL. *Clinical Trials Dictionary, Terminology and Usage Recommendations.* Baltimore, MD: The Johns Hopkins Center for Clinical Trials; 1996.
3. CAPRIE Steering Committee. A randomized, blinded, trial of clopidogrel versus aspirin in patients at risk of ischemic events (CAPRIE). *Lancet.* 1996;348: 1329–1339.
4. Hammer SM, Katzenstein DA, Hughes MD, Gundacker H, Schooley RT, Haubrich RH, et al. A trial comparing nucleoside monotherapy with combination therapy in HIV-infected adults with CD4 cell counts from 200 to 500 per cubic millimeter. *N Engl J Med.* 1996;335:1081–1090.
5. Ast DB, Finn SB, McCaffrey I. The Newburgh-Kingston caries fluorine study. *Am J Public Health.* 1950;40:716–724.
6. Hayes R, Mosha F, Nicoll A, Grosskurth H, Newell J, Todd J, et al. A community trial of the impact of improved sexually transmitted disease treatment on the HIV epidemic in rural Tanzania: 1. Design. *AIDS.* 1995;9:919–926.
7. Weitzman M, Aschengrau A, Bellinger D, Jones R, Hamlin JS, Beiser A. Lead-contaminated soil abatement and urban children's blood lead levels. *JAMA.* 1993;269:1647–1654.
8. Greenwald P, Kelloff G, Burch-Whitman C, Kramer BS. Chemoprevention. *CA Cancer J Clin.* 1995;45:31–49.
9. Multiple Risk Factor Intervention Trial Research Group. Multiple Risk Factor Intervention Trial: risk factor changes and mortality rates. *JAMA.* 1982;248: 1465–1477.
10. COMMIT Research Group. Community intervention trial for smoking cessation (COMMIT): I. Cohort results from a four-year community intervention. *Am J Public Health.* 1995;85:183–192.
11. Heinonen A, Kannus P, Sievanen H, Oja P, Pasanen M, Rinne M, et al. Randomised controlled trial of effect of high-impact exercise on selected risk factors for osteoporotic fractures. *Lancet.* 1996;348:1343–1347.
12. Miller RL. Assisting gay men to maintain safer sex: an evaluation of an AIDS service organization's safer sex maintenance program. *AIDS Educ Prev.* 1995; 7:48–63.
13. Finnegan LP. The NIH Women's Health Initiative: its evolution and expected contributions to women's health. *Am J Prev Med;* 1996;12:292–293.
14. Fisher B, Constantino JP, Wickerham DL, Redmond CK, Kavanah M, Cronin WM, et al. Tamoxifen for prevention of breast cancer: report of the National Surgical Adjuvant Breast and Bowel Project P-1 Study. *J Natl Cancer Inst.* 1998; 90:1371–1388.
15. MacMahon B. Overview of studies on endometrial cancer and other types of cancer in humans: perspectives of an epidemiologist. *Semin Oncol.* 1997; 24(1S1):122–139.
16. Prentice RL. On the role, design, and analysis of disease prevention trials. *Control Clin Trials.* 1995;16:249–258.
17. McGuire WP, Hoskins WJ, Brady MF, Kucera PR, Partridghe EF, Look KY, et al. Cyclophosphamide and cisplatin compared with paclitaxel and cisplatin

in patients with stage III and stage IV ovarian cancer. *N Engl J Med.* 1996; 334:1–6.

18. Kaufman D. Cancer therapy and randomized clinical trial: good medicine? *CA Cancer J Clin.* 1994;44:109–114.

19. Ellenberg SS, Foulkes MA. The utility of large simple trials in the evaluation of AIDS treatment strategies. *Stat Med.* 1994;13:405–415.

20. Buring JE, Hennekens CH. Randomized trials of primary prevention of cardiovascular disease in women: an investigator's view. *Ann Epidemiol.* 1994; 4:111–114.

21. Connor EM, Sperling RS, Gelber R, et al. Reduction of maternal-infant transmission of human immunodeficiency virus type 1 with zidovudine treatment. *N Engl J Med.* 1994;331:1173–1180.

22. Gorkin L, Schron EB, Handshaw K, Shea S, Kinney MR, Branyon M, et al. Clinical trial enrollers vs. nonenrollers: the cardiac arrhythmia suppression trial (CAST) recruitment and enrollment assessment in clinical trials (REACT) project. *Control Clin Trials.* 1996;17:46–59.

23. Last JM. *A Dictionary of Epidemiology.* 3rd ed. New York, NY: Oxford University Press; 1995.

24. Moher D, Dulberg CS, Wells GA. Statistical power, sample size, and their reporting in randomized controlled trials. *JAMA.* 1994;272:122–124.

25. Colton T. *Statistics in Medicine.* Boston, MA: Little, Brown and Company; 1974.

26. Nowak R. Problems in clinical trials go far beyond misconduct. *Science.* 1994; 264:1538–1541.

27. Zerbib M, Steg A, Conquy S, Martinache PR, Flam TA, Debre B. Localized hyperthermia versus sham procedure in obstructive benign hyperplasia of the prostate: a prospective randomized study. *J Urol.* 1992;147:1048–1052.

28. Fisher B, Anderson S, Redmond CK, Wolmark N, Wickerham DL, Cronin WM. Reanalysis and results after 12 years of follow-up in a randomized clinical trial comparing total mastectomy with lumpectomy with or without irradiation in the treatment of breast cancer. *N Engl J Med.* 1995;333:1456–1461.

29. Michael M, Boyce WT, Wilcox AJ. *Biomedical Bestiary: an Epidemiologic Guide to Flaws and Fallacies in the Medical Literature.* Boston, MA: Little, Brown and Company; 1984.

30. Friedman LM, Furberg CD, DeMets DL. *Fundamentals of Clinical Trials,* 2nd ed. Littleton, MA: PSG Publishing Co. Inc; 1985.

31. The Steering Committee of the Physicians' Health Study Research Group. Preliminary report: findings from the aspirin component of the ongoing Physicians' Health Study. *New Engl J Med.* 1988;318:262–264.

32. Hofstad B, Vatn M, Hoff G, Larsen S, Osnes M. Growth of colorectal polyps: design of a prospective, randomized, placebo-controlled intervention study in patients with colorectal polyps. *Eur J Cancer Prev.* 1992;1(no6):415–422.

33. Fleming TR. Surrogate markers in AIDS and cancer trials. *Stat Med.* 1994;13: 1423–1435.

34. Newell DJ. Intention-to-treat analysis: implications for quantitative and qualitative research. *Int J Epidemiol.* 1992;21:837–841.

35. Anonymous. Influence of adherence to treatment and response of cholesterol on mortality in the coronary drug project. *N Engl J Med.* 1980; 303: 1038–1041.

36. NIH Revitalization Act, Subtitle B, Part 1, Sec. 131-133. June 10, 1993.

37. Simon R. Randomized clinical trials in oncology: principles and obstacles. *Cancer.* 1994;74:2614–2619.

38. The Steering Committee of the Physicians' Health Study Research Group. Final report on the aspirin component of the ongoing Physicians' Health Study. *New Engl J Med.* 1989;321:129–135.

39. Rothman KJ, Michels KB. The continued unethical use of placebo controls. *N Engl J Med.* 1994;331:394–398.

40. Fabre LF. Buspirone in the management of major depression: a placebo controlled comparison. *J Clin Psych.* 1990;51:55–61.

41. *The Internist's Compendium of Drug Therapy.* Lawrenceville, NJ: Core Publishing Division, Exerpta Medica, Inc; 1990.

EXERCISES

1. Briefly define each of the following terms that are associated with experimental studies:
   A. Randomization
   B. Reference population
   C. Single-masked study
   D. Run-in period
   E. Placebo and sham procedure
   F. Equipoise

2. State the main difference between each of the following:
   A. Individual and community trials
   B. Preventive and therapeutic trials

3. Each of the following problems represents a major threat to the validity of an experimental study. Briefly describe one method for avoiding these problems.
   A. Low compliance
   B. Lack of baseline comparability Randomitee
   C. Biased information on the outcome Mask

4 Describe the essential feature and purpose of an intent-to-treat analysis.

5. What distinctive features of experimental studies enhance their ability to produce scientifically rigorous results?

6. Why are experimental studies difficult to conduct?

8

Cohort Studies

LEARNING OBJECTIVES

By the end of this chapter, the reader will be able to:

- Distinguish between the various types of cohort studies, including open, fixed, closed, retrospective, prospective, and ambidirectional designs.

- Describe the key features of conducting cohort studies, including the selection of the exposed and unexposed populations; the sources of information on the exposure, outcomes, and other key variables; approaches to follow-up; calculating person-time; and data analysis.

- Discuss the strengths and limitations of cohort studies.

Introduction

Although experimental studies are scientifically rigorous, they are often infeasible because of difficulties enrolling participants, high costs, and thorny ethical issues. For example, an experimental study of a substance that increases a person's risk of developing a disease is infeasible because it is unethical to give a potentially harmful substance to a healthy person. Consequently, epidemiologic research consists mainly of observational studies. These studies are considered "natural" experiments, because the investigator acts as a disinterested observer merely letting nature take its course. Observational studies take advantage of the fact that people expose themselves to noxious or healthy substances through their personal habits (such as by drinking alcoholic beverages or taking vitamins), choice of occupation (such as asbestos insulation worker), place of residence (for example, near a lead smelter), and so on. Consequently, many issues that make it infeasible to conduct an experimental study—particularly those related to ethics—are mitigated in an observational study. For example, although it is unethical to conduct an experimental study of the impact of cigarette smoke on the developing fetus by randomly assigning newly pregnant women to either a smoking or nonsmoking group, it is perfectly ethical to conduct an observational study by comparing women who choose to smoke during pregnancy with those who choose not to do so.

As described in Chapter 6, the cohort study is one of the two principal types of observational studies. (The other type, the case–control study, is covered in Chapter 9.) A classical cohort study examines one or more health effects of a single exposure. Subjects are defined according to their exposure status and followed over time to determine the incidence of the health outcomes. This chapter describes the design, conduct, and analysis of cohort studies. First, cohort study terms are defined, and then a detailed discussion of each aspect of these studies is provided. Many design features of cohort studies emulate those of well-done experimental studies, because the goal of both types of studies is to obtain high-quality results.

Cohort Study Definitions and Overview

The term *cohort* comes from the Latin word *cohors,* meaning a group of soldiers.[1(p359)] In ancient Rome, a cohort was one of 10 divisions of a legion, the major unit of the Roman army. Once a cohort was formed, no new soldiers were added, and so soldiers remained in the same cohort for the duration of their service. Attrition occurred mainly through death.

Today, we use the word cohort to characterize "any designated group of persons who are followed or traced over a period of time."[2(p31)] The term is also used to describe a group of individuals with a common characteristic or experience. For example, a birth cohort consists of individuals who are born during a particular year or period, and so share many similar experiences (such as "baby boomers"). Although *cohort study* is the standard term used to describe an epidemiologic investigation that follows groups with common characteristics, some investigators use the terms *follow-up, incidence,* and *longitudinal* study.

Several additional terms are used to describe cohort studies. These terms are related to: the characteristics of the population from which the cohort is derived, whether the exposure changes over time, and whether there are losses to follow-up (see Table 8–1).

Types of Population Studied

The first type of cohort is conducted in an *open* or *dynamic* population. Individuals in an open population may enter or leave at any time because its membership is defined by a changeable characteristic such as smoking

TABLE 8-1 Characteristics of Cohort Studies

Type of population studied	Defined by	Follow-up	Appropriate measure of disease frequency
Open or dynamic	Changeable characteristic	Members come and go; losses may occur	Incidence rate
Fixed	Irrevocable event	Does not gain members; losses may occur	Incidence rate
Closed	Irrevocable event	Does not gain members; no losses occur.	Cumulative incidence

cigarettes, drinking alcohol, having a certain occupation, or living in a specific geographic area. For example, a person is a member of the open population of New York City residents only as long as he or she lives in New York City. Cohort studies that are conducted in an open population usually take into account population changes such as in- and outmigration, and so the incidence rate is the most suitable measure of disease frequency for monitoring health outcomes in this setting. A cohort study of cancer incidence was recently conducted among never-married men who were aged 25 to 54 years and resided in San Francisco, California, from 1973 to 1990.[3] These eligibility criteria were selected in order to identify a population with a high prevalence of HIV infection. This group is considered an open population because it is defined by the changeable characteristics of marital status, age, and place of residence. If a man got married, aged beyond 54 years, or moved away from San Francisco, his membership in the population ended and he was no longer eligible for the study. The study investigators monitored these eligibility changes among the men enrolled in the study, and an estimated 1,390,000 person-years of observation was accrued during the follow-up period (see Chapter 2 for more details about person-time calculations). The person-time data were used as the denominators for the incidence rates of non-Hodgkin's lymphoma and other cancers. The study found that the incidence of non-Hodgkins lymphoma increased 20-fold from 1973 to 1990, while that of anal cancer did not increase. These findings suggest that the causal mechanisms of HIV-related cancer differ for specific cancers.

Cohorts may also be formed on the basis of inalterable characteristics (see Table 8–1). A *fixed cohort* is defined by an irrevocable event—for example, undergoing a medical procedure, giving birth to a child, serving in the military, eating contaminated food at a picnic, or being present at a man-made or natural disaster. Thus, exposures in a fixed cohort do not change over time. In addition, the groups are followed from a defined starting point (usually marked by the event) to a defined ending point. The World War II atomic bomb survivors from Hiroshima and Nagasaki, Japan, comprise one of the best known fixed cohorts to be studied for biological effects of acute radiation exposure.[4] For nearly half a century, researchers have monitored mortality and cancer incidence rates among approximately 94,000 exposed residents who survived the bombings and 27,000 unexposed residents who were outside the city when the bombs were dropped. The incidence rates of various outcomes have been periodically compared between these two groups during the 50-year follow-up period. Incidence rates are the appropriate measure of disease frequency in a fixed cohort when the population experiences losses to follow-up. (Loss to follow-up means that investigators are unable to trace all members of a cohort to determine if they became ill or died.)

The third type of cohort is the *closed cohort*. Like the fixed cohort, a closed cohort is defined by an irrevocable event and has defined starting and ending points for follow-up. The difference between the two is that a closed cohort has no losses to follow-up. For example, a closed cohort study might be conducted among people who attended a party to determine if eating certain foods increased the risk of gastroenteritis during the week following the party. Thus, everyone who attended the party is a member of the closed population who is eligible for the study. Follow-up would start at the end of the party (assuming that all of the contaminated food was eaten by then, and that the illness could occur immediately after ingesting the contaminated food), and it would end 7 days later. No members of the population would be lost, because the observation period is short. Cumulative incidence or average risk is typically used as the measure of disease frequency in this setting, because there are no losses to follow-up.

Characterization of Exposure

Regardless of what type of cohort study is conducted, participants are grouped according to their exposure and followed over time in order to compare the incidence of symptoms, disease, or death. Usually two groups are compared, such as an exposed and unexposed group. The exposed group is called the *index group*, and the unexposed group is termed the *referent* or *comparison group*. It is necessary for the investigator to specify a minimum amount of exposure to qualify for the exposed group. For example, studies of cigarette smoking may use a lifetime history of smoking at least 100 cigarettes to qualify for membership in the exposed smoking group. In addition, when investigators are unable to find truly unexposed people to serve in the comparison group, people with low exposure are selected.

It can be difficult to classify the exposure status of subjects, particularly when the exposure changes over time. For example, a woman might begin smoking as a young adult, smoke cigarettes for a few years, stop while she is pregnant, and then return to smoking after giving birth. Thus, depending on the period, this woman could be considered a nonsmoker, smoker, or ex-smoker. The investigator might decide to consider a women exposed if she ever smoked cigarettes at any time in the past. However, such a simplistic exposure definition might miss an association that is confined to certain aspects of the exposure. For example, the association may only be present for high-intensity smoking (for example, more than two packs per day) or long-duration smoking (for example, more than 10 years).

Thus, whenever possible, investigators divide the exposed group into levels (for example, high, medium, and low exposure) enabling investigators to assess the presence of a dose-response relationship. A dose-response relationship means that the risk of disease increases as the intensity or duration of exposure increases. This categorization can be complicated, because there are many ways to characterize an exposure level. For example, one could use the maximum level ever experienced by the individual, the cumulative level as of a certain date, or the average exposure level over a time period. Exposure to cigarette smoke is often characterized by the number of pack-years that the person has accumulated. This composite measure is calculated by multiplying the average number of packs smoked per day by the number of years smoked at that intensity. Thus, a person who has smoked two packs a day for 20 years has accumulated 40 pack-years of exposure.

Follow-up and Outcome Assessment

During the follow-up period, the exposed and unexposed groups are monitored for the outcomes under study. As in experimental studies, more than one outcome is typically investigated. The outcomes of interest depend on the research question and may include precursors or first occurrence of disease, disease recurrence, or death. For example, a cohort study of U.S. pulp and paper mill workers examined all causes of death.[5] As another example, a cohort study of Canadian farm couples examined their fecundability, that is the monthly probability of becoming pregnant.[6]

At the start of follow-up, members of the cohort are at risk for but have not yet experienced the outcome(s) of interest. By the end of the follow-up period, a proportion of the cohort (up to 100%) will have experienced the outcome(s) under study. The length of the follow-up period can range from a few hours for infectious diseases to several decades for diseases such as cancer or cardiovascular disease. The longer the follow-up period, the more difficult it is to trace and maintain contact with study subjects and the more expensive the study. Although follow-up has become even more difficult in recent years because of increased population mobility, newly available resources such as those on the Internet have helped to offset these difficulties. Follow-up rates should be as high as possible in order to ensure the validity of the study. If the health outcomes of those who are lost to follow-up are different from those who are not lost, the study results may be biased. There is no magical follow-up rate that guarantees the validity of a study (other than 100%), but most epidemiologists are satisfied with follow-up rates higher than 90%.

Timing of Cohort Studies

Three terms are used to describe the timing of events in a cohort study: (1) *prospective*, meaning to look forward in time; (2) *retrospective*, meaning to look back in time; and (3) *ambidirectional*, meaning to look both ways (see Figure 8–1). In order to avoid confusion with other types of studies, the terms retrospective, prospective, and ambidirectional should always modify the word *cohort* and never be used alone.

In a *prospective cohort study,* participants are grouped on the basis of past or current exposure and are followed into the future in order to

Prospective Cohort Study

*——————— Exposure ——————— *

                    *——————— Disease ——————— *

∧

Study Starts

Retrospective Cohort Study

*——————— Exposure ——————— *

                    *——————— Disease ——————— *

                                           ∧

                                   Study Starts

Ambidirectional Cohort Study

*——————— Exposure ——————— *

                    *——————— Disease ——————— *

                   ∧

                 Study Starts

Time ————————————————————————→

FIGURE 8–1. Timing of Cohort Studies

observe the outcome(s) of interest. When the study commences, the outcomes have not yet developed and the investigator must wait for them to occur. The timing of prospective cohort studies is similar to that of experimental studies. For example, a prospective cohort study was conducted to investigate the effect of low-level lead exposure on intelligence and academic achievement among children.[7] Investigators enrolled children at birth and followed them until they were 10 years old. Investigators obtained the children's blood lead levels at birth and several times thereafter. When the children reached 10 years of age, investigators conducted development assessments to determine if prior lead exposure was associated with IQ and school performance.

In a *retrospective cohort study,* both the exposures and outcomes have already occurred by the time the study begins. This type of investigation studies only prior outcomes and not future ones. In fact, retrospective cohort studies often evaluate diseases that occurred many years ago. For example, in the 1990s, Swedish investigators undertook a nationwide retrospective cohort study to evaluate the association between breast implants and connective tissue disorders.[8] The study included more than 7000 women who had undergone breast implant surgery from 1964 through 1993 for cosmetic reasons or for reconstruction after breast cancer. Investigators collected data on the occurrence of connective tissue disorders following the implant surgery. Thus, the surgery and all of the outcomes under study had occurred by the time the investigators began the study. The researchers found no association between breast implants and connective tissue disease.

An *ambidirectional cohort study* has both prospective and retrospective components. For example, the Air Force Health Study is an ambidirectional study of the men who were involved in aerial spraying of herbicides (including the dioxin-contaminated Agent Orange) during the Vietnam War.[9] The purpose of the Ranch Hand Study is to determine if these men have an increased risk of adverse health and reproductive outcomes. The retrospective portion of the study conducted analyses of cancer and mortality that occurred from the men's first tour of duty in Vietnam through the 1980s.[10,11] The prospective component will monitor the health of these men for many years to come.

How does an epidemiologist decide whether to conduct a prospective, retrospective, or ambidirectional cohort study? The answer often depends on the research question, the practical constraints of time and money, and the availability of suitable study populations and records. In addition, the decision usually takes into account the complementary advantages and disadvantages of retrospective and prospective cohort studies. For example, retrospective cohort studies are more efficient (they take less time and money) than prospective studies for investigating diseases that take a long time to develop and come to diagnosis. This is because the disease and exposure have already occurred.

Minimal information is usually available on the exposure, outcome, and other key variables in retrospective cohort studies, because these studies typically rely on existing records that were not designed for research purposes. For example, a retrospective cohort study of men who worked in a chemical factory in the 1950s might have to depend on employment records to identify exposed and unexposed cohort members. These records may only contain the person's name, date of birth, department, job title, and years of employment. A detailed picture of that person's actual job duties and chemical exposures and information on important habits such as cigarette smoking may be missing. In addition, follow-up and ascertainment of the outcomes may be hampered because the historical records may not have information to facilitate locating the study subjects many years later.

In contrast, investigators in a prospective cohort study can usually obtain more detailed information on exposures and other key variables because they have more control of the data collection process and can gather information directly from the participants. Follow-up may also be easier, because the investigator can obtain tracing information from participants and can maintain periodic contact with subjects. In addition, prospective cohort studies are considered less vulnerable to bias because the outcomes have not occurred when the cohort is assembled and the exposures are assessed.

Issues in the Selection of Cohort Study Populations

Emulation of Experimental Studies

The investigator in an experimental study assigns participants to the experimental or comparison group. When the assignment is made randomly and the sample size is sufficiently large, these groups will have nearly identical distributions of baseline characteristics. In contrast, participants in cohort studies enter the exposed and unexposed groups usually on the basis of self-determined behaviors and events. Consequently, the results of cohort studies may be difficult to interpret because of differences between the exposed and unexposed groups that influence the risk of developing the disease. Consider, for example, a cohort study of the effect of maternal cigarette smoking during pregnancy on the risk of birth defects among the offspring. Women who smoke cigarettes during pregnancy are more likely to consume alcoholic beverages than women who do not smoke.[12] Because heavy consumption of alcoholic beverages increases the risk of having a baby with congenital anomalies regardless of whether a woman smokes cigarettes,[13] an association between cigarette smoking and birth defects might really be due to the alcohol consumption.

Epidemiologists try to minimize these types of problems by translating the key features of experimental studies to cohort studies. First, even though it is not possible to randomly assign exposures in cohort studies, differences between groups can be minimized by carefully selecting the exposed and unexposed groups to be as similar as possible. In fact, the ideal comparison group would consist of exactly the same individuals had they not been exposed. For example, the Air Force Health Study compared an exposed group of 1300 Air Force servicemen who flew herbicide spraying missions during the Vietnam War with an unexposed group of Air Force servicemen who flew cargo missions in Southeast Asia during the war that did not involve handling or spraying herbicides.[10] The baseline demographic characteristics and health status of the exposed and unexposed groups were quite similar, because all the men underwent the same selection procedures for serving in the Air Force and flying missions during the Vietnam War.

A second key feature of experimental studies that is translated in cohort studies is the use of placebos. Recall that placebos are used in experimental studies to match as closely as possible the experiences of the experimental and comparison groups and to permit masking of the study investigators (among others). Although cohort studies cannot use placebos, they can match the experiences of the exposed and unexposed groups by selecting individuals with similar characteristics. Investigators sometimes enhance this process by using special matching criteria when selecting unexposed subjects. For example, if investigators want to ensure that the groups are comparable with respect to age, gender, and race, they would employ a technique known as individual matching. For example, they would select an unexposed 50-year-old white male for every exposed 50-year-old white male in the study. Even without placebos, it is relatively easy to mask investigators to the subjects' exposure status during follow-up and outcome ascertainment in a cohort study. One merely keeps this information from the study staff involved in these tasks. Masking guarantees comparable follow-up efforts and outcome ascertainment, which—in turn—help ensure valid results.

The third key feature of experimental studies emulated by cohort studies is the method for determining the overall sample size as well as the relative size of the exposed and unexposed groups. Like experimental studies, cohort studies must include an adequate number of individuals in order to have sufficient statistical power to detect an association if it truly exists. Investigators determine the sample size by taking into account the

TABLE 8–2 Similarities and Differences Between Experimental and Cohort Studies

Similarities
- Both make comparisons across two or more exposure groups.
- Both follow participants to monitor outcome rates.
- Both usually monitor more than one outcome.
- Both select groups to achieve comparability and efficiency.
- Relative proportion of subjects in compared groups do not reflect that of the general population.

Differences
- Experimental study investigators allocate exposure to exposure groups. Cohort study participants choose exposures themselves.
- Experimental studies can use randomization to achieve baseline comparability. Cohort study investigators must carefully select groups to achieve comparability.
- Experimental studies can use placebos to match the groups' experiences and permit masking. Cohort study investigators carefully select groups to match as closely as possible. Cohort studies also use masking.
- Experimental studies are prospective. Cohort studies may be prospective, retrospective, or ambidirectional.

anticipated difference between compared groups, the background rate of the outcome, and the probability of making statistical errors.[14(pp142–146)] The relative sizes of the exposed and unexposed groups are chosen to maximize the power of the study. They are not intended to mimic the frequencies in the general population. For example, an exposure may occur rarely in the general population (for example, 1 exposure per 1000 population), but the frequency in a study population may be 50% (for example, 1000 exposed and 1000 unexposed individuals). The similarities and differences between experimental and cohort studies described so far are summarized in Table 8–2.

Selection of the Exposed Population

The choice of the exposed group in a cohort study depends on the hypothesis under study, the exposure frequency, and feasibility considerations such as the availability of records and ease of follow-up. The two main types of cohorts—special cohorts and general cohorts—are distinguished by the exposure frequency. *Special cohorts* are assembled to study the health effects of rare exposures such as uncommon occupational chemicals, unusual diets or lifestyles, natural or man-made disasters, or medical procedures. *General cohorts* are typically assembled for common exposures such as use of oral contraceptives, dietary factors such as vitamin use, and habits such as cigarette smoking and alcohol consumption. General cohorts are often selected from professional groups such as doctors and nurses, volunteers, or residents in well-defined geographic areas in order to facilitate follow-up and accurate ascertainment of the outcome(s) under study.

When assembling a special cohort, epidemiologists must go to the settings where the exposure has, is, or will occur in order to identify the exposed population. For example, workplace sites such as factories and organizations such as unions frequently serve as sources of individuals for occupational cohort studies. Because workers often have more intense and sustained exposures than the general population, cohort studies of occupational groups are an important component of identifying the causes of disease. For example, an occupational cohort study was conducted among 21,863 male and female workers from 12 countries whose jobs involved producing or spraying phenoxy herbicides and chlorophenols to determine if these workers had an increased risk of cancer deaths.[15] Epidemiologists identified subjects for the cohort study by reviewing employment and other records in businesses involved in manufacturing and spraying these chemicals.

Epidemiologists have conducted special cohort studies among individuals undergoing a medical procedure or treatment involving potentially noxious exposures. For example, important data on the risk of cancer following radiation have come from cohort studies of patients with ankylosing spondylitis (a spinal disorder), who were treated with radiation therapy.[16] Records of 87 radiotherapy centers in Great Britain and Northern Ireland were reviewed to identify more than 14,000 patients treated from 1935 to 1954. Investigators found that ankylosing spondylitis patients were more likely than expected to have leukemia and cancers of the lung, bone, and esophagus.

Epidemiologists have conducted cohort studies among groups with unusual diets or lifestyles such as Seventh Day Adventists and Mormons. For example, Seventh Day Adventists do not consume tobacco, alcohol, or pork, and about 50% follow a lacto-ovovegetarian diet. The Adventist Study has monitored the morbidity and mortality experience of approximately 34,000 Seventh Day Adventists in California for several years.[17] The study has found, for example, that male Adventists have lower overall cancer incidence but a higher incidence of prostate cancer than the general population.

As stated previously, epidemiologists assemble a general cohort from professional groups or residents in well-defined geographic areas in order to study common exposures. One of the best known cohort studies based upon the general population is the Framingham Study. Begun in 1948 and still continuing today, its main purpose is to determine the causes of cardiovascular disease.[18(pp14–29)] The risk factors that have been studied include high blood pressure, high blood cholesterol, physical inactivity, obesity, and smoking—all fairly common exposures. Investigators initially enrolled about 5000 healthy adult residents in Framingham, Massachusetts, a town located about 18 miles west of Boston. In 1948, Framingham was a self-contained community of about 28,000 residents who obtained their medical care from local physicians and two hospitals near the center of town. Framingham residents were considered an excellent population for a long-term epidemiologic study because (1) the town's population was stable, (2) the investigators could identify a sufficient number of people with and without risk factors for heart disease (for example, they expected sufficient numbers of smokers and nonsmokers), and (3) local medical doctors were "highly cooperative and well-informed" and wanted to help investigators recruit subjects for the study. All of these factors have contributed to the study's low dropout rate (only 5% after 50 years) and to its numerous important contributions to our understanding of the etiology of heart disease.

Selection of Comparison Group

In a cohort study, the ideal comparison group would consist of exactly the same individuals in the exposed group had they not been exposed. This theoretical concept is known as the "counterfactual ideal."[19(pp49–50)] Because it is impossible for the same person to be exposed and unexposed simultaneously, epidemiologists must select different sets of individuals for the exposed and comparison groups. Even though different people form each group, the investigator chooses groups as similar as possible on characteristics that influence getting the disease. For example, if gender were related to the risk of the disease (that is, if men had a higher risk than women or vice versa), it would be important for the exposed and unexposed groups to have the same proportion of males and females. The rate of disease in the exposed and comparison groups should be identical if the exposure has no effect on disease occurrence.

The three sources for the comparison group in a cohort study are (1) an internal comparison, (2) the general population, and (3) a comparison cohort (see Table 8–3). An internal comparison group is comprised of unexposed members of the same cohort. For example, Boice and Monson conducted a retrospective cohort study to determine the risk of breast cancer among female tuberculosis patients who had undergone repeated fluoroscopic x-ray examination of the chest during air collapse therapy.[20] This treatment resulted in considerable radiation exposure to the breast. The comparison group consisted of other female tuberculosis patients who

TABLE 8-3 Types of Comparison Groups in Cohort Studies

Type of comparison group	Strengths	Weaknesses
Internal	Most comparable to exposed group	May be difficult to identify
General population	Accessible, stable data	Lack of comparability with exposed group; results may suffer from healthy worker effect; data on key variables may be missing
Comparison cohort	Fairly comparable	Results are often difficult to interpret because comparison cohort often has other exposures

received treatments that did not require fluoroscopic x-ray examinations. Like the exposed group, the women who comprised the internal comparison group were tuberculosis patients at Massachusetts hospitals during the years 1930 to 1954. The study found a 1.8-fold excess of breast cancer cases among the exposed group; however, the risk was higher among women exposed before age 20 years.

When the general population is the source of the comparison group, preexisting available data on disease occurrence and death in a population are the basis for comparison. In the United States, such data are available from the National Center for Health Statistics. Internationally, excellent mortality statistics are compiled by the World Health Organization. Often when the comparison group is composed of the general population, the standardized mortality ratio (SMR) is used as the measure of association. The SMR is the ratio of the observed number of cases of disease or death to the expected number based on general population rates. SMRs usually "standardize" or control for age, gender, race, and calendar time, and are interpreted like relative risks.

For example, the retrospective cohort study described earlier among workers involved in manufacturing or spraying herbicides compared the cancer mortality experience of 21,863 male and female workers to national mortality data while controlling for sex, age, and calendar time.[15] Because the workers came from 12 countries, mortality data collected by the World Health Organization were used to compute the expected number of deaths. Investigators found 1083 deaths due to cancer among the male workers, while 1012 were expected. These findings resulted in an SMR of 1.07. No increase in cancer mortality rates was seen in female workers.

The general population is used as a comparison group when it is not possible to find a comparable internal comparison. This problem is quite common in occupational studies. For example, it is possible that everyone who works in a factory that manufactures herbicides is exposed to a greater or lesser degree. Although office workers, sales representatives, and company officials may be the least exposed, they usually do not comprise a comparable comparison group for production workers because of differences in gender (office workers are mainly female) and socioeconomic status (sales representatives and company officials have higher incomes).

General population comparison groups are commonly used in occupational studies of mortality because these data are quite accessible to researchers. In addition, the data are stable because they are based on large numbers. The assumption that the general population is unexposed is reasonable, because the number of exposed people is generally a small proportion of the total population.

Although there are several advantages to using the general population as a comparison group, there is one main disadvantage. The results are influenced by a form of bias known as the "healthy worker effect." This means that the rates of death and disease among a working population are usually lower than those of the general population. The lower rates of death and disease occur even when a noxious substance is present that elevates certain disease rates. The healthy worker effect occurs because a relatively healthy working population is being compared to the general population, which consists of ill people as well as healthy people. It is well known that there is selective entry of healthy persons and early removal of unhealthy ones from the workforce. In the study of workers exposed to phenoxy herbicides and chlorophenols, subjects had slightly lower than expected overall mortality rates (SMR = 0.97) that stemmed mainly from fewer deaths from circulatory system diseases (SMR = 0.91), and respiratory diseases (SMR = 0.82).[15]

The third type of comparison group, called the comparison cohort, consists of an unexposed cohort from another population. For example, a study compared cardiovascular disease rates among rayon factory workers who were exposed to carbon disulfide with those of paper mill workers who were not exposed to carbon disulfide.[21] Because both groups consisted of blue-collar workers, individual differences in social class and the healthy worker effect were minimized. However, the results of such studies are difficult to interpret because other exposures in the comparison cohort may also influence disease risk. For example, the paper mill workers may be exposed to other chemicals that influence their risk of developing cardiovascular disease.

As an alternative to a single comparison cohort, the Occupational Epidemiology Branch of the National Cancer Institute developed a comparison cohort by pooling data from earlier studies of numerous occupational populations. The assumption is that the population pooled from a variety of occupations and industries will, like the general population, have an average risk of developing particular diseases and that the healthy worker effect will be minimized.[22]

Epidemiologists have found that the internal comparison group is the best type of comparison group to use in a cohort study. If an internal comparison is not available, the general population is the next best option, and the traditional comparison cohort is the option of last resort. The pooled comparison cohort from the National Cancer Institute may change this ranking in the future.

Sources of Information

Sources of Information on Exposures and Other Key Variables

Depending on the hypothesis being tested, cohort study investigators rely on various sources for information on exposures and other important variables. These sources include medical and employment records, interviews, direct physical examinations, laboratory tests, biological specimens, and environmental monitoring. Some of these sources are preexisting, and others are designed specifically for a study. Each has advantages and disadvantages, and so investigators often use several sources to piece together all of the necessary information.

Investigators typically use health care records to describe a participant's exposure history in cohort studies of possible adverse health effects stemming from medical procedures. For example, in Boice and Monson's study of fluoroscopic x-ray exposure during tuberculosis treatment and the subsequent risk of breast cancer, investigators reviewed medical records to identify female patients who had been treated with air collapse and other therapies from 1930 through 1954.[20] The researchers obtained information from the medical record on the stage of the tuberculosis; all treatments received including the number of fluoroscopic x-ray examinations; and key variables such as age, race, religion, and other medical conditions.

The advantages of using medical records as an information source include low expense and a high level of accuracy and detail regarding a disease and its treatment. The medical record may be the best source of information about detailed medical events, particularly those that occurred long ago. For example, it is unlikely that a woman in Boice and Monson's study could recall the number of fluoroscopic x-ray exams that she received 30 years ago.[20] Her medical record could provide this important detail to the investigators to allow them to estimate dose of radiation that the woman received. The main disadvantage of medical records is that information on important variables, apart from basic demographic characteristics, is often missing. For example, Boice and Monson had to send questionnaires to participants to obtain information on breast cancer risk factors such as family history of the disease and age at first birth, menarche, and menopause.

Employment records are used mainly to identify individuals for studies of occupational exposures. Standard data in employment records include job title, department of work, years of employment, and basic demographic characteristics such as gender and date of birth. Like medical records, employment records usually lack data on exposure details and key variables, and so investigators often have to augment them with other sources. For example, in the study of workers exposed to phenoxy herbicides and other chemicals, investigators identified cohort members not only by reviewing individual job records, but also by sending questionnaires to companies about the work environment and types of products manufactured, and by measuring chemical levels in workers' blood and fat tissue.[15] Even with all these sources, the study investigators acknowledged that the exposure assessment was imperfect and that some exposed individuals may have been erroneously classified as unexposed and vice versa. Furthermore, none of the sources had information on variables such as smoking, alcohol use, and other workplace exposures such as asbestos.

Because existing records have their limitations, many studies are based solely on data collected specifically for the investigation. Data collection sources include questionnaires, physical examinations, laboratory tests, biological specimens, and environmental monitoring. For example, Framingham Study participants have undergone interviews, physical exams, laboratory tests, and other tests every 2 years for the last 50 years.[18] The interviews have gathered information on each person's medical history, cigarette smoking, alcohol use, physical activity, dietary intake, and emotional stress. The physical exam and laboratory tests have measured, among other things, height and weight; blood pressure; vital signs and symptoms; and cholesterol, hemoglobin, and glucose levels. The biennial exams and interviews allow investigators to update changes in each person's habits and health.

Study interviews are most often administered by trained personnel either in person or over the telephone. Sometimes self-administered questionnaires are used. Interviews and questionnaires are particularly useful for obtaining information on lifestyle characteristics that are not routinely or consistently recorded in medical and other records (such as alcohol intake, sexual activity, and physical activity). Although these data tend to be better than existing records, questionnaires and interviews must still rely on the ability of participants to know and recall information. Certainly, participants have the ability to recall important characteristics and events (such as history of cigarette smoking or family history of breast cancer), but it may be difficult for them to recall other types of information. For example, many individuals in occupational settings are not aware of the precise chemicals to which they are exposed at their job sites.

Epidemiologic studies of environmental pollution typically must conduct environmental monitoring to determine a participant's exposure. For example, investigators in the Six Cities Study, a prospective cohort study of the effect of air pollution on mortality, collected data on outdoor air concentrations of total suspended particulate matter, sulfur dioxide, ozone, and suspended sulfates from monitoring stations centrally located in the communities where the participants resided.[23]

When possible and appropriate, epidemiologists also gather exposure data using biological measurements in participants' blood, urine, bone, and toenails. These measurements are known as biomarkers of exposure. These markers can not only provide measures of the exposure but also provide markers of internal organ dose. For example, a prospective cohort study of the health effects of lead exposure tested children's blood lead levels at birth and several times thereafter.[7] The blood lead data provided an integrated assessment of each child's exposure over the previous 6 weeks. In another cohort study, investigators collected toenail clippings from study subjects in order to obtain an integrated measure of selenium intake over the previous 26 to 52 weeks.[24]

Data collected specifically for a study are of higher quality than those in existing records, but they are more expensive to obtain. For example, a 30-minute telephone interview used in a 1998 study to collect information on environmental exposures and confounders cost approximately $100 to $200 per participant.[25] In-person interviews, which were conducted when the subject was too ill to be interviewed by phone, were even more expensive because they involved travel time to the participant's home. Laboratory tests of biological and environmental samples can also be quite expensive. For example, analysis of polychlorinated biphenyls, dioxin, and metabolites of DDT in serum can cost about a thousand dollars per sample.

Sources of Outcome Information

The sources of outcome information in a cohort study are similar to the sources of exposures information: interviews, self-administered questionnaires, physical examinations, biological specimens, laboratory tests, and medical records. Although accuracy is the primary consideration when selecting a source of outcome data, cost and practical considerations are also important. Investigators often rely on several sources to gather the information because of the advantages and disadvantages described earlier.

For example, the Framingham Study used a combination of interviews, physical examinations, and laboratory tests to gather information on the incidence and precursors of coronary heart disease, stroke, and peripheral artery disease.[18] Medical records and laboratory tests were used to confirm information that was reported in the interview. For example, heart attacks reported by Framingham Study participants were confirmed by electrocardiographic (ECG) changes and enzyme changes diagnostic of the disorder. The presence of Q waves not previously seen was considered definitive evidence that a heart attack had occurred. The ECG evidence was useful in improving the accuracy of the heart attack data; investigators excluded about 20% of heart attacks reported by participants because of equivocal evidence.[18]

Biological specimens provided by the participant can also provide early evidence of disease. A biological marker is often considered an intermediate outcome because it is on the pathway from exposure to the appearance of clinical disease. For example, CD4 lymphocyte counts are markers of HIV-1 infection and AIDS disease progression. A rapid decline in CD4 counts occurs shortly after infection and continues over time through the onset of clinical disease to death.

Outcome information can be gathered from state and national disease registries (most commonly for cancer occurrence) and departments of vital records (for mortality information). Investigators can collect this type of data without directly involving the participant, which reduces study costs. In fact, mortality data are relatively easy to obtain now that the National Death Index (NDI) is available for medical research. Compiled by the U.S. National Center for Health Statistics, the NDI is a computerized central file of death record information beginning with deaths in 1979. Investigators submit identifying information to the NDI staff, who search their database for a match. The more information submitted, the greater the likelihood that an accurate match will be found. However, although mortality data are readily accessible and complete, their accuracy is often questioned because there are no strict criteria to guide physicians who are completing cause-of-death information on death certificates.

Whatever the source, it is important to follow comparable procedures for determining the outcomes among the exposed and unexposed groups. Investigators' use of differing sources and procedures may lead to inaccurate results. Thus, all resources used for one group must be used for the other. In addition, investigators should be masked to the exposure status of subjects so that they make unbiased decisions when assessing the outcomes. For example, an investigator might have to decide if an interview report of a "breast tumor" is a malignant or benign tumor. Masking the investigator will ensure that the decision, whatever it is, is unrelated to the participant's exposure status. In addition, investigators should develop standard outcome definitions to guarantee accuracy and comparability. These definitions should be based on information that is readily available from acceptable and accessible procedures. Furthermore, diagnostic criteria should be both sensitive (able to pick up cases of disease) and specific (able to exclude individuals without disease). For example, the diagnosis of angina pectoris might include clinical symptoms such as dull, heavy discomfort in the substernal area, particularly after a meal and with exertion or emotional distress, and evidence of ECG abnormalities at rest and with exercise.

Approaches to Follow-up

Loss to follow-up occurs either when a participant no longer wishes to take part in a study or when he or she cannot be located. Minimizing these losses is crucial for two reasons. First, losses to follow-up effectively decrease the sample size and reduce the ability of the study to detect an association, if one is present. Second, those who are lost to follow-up may differ in important ways from those who are successfully traced. Of particular concern is that lost individuals are more likely to have developed the disease under study. If lost individuals are more or less likely to be exposed than those successfully traced, the study results may suffer from a form of bias known as information bias (see Chapter 10 for more details).

Because high rates of follow-up are critical to the success of a cohort study, investigators have developed a variety of methods to maximize retention and trace study members.[26] For prospective cohort studies, strategies include collection of baseline information that helps to locate participants as the study progresses. This information usually includes the participant's full name; current address; telephone number; Social Security number; date and place of birth; and the names, addresses, and phone numbers of physicians, friends, and relatives who will always know where the participant is living.

Another recommended strategy for prospective studies is regular mail or personal contact with participants. These contacts might involve requests for up-to-date outcome information or newsletters describing the study's progress and findings. The mailing is used to help participants "bond" with the study and to obtain address corrections from the U.S. Postal Service.[26]

Additional mailings are the best strategy to use when participants do not initially respond. Investigators typically send at least two follow-up letters or postcards by first class or certified mail, emphasizing the importance of the request. If additional mailings are unsuccessful, investigators use telephone calls and even home visits to contact nonrespondents.

When participants are truly lost to follow-up, researchers use a number of additional strategies.[26] Usually the simplest and least expensive ones are used first and more difficult and expensive ones are used later. In the early stages of follow-up, letters are sent to the last known address with "Address Correction Requested." In addition, investigators check telephone directories, directory assistance, and Internet resources such as the "White Pages." An increasingly popular resource is the U.S. Postal Service's National Change of Address (NCOA) system, which has up-to-date change-of-address data for almost the entire country.

If these steps prove unsuccessful, investigators contact relatives, friends, or physicians who were identified at baseline. If this step is unsuccessful, investigators can turn to many local, state, and national resources including state vital statistics records (for births, marriages, divorces, and deaths); driver's license, voter registration, and public utility records; the National Death Index; the Social Security Administration; the Centers for Medicare and Medicaid Services; credit bureaus; and commercial companies that specialize in tracing individuals.

Tracing is a laborious and challenging process. It has become even more difficult today because of increased population mobility. However, newly available resources such as those on the Internet offset these difficulties to some degree. The time and monetary investment in follow-up is worthwhile because it helps secure the success of the study.

Analysis of Cohort Studies

The primary objective of the analysis of cohort study data is to compare disease occurrence in the exposed and unexposed groups. Disease occurrence is usually measured using cumulative incidence or incidence rates, and the relationship between exposure and disease occurrence is quantified by the cumulative incidence or incidence rate difference and/or ratio. Although the measures of disease frequency and association are covered in detail in Chapters 2 and 3, the calculation of person-time and the concepts of induction and latent periods are discussed here in the context of cohort study analysis.

Calculating Person-Time

Calculating an incidence rate involves determining the amount of person-time accrued by each study subject. It is important to remember that person-time is, in essence, follow-up time and that follow-up time is calculated only within the context of a study. It is also important to differentiate years of follow-up from years of exposure and years of latency. For example, consider a hypothetical occupational retrospective cohort study in which follow-up starts on January 1, 1950, and ends at the time of death or the closing date of the study (January 1, 1995). Let us consider a hypothetical person who was born on January 1, 1920; started work at age 20 on January 1, 1940; worked for 45 years until 1985; and died at age 70 on January 1, 1990 (see Figure 8–2).

The maximum number of person-years that any individual can accrue in this study is 45 years (C to F). The number of person-years that our hypothetical individual accrued was 40 years (C to E). The total number of person-years that an individual accrues never changes. However, it is often divided among various exposure categories such as age and calendar year when the individual started work, and duration of employment. Note that the number of years that our hypothetical individual worked (B to D) is a measure of exposure duration and is different from the number of person-years that he accrued in the study.

As a real-life example, let us consider Boice and Monson's study of breast cancer after repeated chest fluoroscopies.[20] In this study, years of follow-up were accumulated from the date of the first fluoroscopic examination for exposed women and first sanatorium admission for comparison subjects. Follow-up ended at different points, depending on what happened to the women. For women who developed breast cancer, follow-up ended with the diagnosis date. For women who did not develop breast cancer, it ended with the date of death for those who died, the closing date of the study (July 1, 1975) for those who were still alive at the end of the study, and the date last known to be alive for those who were lost to follow-up. Using these start and end dates, the 1047 women in the exposed group accrued 28,011 person-years of follow-up, and the 717 women in the comparison group accrued 19,025 person-years of follow-up. The maximum possible length of follow-up for any participant was 45 years (from first possible treatment in 1930 to closing date of study in 1975); the average was about 26 years.

	A	B	C	D	E	F
Year	1920	1940	1950	1985	1990	1995
Age (years)	0	20	30	65	70	—
Milestone	Born	Starts work	Follow-up starts	Retires	Dies	Follow-up ends

FIGURE 8–2. Accrual of Person-time

Induction and Latent Periods

The analysis of a cohort study typically considers the length of time between the causal action of an exposure and the eventual diagnosis of disease.[27] The causal action of an exposure occurs when sufficient exposure has accrued. The *induction period* that follows is the interval between the action of a cause and disease onset. An example of disease onset might be the transformation of a normal breast cell into a cancerous one. The *latent period* is the subsequent interval between disease onset and clinical diagnosis. For example, a clinical diagnosis of breast cancer occurs when the tumor becomes large enough to be detected either by screening mammography or physical examination.

Because the time of disease onset is usually not possible to determine, the induction and latent periods are typically merged into the *empirical latent period*. For example, in a study of the relationship between tetrachloroethylene-contaminated drinking water and the risk of breast cancer, investigators hypothesized that the water contaminant might act either as a tumor initiator (early in the carcinogenic process) or as a promoter (late in the process), and so they conducted analyses considering empirical latent periods ranging from 0 to 15 years.[25]

Special Types of Cohort Studies

The comparison group in a cohort study may come from either an internal source, another cohort, or the general population. Two special types of cohort studies—proportional mortality ratio (PMR) and standardized mortality ratio (SMR) studies—are conducted to compare the mortality experience of the exposed group to that of the general population. Both types of studies are common in occupational epidemiology because there is often no truly unexposed group in the workplace.

The difference between PMR and SMR studies is the type of information needed to calculate the measure of association. All of the information for the PMR study comes from death certificates (date, age, cause of death). The observed number of deaths due to a specific cause in the exposed group is compared to the expected number which is derived from the proportion of deaths resulting from that cause in the general population. The resulting PMR, which is interpreted like a relative risk, shows the relative importance of a specific cause of death in relation to all deaths.

For example, investigators compared the mortality patterns of pulp and paper mill workers to those of the U.S. population in a PMR study.[28] The study population consisted of members of the United Paper Workers International Union who died from 1970 through 1984, and were employed for at least 10 years in the industry. Information on year of birth, sex, race, year of death, and cause of death was abstracted from death certificates. For each cause of death, investigators compared the observed number of deaths to the expected number while controlling for sex, race, age, and calendar year of death. The study found a 31% increased risk of deaths from malignant neoplasms, particularly cancer of the lung, lymphopoietic system, and large intestine. A reduced risk of death was observed for cancers of the stomach and pancreas. The largest single category of death, arteriosclerotic heart disease, was neither increased nor reduced.

In an SMR study, investigators need additional information to compare the mortality experience of the exposed group with that of the general population. This is because the SMR compares the mortality rates of the two groups, while the PMR study compares mortality proportions. Thus, information on person-years of follow-up among the study group is needed to calculate the expected number of deaths.

For example, following publication of several PMR studies reporting increased cancer risks, investigators undertook an industry-wide SMR study of pulp and paper workers.[5] The study included 63,025 long-term workers from 51 mills across the United States. The workers were required to be employed for at least 10 years to be eligible. Vital status was identified through the mills, Social Security mortality tapes, and the National Death Index. Investigators calculated SMRs using three comparison populations: the U.S. population, the 20 states in which the mills were located, and the residents of the 330 counties that were within a 50-mile radius of each mill. The latter two comparison populations were used because their demographic characteristics were similar to those of the workers.

A total of 7171 deaths occurred among cohort members through the end of 1991. Person-time of follow-up was calculated for cohort members starting with 10 years after first employment or when the mill was enrolled in the study (whichever came last), and ending with the termination of the study or death. SMRs were calculated that adjusted for age, calendar time, race, and sex. The investigators found that the overall mortality rate of pulp and paper mill workers was significantly lower than that of the U.S. population (SMR=0.74) and that the workers' mortality rate was not elevated for any specific cause of death, including malignancies. However, in a few instances, a higher mortality rate was seen when workers were separated according to the type of pulping process used at their plant.

Because PMR studies take less time and cost less money, they are often done before an SMR study is initiated. However, it is informative to conduct both types of studies in the same population.[29(p131)] Note that SMR studies and, to a lesser extent, PMR studies suffer from the "healthy worker effect."[29(p114)] PMR studies also suffer from the "see-saw effect," in which deficits in one cause of death necessarily result in the study population in corresponding increases in other causes of death. This occurs

TABLE 8–4 Strengths and Weaknesses of Cohort Studies

Strengths
- Efficient for rare exposures
- Good information on exposures (prospective)
- Can evaluate multiple effects of an exposure
- Efficient for diseases with long induction and latent periods (retrospective)
- Less vulnerable to bias (prospective)
- Can directly measure disease incidence or risk
- Clear temporal relationship between exposure and outcome (prospective)

Weaknesses
- Inefficient for rare outcomes
- Poor information on exposures and other key variables (retrospective)
- Expensive and time consuming (particularly prospective)
- Inefficient for diseases with long induction and latent periods (prospective)
- More vulnerable to bias (retrospective)

because the total number of observed deaths in the study population must equal the number of expected deaths derived from the general population.

Strengths and Limitations of Cohort Studies

The goal of every epidemiologic study is to harvest valid and precise information about the relationship between an exposure and a disease in a population. The various study designs merely represent different ways of harvesting this information. Each type of design has strengths and weaknesses (see Table 8–4), which tend to be complementary. For example, the pros and cons of retrospective and prospective cohort studies tend to balance one another. However, under certain circumstances, a cohort study design is clearly indicated. Investigators should use a cohort study when they wish to learn about multiple effects of an exposure or when the exposure is rare, and they should use a retrospective cohort design when the outcome of interest has a long induction and latent period.

Summary

Cohort studies examine the health effects of an exposure by following two or more groups with a common characteristic (exposed and unexposed). Cohort studies may be conducted in populations that are defined by changeable conditions (open or dynamic) or irrevocable events (fixed and closed). The timing of cohort studies can be prospective, retrospective, or ambidirectional. In prospective cohort studies, investigators group participants on the basis of past or current exposure and follow them into the future in order to observe the outcome(s) of interest. In retrospective cohort studies, investigators group participants on the basis of past exposures and evaluate outcomes that have already occurred. Ambidirectional cohort studies have retrospective and prospective components. Retrospective cohort studies are more efficient than prospective ones for studying diseases with long induction and latent periods. However, prospective studies are less vulnerable to bias than retrospective cohort studies.

Several design features of cohort studies emulate those of experimental studies in order to produce high-quality results, including the selection of comparable groups and the masking of investigators to subjects' exposure status during follow-up and outcome ascertainment. Regarding the former, the ideal comparison group would consist of the same individuals in the exposed group had they not been exposed. This is known as the "counterfactual ideal." Because it is impossible for the same individuals to be exposed and unexposed simultaneously, the investigator must select different sets of individuals for comparison. The comparison group can come from an internal comparison group, the general population, or a comparison cohort. An internal comparison group consists of unexposed members of the same cohort. A general population comparison group is selected on the basis of preexisting population data such as mortality rates from the National Center for Health Statistics. A comparison cohort consists of unexposed members of another cohort. The internal comparison group is considered the best of the three because it is most similar to the exposed group.

Depending on the hypothesis being tested, investigators rely on a variety of sources for information on exposures, outcomes, and other key variables. These sources include medical and employment records, interviews, direct physical examinations, laboratory tests, and environmental monitoring. During the follow-up period, the groups are monitored for the outcomes under study. Loss to follow-up occurs when participants no longer wish to participate or when they can no longer be located. Because follow-up losses are a threat to the validity of study, epidemiologists use a variety of methods to maximize retention and tracing of study members, including collection of baseline information to help locate participants as the study progresses.

The main strengths of cohort studies are that they are efficient for studying rare exposures, they allow investigators to evaluate multiple health effects of an exposure, and retrospective cohort studies are efficient for studying diseases with long induction and latent periods. The main weaknesses of cohort studies are that they are inefficient for studying rare outcomes, prospective cohort studies are inefficient for studying diseases with long induction and latent periods, and retrospective cohort studies are vulnerable to bias.

References

1. Pickett JP, exec ed. *The American Heritage Dictionary of the English Language.* 4th ed. Boston, MA: Houghton Mifflin; 2000.
2. Last JM, ed. *A Dictionary of Epidemiology.* 3rd ed. New York, NY: Oxford University Press; 1995.
3. Rabkin CS, Yellin F. Cancer incidence in a population with a high prevalence of infection with human immunodeficiency virus type 1. *J Natl Cancer Inst.* 1994;86:1711–1716.
4. Kodama K, Mabuchi K, Shigematsu I. A long-term cohort study of the atomic bomb survivors. *Int J Epidemiol.* 1996;6:S95–S105.
5. Matanoski G, Kanchanaraksa S, Lees PSJ, Tao XG, Royall R, Francis M, et al. Industry-wide study of mortality of pulp and paper mill workers. *Am J Ind Med.* 1998;33:354–365.
6. Curtis KM, Savitz DA, Arbuckle TE. Effects of cigarette smoking, caffeine consumption, and alcohol intake on fecundability. *Am J Epidemiol.* 1997;146:32–41.
7. Bellinger DC, Stiles KM, Needleman HL. Low level lead exposure, intelligence and academic achievement: a long-term follow-up study. *Pediatrics.* 1992;90: 855–861.
8. Nyren O, Yin L, Josefsson S, McLaughlin JK, Blot WJ, Engqvist M, et al. Risk of connective tissue disease and related disorders among women with breast implants: a nation-wide retrospective cohort study in Sweden. *Br Med J.* 1998; 316:417–422.
9. Lathrop GD, Wolfe WH, Albanese RA, Moynahan PM. *An Epidemiologic Investigation of Health Effects in Air Force Personnel Following Exposure to Herbicides. Baseline Morbidity Results.* Washington, DC: US Air Force; 1984.
10. Wolfe WH, Michalek JE, Miner JC, Rahe A, Silva J, Thomas WF, et al. Heath status of Air Force veterans occupationally exposed to herbicides in Vietnam I. Physical health. *JAMA.* 1990;264:1824–1831.
11. Michalek JE, Wolfe WH, Miner JC. Health status of Air Force veterans occupationally exposed to herbicides in Vietnam II. Mortality. *JAMA.* 1990;264: 1832–1836.
12. Vega WA, Kolody B, Hwang J, Noble A. Prevalence and magnitude of perinatal substance exposures in California. *N Engl J Med.* 1993;329:850–854.
13. Streissguth AP. Fetal alcohol syndrome: an epidemiologic perspective. *Am J Epidemiol.* 1978;107:467–478.
14. Colton T. *Statistics in Medicine.* Boston, MA: Little, Brown, and Co; 1974.
15. Kogevinas M, Becher H, Benn T, Bertazzi PA, Boffetta P, Bueno-de-Mesquita HB, et al. Cancer mortality in workers exposed to phenoxy herbicides, chlorophenols, and dioxins: an expanded and updated international cohort study. *Am J Epidemiol.* 1997;145:1061–1075.
16. Darby SC, Doll R, Gill SK, et al. Long term mortality after a single treatment course with x-rays in patients treated for ankylosing spondylitis. *Br J Cancer.* 1987;55:179–190.
17. Mills PK, Beeson WL, Phillips RL, Fraser GE. Cancer incidence among California Seventh-Day Adventists, 1976–1982. *Am J Clin Nutr.* 1994;59: 1136S–1142S.

18. Dawber TR. *The Framingham Study: The Epidemiology of Atherosclerotic Disease.* Cambridge, MA: Harvard University Press; 1980.
19. Rothman KJ, Greenland S. *Modern Epidemiology.* 2nd ed. Philadelphia, PA: Lippincott-Raven Publishers; 1998.
20. Boice JD, Monson RR. Breast cancer in women after repeated fluoroscopic examination of the chest. *J Natl Cancer Inst.* 1977;59:823–832.
21. Hernberg S, Partenen T, Nordman C-H, Sumari P. Coronary heart disease among workers exposed to carbon disulfide. *Br J Ind Med.* 1970;27:313–325.
22. Computerized Occupational Referent Population System (CORPS). Available at: http://dceg.cancer.gov/ebp/oeb/AvailRes.html. Accessed January 2003.
23. Dockery DW, Pope CA, Xu Spengler JD, Ware JH, Fay ME, et al. An association between air pollution and mortality in six US Cities. *N Engl J Med.* 1993; 329:1753–1760.
24. Yoshizawa K, Willett WC, Morris SJ, Stampfer MJ, Spiegelman D, Rimm EB. Study of prediagnostic selenium level in toenails and the risk of advanced prostate cancer. *J Natl Cancer Inst.* 1998;90:1219–1224.
25. Aschengrau A, Paulu C, Ozonoff D. Tetrachloroethylene-contaminated drinking water and the risk of breast cancer. *Environ Health Perspect.* 1998; 106:947–953.
26. Hunt JR, White E. Retaining and tracking cohort study members. *Epidemiol Rev.* 1998;20:57–70.
27. Rothman KJ. Induction and latent periods. *Am J Epidemiol.* 1981;114:253–259.
28. Solet D, Zoloth SR, Sullivan C, Jewett J, Michaels DM. Patterns of mortality in pulp and paper workers. *J Occup Med.* 1989;31:627–630.
29. Monson RR. *Occupational Epidemiology.* Boca Raton, FL: CRC Press; 1990.

EXERCISES

1. Briefly define each of the following terms that are associated with cohort studies:
   A. Open or dynamic cohort
   B. Fixed cohort
   C. Retrospective cohort study
   D. Prospective cohort study
   E. Standardized mortality ratio (SMR) study

2. State the main similarity and main difference between cohort and experimental studies.

3. Describe the strengths and weaknesses of the three types of comparison groups used in cohort studies. Which one comes closest to the counterfactual ideal?

4. State whether or not a cohort study is best suited for each of the following scenarios:
   A. When little is known about a rare exposure Y
   B. When little is known about a rare disease N
   C. When the study population will be difficult to follow N
   D. When you want to learn about multiple effects of an exposure Y

5. Why is it important to minimize loss to follow-up?

6. How is person-time calculated within the context of a cohort study?

9

Case–Control Studies

LEARNING OBJECTIVES

By the end of this chapter, the reader will be able to:

- Discuss the traditional and modern views of case–control studies.
- List the settings in which case–control studies are desirable.
- Describe the key features of conducting case–control studies, including the selection of cases and controls, the sources of exposure information, and data analysis.
- Describe the key aspects of case-crossover studies.
- Discuss the strengths and limitations of case-control studies.

Introduction

As in other fields in science and public health, ideas about the theoretical framework underlying epidemiologic research continue to evolve. This is perhaps most true about epidemiologists' views regarding case–control studies, the second principal type of observational study. The goal of a case–control study is identical to that of any other epidemiologic study—the valid and precise measurement of the relationship between an exposure and disease. However, epidemiologists' views about the appropriate way to conceptualize and design this type of study have changed considerably over the past two decades. As a consequence of these changes, epidemiologists have come to realize that the quality of a case–control study can be as high as that of a cohort study.

This chapter presents the traditional view of the case–control study and then describes the conceptual shift that has occurred over the last two decades. Next, the chapter describes specific features of the design, conduct, and analysis of case–control studies, including the selection of cases and controls, measurement of exposure, and calculation of another measure of association termed the odds ratio. Examples are provided to illustrate how case–control studies have been used to answer important public health questions. The chapter concludes with a discussion of the strengths and limitations of case–control studies.

The Changing View of Case–Control Studies

The Traditional View

Traditionally, epidemiologists viewed case-control studies as an alternative to cohort studies. Recall that a cohort study begins with a group of nondiseased people who are categorized according to exposure level and followed to measure the occurrence of disease. In contrast, in the traditional conceptualization of a case–control study, subjects are selected on the basis of whether they have or do not have the disease. Those that have the disease are termed *cases* and those who do not have the disease are termed *controls*. Investigators obtain and compare the exposure histories of cases and controls.

For example, consider a hypothetical case–control study of pesticide exposure and breast cancer from the traditional standpoint. A series of breast cancer cases are identified and enrolled, and a series of control subjects without breast cancer are also identified and enrolled. Investigators obtain pesticide exposure information by interviewing the women about their prior work and leisure activities (for example, they might ask participants if they ever worked on a farm or gardened with pesticides). Next, the investigators compare the exposure histories of the cases and controls. If 75% of breast cancer cases and only 25% of controls have a positive exposure history, the researchers would conclude that there is an association between pesticide exposure and breast cancer.

The central feature of the traditional view is the comparison of the exposure histories of cases and controls. The logic of this approach differs from that of experimental and cohort study designs, in which the key comparison is the disease incidence between the exposed and unexposed (or least exposed) groups. In other words, the traditional view asserts that experimental and cohort studies move from cause to effect, and case–control studies move from effect to cause. Thus, many who espouse the traditional view believe that the logic of a case–control study is backwards.[1] They also believe that case-control studies are much more prone to bias and thus inferior to other designs. In fact, the term "TROHOC" study (COHORT spelled backwards) was coined as a disparaging moniker for case–control studies.

The Modern View

Epidemiologists' view of case–control studies began to change in the 1980s with the work of Miettinen, who argued that it is incorrect to consider a case–control study merely the reverse of a cohort study.[2] He coined the term "TROHOC fallacy" to describe this erroneous thinking. Miettinen argued that a case–control study is an efficient way to learn about the relationship between an exposure and disease. More specifically, he stated that the case–control study is a method of sampling a population in which cases of disease are identified and enrolled and a sample of the source population that gave rise to the cases is also identified and enrolled. The sample of the source population is known as the control group. Its purpose is to provide information on the exposure distribution in the population that produced the cases, so that the disease rates in exposed and nonexposed groups can be compared. Thus, Miettinen asserted, the key comparison in a case–control study is the same as that in a cohort study—a comparison between the exposed and nonexposed groups.

The following hypothetical example illustrates the modern view of the case–control study. Suppose that investigators undertook a prospective cohort study in 1980 to determine the causes of chronic diseases among middle-aged women in the United States. Investigators decided to conduct a general cohort study, and so they assembled a group of 100,000 female teachers aged 45 to 65 years. They planned to examine numerous risk factors (such as use of contraceptives, diet, smoking, alcohol consumption, and environmental exposures), and so they collected data on these characteristics, as well as data on health outcomes and other key variables. Investigators used a combination of periodic interviews, physical exams, and laboratory tests to gather this information. In particular, blood was drawn from all participants at baseline, and these samples were processed and frozen for later use.

In 1999, the study investigators became interested in the hypothesis that pesticides such as DDT increased a woman's risk of breast cancer. Data from other studies suggested that these compounds could increase a woman's risk by mimicking the action of endogenous estrogens.[3] The investigators decided to measure serum levels of DDE (the metabolic byproduct of the pesticide DDT) in the frozen blood samples taken from cohort members in 1980. Even though DDT was banned in 1969,[4(pp275–360)] it is quite persistent and so serum levels taken in 1980 should give a fairly accurate estimate of past exposure.

The investigators sent the 100,000 samples to a laboratory for DDE analysis. Upon receipt of the laboratory results, the investigators characterized the cohort according to DDE level (high or low). In addition, they examined the health outcome data collected so far, and found that 2000 study participants had developed breast cancer since the beginning of the study. The investigators arranged the exposure and outcome data into a two-by-two table (see Table 9–1) and calculated the relative risk in the usual fashion: by comparing the occurrence of breast cancer (here, cumulative incidence of breast cancer) among women with high DDE levels to that among women with low DDE levels. Thus, the relative risk or cumulative incidence ratio was (500/15,000)/(1500/85,000) or 1.89.

Unfortunately there was a major problem in evaluating the hypothesis in this manner: quantifying DDE serum levels was very expensive—about $100 dollars per sample. Thus, ascertaining DDE exposure levels on all 100,000 study subjects cost $10 million dollars.

Note that the cohort study approach in this setting is prohibitively expensive. What would have happened if the investigators used a much less costly approach such as a case–control study nested within the cohort? How would they go about conducting such a study? First, they would analyze the baseline serum samples of all 2000 women who were diagnosed with breast cancer (the cases). Next, they would carefully select a sample of the cohort to be the control group. Let us assume that they decide to select 4000 women for the control group. The results of such a study are shown in Table 9–2.

The investigators could use these data to estimate the relative risk of breast cancer among women with high versus low DDE levels. The estimate would be similar to the relative risk calculated for the entire cohort if certain conditions were met. The most important of these conditions is the

TABLE 9–1   Data from a Hypothetical Cohort Study of Serum DDE Levels and the Risk of Breast Cancer

	Breast Cancer		
DDE Level	Yes	No	Total
High	500	14,500	15,000
Low	1,500	83,500	85,000
Total	2,000	98,000	100,000

TABLE 9–2   Data from a Hypothetical Case–Control Study of DDE Exposure and Breast Cancer Nested within a Cohort

	Breast Cancer		
DDE Level	Yes	No	Total
High	500	600	1,100
Low	1,500	3,400	4,900
Total	2,000	4,000	6,000

proper selection of controls. (Control selection is discussed in more detail later in this chapter.)

Note that the nested case–control study is much more efficient than the cohort study. The cases are the same as those that would be included in the cohort study, and the controls provide a less expensive and faster way of determining the exposure experience in the population that generated the cases.[5(p74)] Certainly, the cost of determining the DDE exposure levels in the nested case–control study would be much less than that of the cohort study ($600,000 versus $10 million). The analysis of both the case–control and the cohort study involves comparing the disease frequency among the exposed and nonexposed groups. The cases in both studies form the numerators of the measures of disease frequency. The denominators are slightly different. The *total* number of persons or person-time forms the denominator in a cohort study, while a sample of persons or person-time forms the denominator in a case–control study. This sample is known as the control group.

Thus, the modern view of a case–control study holds that it is a method of sampling a population, in which investigators identify and enroll cases of disease and identify and enroll a sample of the population that produced the cases. The purpose of the control group is to determine the relative size of the exposed and unexposed denominators in the source population. The sample is an alternative to obtaining exposure information on the entire study population. As in experimental and cohort studies, the essential comparison is between the exposed and unexposed groups.

When Is It Desirable to Use the Case–Control Method?

As described in Chapter 6, epidemiologists consider many factors to determine which type of study design is most appropriate for investigating a particular hypothesis. These factors include the frequency of the exposure and disease, feasibility, costs, and ethical issues. If an observational study is in order, the choice is typically between a cohort and case–control study, but how does an investigator decide which type of study is better?

Epidemiologists prefer the case–control study in five types of situations (see Table 9-3). First, as for the DDE and breast cancer study

TABLE 9–3   Situations in Which a Case–Control Study Is Desirable

- Exposure data are difficult or expensive to obtain.
- The disease is rare.
- The disease has a long induction and latent period.
- Little is known about the disease.
- The underlying population is dynamic.

described earlier, a case–control study is preferable when the exposure data are difficult or expensive to obtain. Collecting exposure data on fewer individuals (typically all of the cases and a sample of the source population) saves both time and money. If control selection is unbiased, the cost savings will not adversely affect the validity of the study.

Second, a case–control study is more efficient than a cohort study when the disease is rare, which is usually defined as a frequency of 20% or less. For example, consider a cohort study of 100,000 subjects examining the relationship between diet and the occurrence of cancer. Although this study would be adequate for examining common types of cancer such as those occurring in the lung, breast, and colon-rectum, it would not be adequate for examining rare ones such as cancer of the gall bladder. The incidence rate of gall bladder cancer is about 1 per 100,000 per year,[6] and so only about 30 cases of this cancer would occur in a 100,000-member cohort after 30 years of follow-up. This yield is meager considering the time and expense of following 100,000 individuals for such a long period of time. Furthermore, in a cohort study with only 30 cases, it is unlikely that investigators would be able to detect an association between disease and diet, unless it were quite strong.

Third, a case–control study is preferable to a cohort study, at least a prospective one, when the disease has a long induction and latent period (that is, when there is a long time between the causal action of an exposure and the eventual diagnosis of disease).[7] For example, cancers involving solid tumors are thought to have induction/latency periods of 15 or more years.[8,9] A prospective cohort study would have to follow participants for a long time in order to observe these types of outcomes. Follow-up is avoided in a case–control study because it is retrospective (that is, both the exposure and the outcome have already occurred at the time the subject is enrolled).

Fourth, case–control studies are preferable when little is known about the disease, because it allows the investigators to evaluate more than one hypothesis. For example, the earliest etiologic studies of acquired immune deficiency disease (AIDS) were case–control studies. Conducted before the human immunodeficiency virus (HIV) was determined to be the cause of AIDS, these studies investigated many possible causes, including illicit drug use, sexual behaviors, and sexually transmitted and viral diseases.[10]

Fifth, case–control studies are desirable when the population under study is dynamic. Recall that the membership of a dynamic population is defined by a changeable state or condition and that its membership continually changes with inflow and outflow (see Chapter 2 for more details). The most common type of dynamic population is defined by residence in a particular geographic area. Inflow occurs when someone moves or is born into the geographic area, and outflow occurs when someone moves away or dies. A case–control study is desirable in this setting because it is difficult for researchers to identify and keep track of a population that is constantly changing.

For example, investigators conducted a case–control study on tetra-chloroethylene-contaminated drinking water and the risk of breast cancer in the Cape Cod region of Massachusetts, the hook-shaped peninsula in the southeastern part of the state.[11] Tetrachloroethylene (also known as PCE) is a solvent that is commonly used in dry cleaning. The substance had leached into the public drinking water supplies in the Cape Cod area from an improperly cured vinyl liner that was placed inside certain water distribution pipes. The Cape Cod population has experienced tremendous changes in the past 20 years. In particular, there has been a large influx of new residents, mainly elderly retirees.[12] In addition, the region has a large part-time summer population. The challenge of enumerating and tracking a cohort under these circumstances was one of several reasons why the investigators chose to conduct a case–control study to test the hypothesis that exposure to PCE-contaminated drinking water increased the risk of breast cancer.

Selection of Cases

Case Definition

All epidemiologic research, including case–control studies, involves com-posing a disease or case definition. This task usually involves dividing subjects into two groups: those who have the disease and those who do not. The criteria that are used to make such decisions are usually based on a combination of signs and symptoms, physical and pathological exami-nations, and results of diagnostic tests. Which and how many criteria are used to define a case has important implications for determining accu-rately who has the disease. If nonspecific criteria are used, most but not all people with the disease will be captured, but many people who do not have the disease will be included erroneously. For example, if only chest pain were used to define cases of myocardial infarction, most but not all heart attack cases would be included (people with "silent" heart attacks would be missed), but people with other conditions that produce chest pain (such as indigestion) would be included mistakenly. If restrictive criteria are used, fewer cases will be eligible for inclusion in the study, so the sample size will be smaller. Nonetheless, if given a choice between being inclusive or restrictive, it is better to be restrictive because it leads to fewer classification errors.[13]

In practice, it is best to use all available evidence to define with as much accuracy as possible the true cases of disease. In addition, cases should be defined with the likely causal mechanism in mind, and cases that are likely to result from the same causal mechanism should be grouped together. This approach might seem paradoxical, since the purpose of the research is usually to identify the causal mechanism. However, existing knowledge, albeit incomplete, can be used as a guide. For example, we currently know enough about the etiology of uterine cancer to separate cancer of the cervix (the neck of the uterus) from cancer of the uterine corpus (the body of the uterus). In addition, we know enough about the formation of the human heart during gestation to separate infants born with a ventricular septal defect (a hole in the wall separating two lower chambers of the heart) from infants born with transposition of the great vessels (reversal of the locations of the aorta and pulmonary artery).

Once a case group is formed, it is always possible to divide the cases according to various criteria such as histologic subtype, severity (for example, mild, moderate, and severe), and the likelihood that the diagnosis is accurate (for example, definite, probable, or possible). These subdivisions usually improve the accuracy of the case definition by reducing classification errors.

Sometimes different criteria are used in different studies because epidemiologists disagree about the best way to define the disease. For example, there are currently at least five classification schemes for defining cases of rheumatoid arthritis.[13] Even when a consensus is reached, disease definitions change over time as more is learned about the condition and its manifestations. For example, the official definition of AIDS has changed several times as epidemiologists have gained knowledge about its cause and natural history (see Chapter 2 for more details). In either case, it is difficult to compare descriptive statistics and study results when the studies use differing criteria or definitions.

Sources of Case Identification

Once investigators have created a case definition, they can begin identifying and enrolling cases. Typical sources for identifying cases are hospital or clinic patient rosters, death certificates, special surveys such as the National Health and Nutrition Examination Survey (NHANES), or special reporting systems, including cancer or birth defects registries. Investigators should consider both accuracy and efficiency when selecting a particular source for case identification. The goal is to identify as many true cases of disease as quickly and cheaply as possible. A variety of data sources that can be used for case identification are described in Chapter 4. The paragraphs that follow focus on two commonly used sources for case–control studies: hospitals and registries.

Virtually all hospitals in developed countries have computerized databases including names, addresses, diagnoses, and treatments for all in- and outpatients. Investigators can acquire access to these databases to identify subjects for a study after gaining approval of a hospital's ethics committee (which reviews all studies to ensure that the research is ethical and scientifically sound). Investigators can review these databases to find cases. Researchers typically try to identify cases soon after diagnosis, and so they review the database frequently. For example, investigators conducted a hospital-based case–control study on the risk of spontaneous abortion following an induced abortion.[14] Women who experienced a pregnancy loss (the cases) were identified each weekday from hospital admissions records so that they could be interviewed before discharge. Women who delivered liveborn infants at the same hospital comprised the control group. They were identified by reviewing delivery logs each weekday—again, in order to be interviewed before discharge. The investigators sought to interview subjects soon after their pregnancy outcomes in order to obtain accurate information on prior exposures.

Registry systems provide a good source of disease cases. These special reporting systems have been developed mainly for cancer and birth defects. For example, the federally funded Surveillance, Epidemiology and End Results (SEER) Program identifies newly diagnosed cases of 36 types of cancer in 11 population-based registries and 3 supplemental registries across the United States.[15] In addition, 34 U.S. states currently have population-based cancer registries.[16] The Massachusetts Cancer Registry is composed of a network of hospital tumor registrars based in more than 100 acute-care hospitals across the state.[17] The registrars review hospital records to identify all newly diagnosed cancers among state residents. When an incident case is found, the registrar reports identifying and demographic information to the central office. This information is confidential, but it can be made available to researchers for epidemiologic studies with approval from the registry's ethics committee.

Birth defects and cancer registries have greatly facilitated the conduct of case–control studies because investigators can identify all newly diagnosed cases, say within a geographic area, using a single source. For example, the case–control study on breast cancer risk in relation to PCE-contaminated drinking water used the Massachusetts Cancer Registry to identify all newly diagnosed breast cancer cases from 1983 through 1986 among residents of five Cape Cod towns.[11] These cases had been diagnosed and treated in more than 25 hospitals across the state. If they had not had access to the cancer registry, the investigators would have had to gain access to and review discharge records in all 25 hospitals in order to identify the cases.

Incident or Prevalent Cases

An important issue in the selection of cases is whether they should be incident or prevalent. Recall that prevalence depends on the rate at which new cases develop as well as the duration that the cases have the disease. Duration starts with diagnosis and ends with cure or death. Researchers who study the causes of disease prefer incident cases because they are usually interested in the factors that lead to developing the disease rather than factors that affect the duration of the disease.

Epidemiologists sometimes have no choice but to rely on prevalent cases. For example, etiologic studies of birth defects have been conducted exclusively on cases identified at birth. Although defects form during the first 3 months of gestation, it is difficult for researchers to identify malformed fetuses that are miscarried or voluntarily aborted, and so they rely on the surviving infants who are born 9 months later. Thus, etiologic studies of birth defects must be interpreted cautiously because it is impossible to determine if the exposure under study is related to the formation of the defect, the survival of the malformed fetus in utero, or a combination of the two.

Complete or Partial Case Ascertainment

There is a common misconception that a case–control study must include all cases of disease occurring within a defined population.[5(pp103–104)] This erroneous thinking arises from a desire to make the study results as generalizable as possible. However, validity is the primary goal of an epidemiologic study, and validity should never be sacrificed for generalizability. Even when no sacrifice is needed, it is unnecessary to include all cases. It is perfectly legitimate to include only a subset of cases. Thus, it is appropriate to conduct a study using cases identified at only one hospital, even when there are many hospitals in the same geographic area. However, regardless of whether ascertainment is complete, one must be able to define the case group's source population so that comparable controls from the same population can be selected. See Table 9–4 for a summary of the important issues in defining and selecting cases for a case–control study.

TABLE 9–4 Important Considerations in Case Definition and Selection

- Criteria for case definition should lead to accurate classification of diseased and nondiseased subjects.
- Efficient and accurate sources should be used to identify cases.
- Incident cases are preferable to prevalent ones for causal research.
- Partial case ascertainment is legitimate as long as the source population can be defined.

Selection of Controls

Controls are a sample of the population that produced the cases. Another term for the control group is *referent group* because it "refers to" the exposure distribution in the source population,[2] and another expression for the source population is *study base*. The guiding principle for the valid selection of cases and controls is that they represent the same base population. If this condition is met, then a member of the control group who gets the disease being studied "would" end up as a case in the study. This concept is known as the "would criterion" and its fulfillment is crucial to the validity of a case–control study.

Another important principle is that controls must be sampled independently of exposure status. In other words, exposed and unexposed controls should have the same probability of selection. This concept is best explained by returning to the hypothetical cohort and case–control studies of serum DDE levels and the risk of breast cancer described earlier in this chapter (see Tables 9–1 and 9–2). Of the 100,000 cohort members, 4000 were selected as controls, and so the overall control sampling fraction was 4000/100,000 or 4%. The 4% sampling fraction was the same for both the exposed and unexposed groups: $15,000 \times 0.04 = 600$ exposed controls, and $85,000 \times 0.04 = 3400$ unexposed controls. Thus, this study follows the principle that control selection should be independent of exposure status.

Sources of Control Identification

Investigators can use several sources to identify controls for case–control studies. They can sample individuals from the general population, individuals attending a hospital or clinic, individuals who have died, or friends or relatives identified by the cases. The following section describes each type of control along with its advantages and disadvantages.

POPULATION CONTROLS When cases are identified from a well-defined population (such as residents of a geographic area), population controls are typically selected as the referent group. Population controls can be identified using a variety of sources, including tax lists, voter registration lists, driver's license rosters, telephone directories, and national identity registries. Another common method for identifying population controls is through random digit dialing (a method for identifying a random sample of telephone subscribers living in a defined geographic area). In the case–control study of PCE-contaminated drinking water and risk of breast cancer, investigators used this method to identify living controls aged 64 years and younger.[11]

Population controls have one principal advantage that makes them preferable to other types of controls. Because of the manner in which the controls are identified, investigators are usually assured that they come from the same base population as the cases.

However, population controls have several disadvantages. First, it is time consuming and expensive to identify them, particularly when investigators use random digit dialing. In the study of PCE-contaminated drinking water and breast cancer, investigators had to call 2236 residential households in order to interview 184 eligible random digit dial controls. Approximately 63% of households did not have any resident who met the eligibility criteria, and 20% never answered the phone after many calls, and about 6% did not respond to the questions that determined eligibility. Ultimately, 249 households were identified with an eligible resident, of whom 184 were interviewed.

Second, it may be difficult to obtain the cooperation of population controls because they usually do not have the same level of interest in participating as do cases and controls identified from other sources. For example, in the study of PCE-contaminated drinking water and breast cancer, investigators interviewed 74% of contacted and eligible random digit dial controls and 90% of contacted and eligible cases. Investigators try to improve response rates by sending an introductory letter to potential subjects that describes the general purpose of the study. However, they cannot use this strategy with random digit dial controls because they usually do not know the names and addresses of the individuals.

The third limitation of population controls concerns their recall of past exposures. Because these investigators are generally healthy, their recall may be less accurate than that of the cases who are likely reviewing their history in search of a reason for their illness.

The use of random digit dial controls has another drawback. Although 94% of households in the United States have telephones, telephone subscribership is related to socioeconomic status, employment status, and race.[18] For example, the 1990 Census found that 53% of American Indians living on reservations had no telephone.[19] Thus, random digit dialing is not a good method for identifying controls in this population.

HOSPITAL OR CLINIC CONTROLS When investigators identify cases using hospital and clinic rosters, they typically identify controls from these same records. Thus, hospital and clinic controls have diseases or have experienced events (such as a car accident) for which they must seek medical care. The most difficult aspect of using these types of controls is determining which diseases or events are suitable for the control group. Two general principles should be followed in this regard. First, the illnesses in the control group should, on the basis of current knowledge, be unrelated to the exposure under study. For example, a case–control study of cigarette smoking and myocardial infarction should not use emphysema patients as controls because cigarette smoking is known to be a cause of emphysema.

Second, the illness of the controls should have the same referral pattern to the health care facility as that of the cases. For example, a case–control study of an acute condition such as a myocardial infarction should identify controls with other acute conditions such as appendicitis or car accident injuries. In theory, following this principle will help ensure that the study base is the same for cases and controls. However, in practice, this strategy may be difficult to implement, particularly given the drastic changes that are now occurring in health care delivery in the United States.

Sometimes hospital and clinic controls have a disease that is quite similar to that of cases. For example, birth defect studies often select case infants with one type of defect and control infants with other types of defects that are unrelated to the exposure under study. Because both the cases and controls are ill, parents' recall of past exposures should be comparable. This strategy minimizes "recall bias," a type of information bias that is discussed in more detail in Chapter 10.

Hospital controls have several advantages including easy identification and good participation rates, and so they are less expensive to identify than population controls. Furthermore, hospital controls are comparable to the cases if they come from the same source population. Finally, their recall of prior exposures is considered comparable to that of cases because they are also ill. Their main disadvantage is the difficulty in determining appropriate illnesses for inclusion. The illness should be unrelated to the exposure under study and should have the same referral pattern as cases.

DEAD CONTROLS In the past, epidemiologists recommended enrolling deceased controls when a portion or the entire series of cases was deceased when data collection began. These controls were usually identified by reviewing death records of individuals who lived in the same geographic area and died during the same time period as the cases. Investigators' rationale for selecting dead controls was to ensure comparable data collection procedures between the two groups. For example, if investigators collected data by interview, they would conduct proxy interviews for the dead cases and dead controls. These interviews were usually conducted with the subject's spouse, child, relative, or friend because these individuals were knowledgeable and willing to participate on behalf of the subject.

Today, most epidemiologists discourage the use of dead controls because these controls may not be a representative sample of the source population that produced the cases (which, by definition, consists of living people). For example, dead controls are more likely than living controls to have an exposure such as smoking because this activity causes death in a large number of people.[20]

FRIEND, SPOUSE, AND RELATIVE CONTROLS In rare circumstances, investigators use a case's friend, spouse, or relative (usually a sibling) as the control. These individuals are usually nominated by cases. They are selected because they are likely to share the cases' socioeconomic status, race, age, and educational level. Furthermore, sibling cases and controls share genetic traits. These individuals are usually willing to participate because they know the cases.

However, several difficulties arise with these controls. First, cases may be unable to nominate people to serve as controls, particularly if they have few appropriate friends, are widowed, or are only or adopted children. Second, cases may be unwilling to nominate anyone because they do not want to reveal their illness or their participation in a study. Third, these controls could possibly share the habits of the cases (such as smoking or drinking), which can lead to biased results if the study hypothesis involves these exposures. For example, in a study of alcohol use and esophageal cancer risk, cases might nominate their drinking partners as controls. This would make the exposure histories of case and controls similar and bias the results toward the null.

Summary

When selecting a source of controls, epidemiologists must always return to the basic purpose of the control group for guidance: to provide information on the exposure distribution in the population that produced the cases. Thus, controls must represent the source population and must be sampled independently of exposure status. In order to determine if the source population of cases and controls is the same, investigators must ask the following question: If a member of the control group actually had the disease under study, would he end up as a study case? The answer to this question should always be yes. These and other important considerations for selecting controls are summarized in Table 9–5.

TABLE 9–5 Important Considerations for Selecting Controls

■ Controls are a sample of the population that gave rise to the cases.

■ The purpose of the control group is to provide information on the exposure distribution in the source population.

■ The "would" criterion should be used to determine if the source population of cases and controls is the same.

■ Several sources are available for identifying controls including the general population; hospital and clinic rosters; death certificates; and cases' friends, spouses, and relatives.

■ Each source has advantages and disadvantages. If available, population controls are preferred because investigators are more confident that they come from the source population that produced the cases, and population controls avoid problems encountered with other types of controls.

Ratio of Controls to Cases

When the number of available cases is limited and controls are relatively plentiful, it is possible to increase the power of the study to detect an association by increasing the size of the control group. Control-to-case ratios of up to four to one help to increase power. Ratios higher than this are not considered worthwhile because of the increased cost of enrolling and gathering data from additional controls.[21] Of course, if the study is based on data that have already been collected, the cost of additional controls is so small that there is no reason to limit the ratio to four to one.

Methods for Sampling Controls

Consider a hypothetical cohort study with 100,000 individuals. Of these, 50,000 are exposed to high arsenic levels in drinking water and 50,000 are exposed to low arsenic levels. Both groups are enrolled in a study in 1990 and are followed for 10 years until 2000. The occurrence of skin cancer is the health outcome of interest. Obtaining a biological measure of arsenic exposure is quite expensive, so the investigator decides to conduct a nested case–control study within this cohort. Recall that the controls should be a sample of the source population that produced the cases. Exactly how should the investigator go about selecting controls?

The investigator could use one of three strategies (see Figure 9–1). In the first strategy, known as *survivor sampling*, the investigator would choose controls from cohort members who never experience skin cancer during the entire follow-up period. In this scenario, the controls would be selected from the "noncases" or "survivors" at the end of follow-up in 2000. Survivor sampling is the predominant method of selecting controls in traditional case–control studies.

The second approach is to sample controls from the population at risk at the beginning of follow-up in 1990. This approach is called *case-base* or *case-cohort* sampling.

The third strategy, known as *risk set sampling*, involves longitudinally sampling controls throughout the 10-year follow-up period. In this approach, the investigator selects a control from the population at risk when a case is diagnosed. Thus, when a skin cancer case is diagnosed, the investigator selects a control from members of the cohort who are at risk of skin cancer at that point in time.

Note that when case-base and risk set sampling methods are used, the control group could include future cases of skin cancer. Although this may seem incorrect, modern epidemiologic theory supports it. Recall that both diseased and nondiseased individuals contribute to the denominators of risks and rates in cohort studies. Thus, it is reasonable for the control group to include future cases of disease because it is merely an efficient way to obtain denominator data.

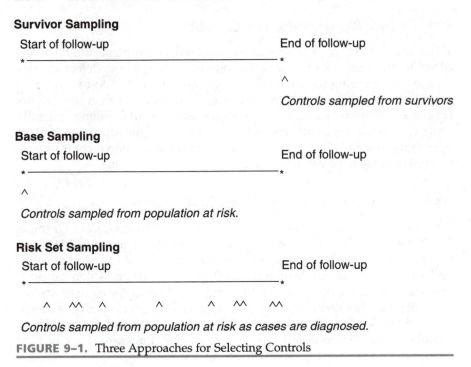

FIGURE 9–1. Three Approaches for Selecting Controls

Sources of Exposure Information

Case–control studies have been used to investigate the risk of disease in relation to a wide variety of exposures, particularly those related to lifestyle, occupation, environment, genes, diet, reproduction, and the use of medications.[22] Most exposures are complex, and so investigators must attempt to obtain sufficiently detailed information on their nature, sources, frequency, and duration during critical periods in a subject's life. A *critical period* is a time when the subject is susceptible to the action of an exposure. The timing and duration of a critical period depend on the particular exposure; it may be lifelong or limited to a narrow window. An example of the latter is the critical exposure period for teratogens that cause structural birth defects. This interval is limited to the first trimester of pregnancy when the fetal organs are forming.[23(pp17–82)]

Investigators can use a variety of sources to obtain exposure data for case–control studies, including in-person and telephone interviews; self-administered questionnaires; preexisting medical, pharmacy, registry, employment, insurance, birth, death, and environmental records; and biological specimens[22] (see Table 9–6). When selecting a particular source, investigators consider availability, accuracy, logistics, and cost.

TABLE 9–6   Sources of Exposure Information

Source	Types	Key characteristics
Questionnaires	Face-to-face, telephone, self-administered	Can obtain information on many exposures with relative ease and flexibility; must be carefully designed and administered to elicit accurate information; expensive
Preexisting records	Administrative, medical, regulatory	May be the only available exposure source; avoids bias; may be incomplete; may lack uniformity and details; inexpensive
Biomarkers	Levels in blood, urine, bone, toenails	Can estimate internal dose; infrequently used because of difficulty identifying valid and reliable markers of exposure to noninfectious agents; expensive

Accuracy is a particular concern in case–control studies because exposure data are retrospective. Relevant exposures may have occurred many years before data collection, making it difficult to gather correct information. For example, a case–control study of active and passive cigarette smoking and the occurrence of breast cancer gathered exposure data from participants' childhood through the present; this approach required most participants to recall their personal exposures over a 50-year span.[24]

In case–control studies, questionnaires serve as the most commonly used source of exposure data.[22] These are usually administered using face-to-face interviews, although telephone interviews (particularly computer-assisted telephone interviews) are becoming increasingly popular. Self-administered questionnaires are used least often, mainly because of poor response rates. However, they are inexpensive and good for socially sensitive topics. Whatever the method of administration, the questionnaire respondent is typically the index subject (that is, the case or control). A surrogate such as a spouse or other relative may be interviewed if the index subject cannot participate.

Questionnaires can elicit detailed information on a wide range of exposures with relative ease and flexibility.[22] However, questionnaires depend on the ability of participants to interpret the questions correctly and to remember and report information accurately. Thus, it is important that questions be worded clearly, placed in logical order, and have appropriate response options. In addition, questionnaires should be pretested to identify problems with comprehension, recall, response formulation, and recording. Memory aids such as a calendar of important life events are recommended to enhance respondents' recall. Furthermore, investigators must incorporate procedures to minimize interviewer bias, which stems from systematic differences in questioning the cases and controls (see Chapter 10). One method for reducing this type of bias is to mask interviewers to the outcome status of the study subjects.

Records collected for medical, administrative, and regulatory purposes are another important source of exposure data.[22] Such records may be the only source of information for certain occupational and environmental exposures. For example, most individuals are unaware of the contaminant levels in their drinking water, particularly levels from the past. Thus, investigators rely on routinely collected water-quality data as the source of exposure information for case–control studies of drinking water contaminants and adverse health outcomes.[25,26] Other reasons for using preexisting exposure data include low cost and lack of bias. Because these data are collected before the outcomes occur, investigators are not faced with systematic differences between cases and controls in data availability and collection methods, so the results are not biased. The principal disadvantages of preexisting exposure data include unavailability of records (particularly records from many years earlier), lack of uniformity, and lack of sufficient detail.[22] For example, data on drinking water contaminants are generally not available for private water supplies and for public supplies before 1974 when the federal Safe Drinking Water Act was passed.[27] Furthermore, water samples are usually collected from public taps (often in a town hall or school) and are assumed, rightly or wrongly, to represent the drinking water quality of all households in the area.

Biomarkers are the third main source of exposure data in case–control studies. These cellular, biochemical, and molecular alterations that indicate exposure are usually based on biological measurements of media such as blood, urine, bone, or nails.[28(p3)] For example, studies have measured urinary cotinine as a measure of exposure to cigarette smoke and urinary alkyl phosphate residues as a measure of organic phosphate pesticide exposure.[28(p8–9)] Although biomarkers have the potential for estimating the internal dose that a person has absorbed and for improving the accuracy of the exposure assessment, they have been used in only a small portion of case–control studies.[22] This is because it is difficult to identify valid and reliable markers for exposure to noninfectious agents. In addition, if the biomarker is collected after the disease has occurred, the presence of the disease and its treatment could affect its accuracy.

It costs more to collect exposure data specifically for a case–control study than to use existing records. A 30-minute telephone interview in the study of PCE-contaminated drinking water and breast cancer cost approximately $150 per participant.[11] In-person interviews, which were conducted when the subject was too ill to be interviewed by phone, were even more expensive because they involved travel to the participant's home. Laboratory tests for biomarkers can also be quite expensive. For example, analysis of polychlorinated biphenyls, dioxin, and metabolites of DDT in serum can cost about a $1000 per sample.[29]

Analysis of Case–Control studies

Calculation of Odds Ratios

Controls are a sample of the population that produced the cases. However, in most instances, investigators do not know the size of the total population that produced the cases. When investigators do not know the sampling fraction, they cannot fill in the total population in the margin of a two-by-two table or obtain rates and risks of disease (see Table 9–7).

When this situation occurs, investigators calculate a number called an *odds,* which functions as a rate or risk in a case–control study. The odds of an event is the probability that it will occur divided by the probability that it will not occur. For example, the probability of getting heads on one coin toss is 0.50, and the probability of not getting heads on one coin toss is also 0.50. Thus, the odds of getting heads on a coin toss is 0.50/0.50 or 1:1. In a case–control study, we calculate the odds of being a case (a/b) among the exposed and the odds of being a case among the nonexposed (c/d) (see Table 9–7). The ratio of these two odds is known as the *disease odds ratio.* The odds ratio is expressed as follows:

$$\frac{a/b}{c/d} \quad \text{or} \quad ad/bc$$

The odds ratio can also be conceptualized in another way: the ratio of the odds of being exposed among the cases (a/c) divided by the odds of being exposed among the controls (b/d). This is known as the *exposure odds ratio,* and it is algebraically equivalent to the disease odds ratio. Sometimes the term *cross-product ratio* is used for both of these odds ratios. In any case, the odds ratio provides an estimate of the relative risk, just as the incidence rate ratio and cumulative incidence ratio do.

Consider the following example. Investigators conducted a case–control study on the risk of spontaneous abortion among women who had a prior induced abortion.[14] Cases consisted of women who were hospital-

TABLE 9–7 Two-by-Two Table in a Case–Control Study

Exposed	Cases	Controls	Total Population
Yes	a	b	?
No	c	d	?

ized at a Boston hospital for a spontaneous abortion through 27 weeks' gestation. Controls consisted of women who delivered liveborn infants at the same hospital within a few days of the case's pregnancy loss. The exposure—prior induced abortion—could have occurred in the preceding pregnancy, in the more distant past, or not at all. The results for first-trimester pregnancy loss are summarized in Table 9–8.

Data from this study can be used to calculate the odds of being a case among women with a history of induced abortion (42/247) and the odds of being a case among women without a history of induced abortion (107/825). Thus, the disease odds ratio was (42/247)/(107/825) = (42×825)/(247×107) = 1.3. These data can also be used to calculate the exposure odds ratio. For cases, the odds of having prior induced abortion was 42/107, and the odds of having a prior induced abortion among controls was 247/825. Thus, the exposure odds ratio was (42/107)/(247/825) = (42×825)/(247×107) = 1.3. The interpretation of both odds ratios is as follows: Women with a prior induced abortion had a 30% increased risk of experiencing a first-trimester spontaneous abortion as compared to women with no such history.

Interpretation of Odds Ratios

Depending on the method of control selection, the odds ratio from a case–control study estimates different relative measures of comparison.[30] When survivor sampling is conducted, the odds ratio estimates the odds ratio in the base population. When case-base sampling is used, the odds ratio estimates the risk ratio in the base population. When risk set sampling is used, the odds ratio estimates the rate ratio in the base population.

Epidemiologists used to think that the "rare disease assumption" was needed for the odds ratio to estimate the measures described above. However, now we realize that none of these estimates requires this assumption.[30] This assumption is only needed when investigators want one measure to approximate another measure. For example, the odds ratio

TABLE 9–8   Results from a Case–Control Study of the Risk of Spontaneous Abortion Following Induced Abortion

Prior induced abortion	Spontaneous abortion (cases)	Delivery (controls)
Yes	42	247
No	107	825

Source: Data from Levin AA, Schoenbaum SC, Monson RR, Stubblefield PG, Ryan KJ, Association of induced abortion with subsequent pregnancy loss. *JAMA*. 1980;243:2495–2499.

calculated from a study that has used survivor sampling will be a good estimate of the risk ratio only when the disease is rare.

Calculation of Attributable Proportion

We cannot obtain the actual rate or risk of disease in the exposed and unexposed groups in a case–control study, except under special circumstances when the sampling fraction of the controls is known. Thus, it is not usually possible to obtain an absolute measure of comparison such as the risk and rate difference. The odds cannot be used as a substitute because the difference between two odds changes as the size of the control group changes. The ratio of two odds does not.

However, it is possible to obtain a measure of the public health impact of the exposure—the *attributable proportion among the exposed* (AP_e)—in case–control studies. This measure estimates the fraction of exposed cases that would be eliminated if the exposure were eliminated or reduced, assuming that the exposure caused the disease (see Chapter 3 for more details). Its formula in case–control studies is as follows:

$$[(OR - 1)/OR] \times 100,$$

where OR is the odds ratio. Thus, the attributable proportion in the spontaneous abortion study described earlier is $[(1.3 - 1)/1.3] \times 100$ or 23%. This means that 23% of the spontaneous abortions among exposed cases would not have occurred if the cases did not have a history of induced abortion. Of course, this calculation assumes that having an induced abortion causes women to miscarry subsequent pregnancies.

The Case-Crossover Study: A New Type of Case–Control Study

The case-crossover study is a new variant of the case–control study that was developed for situations "when brief exposure causes a transient change in risk of a rare acute-onset disease."[31] Thus, a case-crossover study is suitable for examining the risk of acute myocardial infarction immediately following heavy physical exertion,[32] risk of motor vehicle collision while using a cellular telephone,[33] and unsafe sex following the consumption of alcohol.[34] In each of these settings, the risk of the outcome is increased for a brief time after exposure.

The period of increased risk following the exposure is termed the hazard period.[32] In the case-crossover study, cases serve as their own controls and the exposure frequency during the hazard period is compared to that from a control period. The duration of the hazard period depends on the exposure and outcome being studied. For example, the period of increased risk for myocardial infarction following heavy physical activity is less than 1 hour.[35] As its originator states, "The case-crossover design is a scientific way to ask and answer the question clinicians so often ask patients: Were you doing anything unusual just before the episode?"[31]

A somewhat unusual characteristic of the case-crossover study is that cases serve as their own controls. However, this feature is also employed in crossover experimental studies in which the subject receives two treatments in succession and investigators compare outcomes in the same subject.[36] Because each person's response to one treatment is compared to his response to the other treatment, the influence of fixed personal characteristics (such as race and sex) is eliminated from the comparison. The notion of cases serving as their own controls also harkens back to the "counterfactual ideal" as described in Chapter 8. Recall that the counterfactual ideal means that the perfect comparison group for a group of exposed individuals consists of exactly the same individuals had they not been exposed.

The case-crossover method was first used to study the risk of myocardial infarction following heavy physical exertion and other activities.[32] The investigators interviewed 1228 myocardial infarction patients aged 22 to 92 years within 30 days of their heart attack. The interview obtained detailed data on physical exertion for the 26-hour period before the onset of heart attack symptoms, and the usual frequency of physical exertion during the previous year. A person was considered exposed if his or her physical exertion included, for example, jogging, tennis, fast biking, heavy gardening, heavy or deep snow shoveling, or ladder or stair climbing with a 50-pound load. The hazard period was defined as the 1-hour interval immediately before the start of the heart attack.

Control information was based on the case's exposures before the hazard period. In fact, the investigators made several comparisons. First, investigators compared the frequency of heavy exertion during the hazard period to a 1-hour control period at the same time of day on the day before the heart attack. Second, investigators examined the frequency of heavy exertion for several 1-hour control periods during the 25 hours preceding the hazard period. Third, they contrasted the exposure during the hazard period with the individual's usual exposure frequency over the previous year. The investigators obtained similar results, regardless of which control period was used. They found that the risk of myocardial infarction was approximately five to seven times higher following heavy exertion than following light or no exertion.

The case-crossover design was used to investigate the association between cellular-telephone calls and motor vehicle accidents.[33] The investigators studied 699 drivers who had cellular phones and were involved in motor vehicle collisions resulting in considerable property damage but no personal injury. Investigators interviewed the subjects and reviewed records of the accident and cellular telephone billing accounts. The hazard period was defined as the 10-minute interval before the time of the accident. Investigators compared the phone activity during the hazard period to a control period at the same time 1 week before the collision. The risk of collision was four times higher when a cellular phone was being used than when it was not in use. Increased relative risks were seen for both men and women, for drivers of all ages, and for drivers with all levels of experience.

Thus, the case-crossover study is a useful design for studying the influence of brief exposures on the risk of onset of acute incidents.[32] Because cases serve as their own controls, these studies have several advantages over traditional case–control studies. First, they are immune to a type of bias (called control selection bias) that arises from the selection of controls that are unrepresentative of the base population that produced the cases. Second, cases and controls have many identical characteristics (such as race and gender). Finally, they are more efficient and require fewer subjects than traditional case–control studies because variability is reduced. The chief features of case-crossover studies are summarized in Table 9–9.

Applications of Case–Control Studies

Case–control studies are currently being used for determining the causes of disease and for numerous "problem solving activities within the practice of public health and medicine."[37] These problem-solving activities include evaluating the effectiveness of vaccines, evaluating treatment and prevention programs,[38,39] and investigating outbreaks of disease.[40] Examples of these applications are described in the sections that follow.

Evaluation of Vaccine Effectiveness

Epidemiologists conducted a case–control study in Cali, Colombia, to determine the effectiveness of the BCG vaccine in preventing tuberculosis.[41] A citywide policy had been in place since 1973 to vaccinate all newborns and children under the age of 10 years. However, the 1980 incidence rate among children was 66.6 per 100,000 persons. The investigators conducted a case–control study instead of a prospective cohort or experimental

TABLE 9–9   Key Aspects of Case-Crossover Studies

- The purpose is to study the effect of transient exposures on the risk of acute events.
- Cases serve as their own controls.
- The brief period of increased risk following a transient exposure is termed the hazard period.
- The exposure frequency during the hazard period is compared to a control period.

study because it was less expensive, would take less time, and would provide clues about variability of vaccine effectiveness.

Cases included children under 15 years of age who had contracted tuberculosis from 1977 through 1982. Controls included similarly aged children who lived in the same households as the cases. None of the controls had ever shown symptoms or x-ray evidence of tuberculosis. The investigators stated that they decided to use a household control group because "it represented an easily accessible group with economic status and environmental exposure comparable to the children in treatment" (the cases). Exposure to the vaccine was determined by direct observation of the BCG scar on the children's backs or arms. In addition, the investigators obtained vaccination dates from parents and confirmed them by reviewing health center records. The exposure was defined as a positive history of BCG vaccination at birth.

The investigators found that vaccinated children had an overall 16% reduced risk of tuberculosis than did nonvaccinated children. However, there was a large risk reduction for children who were vaccinated during the early period of the program (the odds ratios ranged from 0.40 to 0.18), and those vaccinated during the latter part of the program derived no benefit. The authors hypothesized that the difference in effect stemmed from the use of different vaccine strains in the earlier and later parts of the program.

Evaluation of a Prevention Program

Investigators used a case–control study to evaluate the role of bicycle helmets in preventing head injuries during bicycle accidents.[42] Cases included 235 individuals who sought medical care for a bicycle-related head injury at one of five urban emergency departments in 1986 and 1987. A head injury was defined as an injury to the part of the head that a helmet would likely protect—the forehead, scalp, ears, skull, brain, and brain stem.

The investigators used two control groups: (1) 433 individuals seen at the same emergency departments for bicycle-related injuries not involving the head, and (2) 558 members of a health maintenance organization who reported having bicycle accidents in the past year. The latter group, which was a sample of the population at risk for bicycle injuries, consisted of cyclists who had experienced accidents, regardless of whether they were hurt or sought medical treatment.

Of the cases, 7% were wearing helmets when they were injured; 24% of the emergency room control group and 23% of the health maintenance organization controls were wearing helmets when their accidents occurred. After controlling for differences between cases and controls, the investigators found an 85% reduction in the risk of head injuries among those who used bicycle helmets (the odds ratio was 0.15). They concluded that bicycle helmets were very effective in preventing head injuries and recommended a major campaign to increase their use.

Investigation of an Outbreak of Disease

The first case reports of toxic shock syndrome (TSS) were reported in the medical literature in 1978.[43] TSS is a "severe, acute disease associated with strains of staphylococci of Phage Group 1 that produce[s] a unique epidermal toxin."[44] Little was known about its risk factors, but the case report data suggested that menstruation was associated with its onset. Thus, investigators undertook a case–control study to describe menstrual risk factors for TSS.[44]

The case group consisted of 35 premenopausal, nonpregnant women who were diagnosed with TSS in Wisconsin from 1975 through 1980. The case definition was quite restrictive and included numerous signs, symptoms, and laboratory test results. Controls were selected from a population of premenopausal, nonpregnant women who attended a Wisconsin gynecology clinic for routine care. Three age-matched controls were selected for each case. Cases and controls were interviewed to obtain data on their age, marital status, the intensity and duration of their menstrual flow, pattern of tampon and napkin use, preferred brands, birth control methods, vaginal infections, and sexual activities.

The investigators found that 97% (34/35) of the cases used tampons during the menstrual period near the onset of TSS, and 76% (80/105) of the controls always used tampons during their menstrual periods. Thus, there was almost an 11-fold increased risk of TSS associated with tampon use $[(34{\times}25)/80{\times}1) = 10.6]$. Although they were unsure of the exact role of the tampon in the pathogenesis of the disease, the investigators hypothesized that the highly absorbent tampon fibers might produce mucosal drying and micro ulcerations that could become infected with *Staphylococcus aureus*, a bacterium commonly isolated from the vagina or cervix of TSS patients.

Strengths and Limitations of Case–Control Studies

The main strength of case–control studies is their efficiency. They take less time and cost less money to conduct than cohort or experimental studies, primarily because the control group is a sample of the source population. Case–control studies are particularly efficient for studying rare diseases because fewer subjects are needed than for cohort studies, and for studying diseases with long induction and latent periods because long-term prospective follow-up is avoided. Another strength is their ability to provide information on a large number of possible risk factors, which makes case–control studies particularly useful for studying diseases whose etiology is largely unknown.

The main limitation of case–control studies is the increased possibility of bias because of the retrospective nature of the data collection. In fact, some epidemiologists have argued that case–control studies are not well suited for detecting weak associations—odds ratios less than 1.5—because of the likelihood of bias.[45] Although bias is unlikely to be entirely account-able for a strong association, it may entirely account for a weak association. (This phenomenon is discussed in more detail in Chapter 10.) In addition, because case–control studies rely on retrospective data collection, it is dif-ficult to establish a clear temporal relationship between the exposure and disease. As is discussed in Chapter 15, one of the most important guide-lines for inferring causation is establishing that the exposure preceded the disease. The strengths and weaknesses of case–control studies are summa-rized in Table 9–10.

Summary

Over the past 20 years, epidemiologists' view of the case–control study has changed dramatically. The case–control study is no longer seen as an inferior alternative to a cohort study, but rather it is regarded as a highly efficient design for learning about exposure–disease relationships. Case–control studies are particularly desirable when: (1) the exposure data are difficult or expensive to obtain, (2) the disease is rare or has a long latent and induction period, (3) little is known about the disease, or (4) the under-lying population is dynamic. In addition, the case-crossover study, a new variant of the case–control study, was designed to study the acute effects of transient exposures.

Case selection includes composing an accurate disease definition and determining accurate and efficient sources for identifying cases such as hospital or clinic patient rosters, death certificates, and special reporting

---

TABLE 9–10   Strengths and Weaknesses of Case–Control Studies

Strengths

- Efficient for rare diseases
- Efficient for diseases with long induction and latent periods
- Can evaluate multiple exposures in relation to a disease, so good for diseases about which little is known

Weaknesses

- Inefficient for rare exposures
- May have poor information on exposures because retrospective
- Vulnerable to bias because retrospective
- Difficult to infer temporal relationship between exposure and disease

systems. Incident cases are preferable over prevalent ones for causal research because investigators are usually interested in factors that lead to developing the disease rather than factors that affect the disease duration.

Controls are a sample of the population that produced the cases whose purpose is to provide information on the exposure distribution in the source population. The guiding principle for selecting controls is that they must represent the same base population as the cases and thus satisfy the "would criterion." Several sources are available for identifying controls including the general population (for example using random digit dialing); hospital or clinic rosters; death certificates; and friends, spouses, and relatives of cases. One of three sampling frames are used to select controls: noncases at the end of the observation period, the population at risk at the beginning of the observation period, or the population at risk when each case is diagnosed.

Because exposures are complex, sufficiently detailed information must be obtained on their nature, sources, frequency, and duration. Sources of exposure data include in-person and telephone interviews, self-administered questionnaires, preexisting records, and biological specimens. When selecting a particular source, investigators consider availability, accuracy, logistics, and cost. The analysis of case–control studies involves calculating a measure of association termed the odds ratio. This measure is used because disease rates cannot be calculated in most case–control studies.

The main advantages of case–control studies are efficiency and informativeness. Their main disadvantages include an increased possibility of bias and difficulty in establishing a clear temporal relationship between the exposure and disease because of the retrospective nature of the data.

References

1. Feinstein AR. Clinical biostatistics XX. The epidemiologic trohoc, the ablative risk ratio, and "retrospective" research. *Clin Pharmacol Ther.* 1973;14: 291–307.
2. Miettinen OS. The "case–control" study: valid selection of subjects. *J Chron Dis.* 1985;38:543–548.
3. Davis DL, Bradlow HL, Wolff M, Woodruff T, Hoel DG, Anton-Culver H. Medical hypothesis: xenoestrogens as preventable causes of breast cancer. *Environ Health Perspect.* 1993;101:372–377.
4. Levine R. Recognized and possible effects of pesticides in humans. In: Hays WJ Jr, Laws ER JR, eds. *Handbook of Pesticide Toxicology.* Vol 1. *General Principles.* San Diego, CA: Academic Press; 1991.
5. Rothman KJ, Greenland S. *Modern Epidemiology.* 2nd ed. Philadelphia, PA: Lippincott-Raven; 1998.
6. Ries LAG. Rates. In: Harras A, Edwards BK, Blot WJ, Ries LAG, eds. *Cancer Rates and Risks.* NIH pub no 96-691, pp 9–54. Bethesda, MD: National Cancer Institute; 1996.

7. Rothman KJ. Induction and latent periods. *Am J Epidemiol.* 1981;114:253–259.

8. National Academy of Sciences. Committee on the Biological Effects of Radiation (BEIR). *Health Effects of Low Levels of Ionizing Radiation, BEIR V.* Washington, DC: National Academy Press; 1989.

9. Schottenfeld D, Haas JF. Carcinogens in the workplace. *CA Cancer J Clin.* 1979; 29:144–168.

10. Jaffe HW, Choi K, Thomas PA, et al. National case–control study of Kaposi's sarcoma and *Pneumocystis carinii* pneumonia in homosexual men: part 1. Epidemiologic results. *Ann Intern Med.* 1983;99:145–151.

11. Aschengrau A, Paulu C, Ozonoff D. Tetrachloroethylene-contaminated drinking water and the risk of breast cancer. *Environ Health Perspect.* 1998;106: 947–953.

12. Cape Cod Commission. Cape Cod demographic and economic trends 1998. *CapeTrends.* 5th ed. Barnstable, MA: Cape Cod Commission; 1999.

13. Lasky T, Stolley PD. Selection of cases and controls. *Epidemiol Rev.* 1994; 16:6–17.

14. Levin AA, Schoenbaum SC, Monson RR, Stubblefield PG, Ryan KJ. Association of induced abortion with subsequent pregnancy loss. *JAMA.* 1980; 243:2495–2499.

15. National Cancer Institute. Available at: http://seer.cancer.gov/About SEER.html. Accessed August 2000.

16. Centers for Disease Control and Prevention. Available at: http:// www.cdc.gov/cancer/npcr/register.htm. Accessed September 2000.

17. Commonwealth of Massachusetts. Executive Office of Health and Human Services. Department of Public Health. *Cancer Incidence in Massachusetts 1982–1992: City/Town Supplement.* Boston, MA: The Commonwealth of Massachusetts; November 1995.

18. Telephone subscribership in the United States. Federal Communications Commission, Common Carrier Bureau. June 2000. Available at: http:// www.fcc.gov/ccb/stats. Accessed October 2000.

19. U.S. Department of Commerce, Bureau of Census. *Detailed Housing Characteristics, American Indian and Alaska Native Areas.* Series 1900 CH-2-1A. Washington DC: U.S. Government Printing Office; 1992.

20. McLaughlin JK, Blot WJ, Mehl ES, Mandel JS. Problems in the use of dead controls in case–control studies. I. general results. *Am J Epidemiol.* 1985;121: 131–139.

21. Gail M, Williams R, Byar DP, et al. How many controls? *J Chronic Dis.* 1976; 29:723–731.

22. Correa A, Stewart WF, Yeh H-C, Santos-Burgoa C. Exposure measurement in case–control studies: reported methods and recommendations. *Epidemiol Rev.* 1994;16:18–32.

23. Langman J. *Medical Embryology.* 4th ed. Baltimore, MD: Williams and Wilkins; 1981.

24. Lash TL, Aschengrau A. Active and passive cigarette smoking and the occurrence of breast cancer. *Am J Epidemiol.* 1999;149:5–12.

25. Aschengrau A, Zierler S, Cohen A. Quality of community drinking water and the occurrence of late adverse pregnancy outcomes. *Arch Environ Health.* 1993; 48:105–113.

26. Fagliano J, Barry M, Bove F, et al. Drinking water contamination and the incidence of leukemia. *Am J Public Health.* 1990;80:1209–1212.

27. Safe Drinking Water Act: Overview. Available at: http://www.iet.msu.edu/regchrt/ sdwaover.htm. Accessed 1999.

28. Hulka BS, Wilcosky TC, Griffin JD. *Biological markers in epidemiology.* New York, NY: Oxford University Press; 1990.

29. Glynn AW, Willett LB. Food frequency questionnaires as a measure of exposure to organochlorines in epidemiological studies. *Ohio State University Bulletin. Special Circular 163-99.* 19991–7.

30. Pearce N. What does the odds ratio estimate in a case-control study? *Int J Epidemiol.* 1993;22:1189–1192.

31. Maclure M. The case-crossover design: a method for studying transient effects on the risk of acute events. *Am J Epidemiol.* 1991;133:144–153.

32. Mittleman MA, Maclure M, Robins JM. Control sampling strategies for case-crossover studies: an assessment of relative efficiency. *Am J Epidemiol.* 1995;142:91–98.

33. Redelmeier DA, Tibshirani RJ. Association between cellular-telephone calls and motor vehicle collisions. *N Engl J Med.* 1997; 336:453–458.

34. Seage GR, Holte S, Gross M et al. Case–crossover study of partner and situational factors for unprotected sex. J Acquir Immune Defic Syndr. 2002; 432–439.

35. Mittleman MA, Maclure M, Tofler GH, et al. Triggering of acute myocardial infarction by heavy exertion: protection against triggering by regular exertion. *N Engl J Med.* 1993;329:1677–1683.

36. Louis TA, Lavori PW, Bailar JC, Polansky M. Crossover and self-controlled designs in clinical research. *N Engl J Med.* 1984;310:24–31.

37. Armenian HK, Lillienfeld DE. Overview and historical perspective. *Epidemiol Rev.* 1994;16:1–5.

38. Comstock GW. Evaluating vaccination effectiveness and vaccine efficacy by means of case–control studies. *Epidemiol Rev.* 1994;16:77–89.

39. Selby JV. Case-control evaluations of treatment and program efficacy. *Epidemiol Rev.* 1994;16:90–101.

40. Dwyer DM, Strickler H, Goodman RA, Armenian HK. Use of case–control studies in outbreak investigations. *Epidemiol Rev.* 1994;16:109–123.

41. Shapiro C, Cook N, Evan D, et al. A case–control study of BCG and childhood tuberculosis in Cali, Colombia. *Int J Epidemiol.* 1985;14:441–446.

42. Thompson RS, Rivara FP, Thompson DC. A case–control study of the effectiveness of bicycle safety helmets. *N Engl J Med.* 1989;320:1361–1367.

43. Todd J, Fishaut M, Kapral F, Welch T. Toxic-shock syndrome associated with phage-group-I staphylococci. *Lancet.* 1978;2:1116–1118.

44. Davis JP, Chesney PJ, Wand PJ, LaVenture M, and the Investigation and Laboratory Team. Toxic-shock syndrome. Epidemiologic features, recurrence, risk factors, and prevention. *N Engl J Med.* 1980;303:1429–1435.

45. Austin H, Hill HA, Flanders WD, Greenberg RS. Limitations in the application of case–control methodology. *Epidemiol Rev.* 1994;16:65–76.

EXERCISES

1. Define each of the following terms:
   A. TROHOC and TROHOC fallacy
   B. Odds ratio
   C. Case-crossover study

2. Describe the situations in which it is desirable to conduct a case–control study.

3. Suppose that a case–control study was conducted among men in the United States in order to find out whether a mother's use of hormones during pregnancy influenced her son's risk of developing testicular cancer later in life. Investigators selected 500 cases who were hospitalized for testicular cancer and 1000 controls. The study found that 90 cases' mothers and 50 controls' mothers had used hormones during pregnancy.
   A. Set up the two-by-two table for these data.
   B. Calculate the odds ratio.
   C. State in words your interpretation of this odds ratio.
   D. Suppose that the investigators hire you as an epidemiologic consultant to help them design this study. They ask you what type of control group is most appropriate for the study. Briefly describe the control group that you would advise them to select and justify your choice.
   E. The investigators also ask you to describe the purpose of the control group in a case–control study. What would you tell them?
   F. In this study, you have a choice between choosing incident and prevalent cases of testicular cancer. Which would you choose? Give two reasons to justify your answer.

4. Describe one advantage and one disadvantage of using population controls in a case–control study.

5. State the main advantages and disadvantages of case–control studies.

10

Bias

LEARNING OBJECTIVES

By the end of this chapter, the reader will be able to:

- Describe the key features and provide examples of selection bias including control selection bias; self-selection bias; and differential surveillance, diagnosis, or referral.

- Describe the key features and provide examples of observation bias including recall bias, interviewer bias, loss to follow-up, and differential and nondifferential misclassification.

- Discuss how the magnitude and direction of bias can affect study results.

- List the ways that selection and observation bias can be avoided or minimized.

Introduction

Epidemiologic studies generally compare the frequency of disease in two (or more) groups according to a characteristic of interest. The characteristic is usually called the exposure. Those who have it form the exposed group, and those who do not have it form the unexposed group. Epidemiologists compare measures of disease frequency in two ways: (1) absolute comparisons such as risk or rate differences and (2) relative comparisons such as risk ratios, rate ratios, and odds ratios. These comparisons are commonly called measures of association or measures of effect. The particular measure that is calculated depends on the study design, the type of data, and the goal of the comparison. Absolute measures typically describe the public health impact of an exposure, and relative measures describe the strength of the causal relationship between an exposure and a disease.

After investigators calculate the measure of association, they must evaluate whether or not the observed result is true. That is, they must assess the internal validity of the study results. A study is considered valid only when the following three alternative explanations have been eliminated:

1. *Bias.* A systematic error in the design or conduct of study that leads to an erroneous association between the exposure and disease.

2. *Confounding.* The mixing of effects between the exposure, the disease, and a third variable that is termed a confounder. Like bias, confounding distorts the relationship between an exposure and disease.

3. *Random error.* The probability that the observed result is due to "chance," an uncontrollable force that seems to have no assignable cause.[1(p309)]

If systematic bias, confounding, and random error have been ruled out as alternative explanations, the investigator may conclude that the association is true, and that the study has internal validity. Only after an observed study result is deemed valid is it appropriate to assess whether the exposure has actually caused the outcome. As is discussed in Chapter 15, making causal inferences is a complicated judgment.

In addition, internal validity must be established before the study results can be generalized to populations beyond the study subjects. The evaluation of generalizability or "external validity" requires review of the study methods, the makeup of the study population, and subject-matter knowledge such as the biological basis of the association. For example, a valid study of risk factors for coronary artery disease among middle-aged American men might be applicable to middle-aged European men but not middle-aged American or European women because of biological differences between the sexes. On the other hand, an invalid study of coronary artery disease among middle-aged American men is generalizable to no one.

This chapter discusses bias in general terms and then focuses on the two main forms of bias in epidemiologic research: selection bias and observation bias. Following a definition of each type of bias, the chapter describes the ways in which they arise and methods for avoiding or minimizing them. Chapters 11 and 12 define and describe methods of assessing and controlling the other two alternative explanations for study findings: confounding and random error.

Overview of Bias

Epidemiologists define bias as a systematic error that results in an incorrect or invalid estimate of the measure of association. Bias can be introduced at any stage of a study—during the design, data collection, analysis, or even publication stages. An epidemiologist's definition of bias differs from another common definition of the term: "preference or inclination, especially one that inhibits impartial judgement" or "prejudice."[1(p176)] In epidemiologic studies, bias does not usually occur because the investigator is "prejudiced," but rather because of ignorance or unavoidable decisions made during the course of a study.

Bias can occur in all types of epidemiologic studies. However, retrospective studies are more susceptible to bias than prospective ones because of differences in the timing of the study. The two main types of bias are selection bias, which can occur during the selection of study participants, and observation or information bias, which can occur during data collection.

When evaluating a study for the presence of bias, investigators must: (1) identify its source, (2) estimate its magnitude or strength, and (3) assess its direction. Recognizing and carefully dissecting the source of the bias is a prerequisite for assessing its strength and direction. Regarding its magnitude, a small amount of bias does not usually have a major impact on the study results; however, a large amount of bias can completely alter the study findings. For example, consider a true relative risk of 2.5. A small amount of bias might alter the estimate of the true relative risk slightly, say to 2.3 or 2.8. Even though some bias is present, the conclusion that there is a moderate association is still correct. However, a large amount of bias could alter the estimate of the true relative risk a great deal, say to 1.0 or 5.0, and lead to an incorrect conclusion.

The impact of bias also depends on the size of the true measure of association. Bias can account entirely for a weak association, but it is unlikely to account entirely for a strong one. This is one reason why epidemiologists have greater confidence that strong associations are valid.

Regarding the direction of the bias, a systematic error can pull the estimate either toward the null or away from the null. Stated another way, it can either underestimate or overestimate the true measure of association. When the direction of the bias is toward the null, it means that the error is obscuring an association that is truly present. For example, if the true relative risk is 2.0, the observed relative risk will be lower, say 1.5. On the other hand, bias can create a spurious or false association when none exists. If the true relative risk is null, the observed relative risk will be either greater than 1 or less than 1 (say 1.5 or 0.5).

Unfortunately, little can be done to fix or remove a bias once it has occurred. Thus, investigators must attempt to avoid bias by carefully designing and conducting the study. For example, epidemiologic studies include features such as masking in order to avoid bias. Key facts about bias are summarized in Table 10–1.

TABLE 10–1 Key Facts about Bias

- An alternative explanation for an association.
- Usually does not result from a "prejudiced" investigator.
- Can pull an association either towards or away from the null.
- Amount of bias can be small, moderate, or large.
- Is avoided when the study is carefully designed and conducted.

Selection Bias

Selection bias is "an error due to systematic differences in characteristics between those who are selected for study and those who are not."[2(p153)] Thus, selection bias results from procedures used to choose study subjects that give a result among participants that is different from the result that would occur among individuals who were eligible but not included in the study. This type of bias is more likely in case–control and retrospective cohort studies because both the exposure and outcome have occurred by the time the subjects are selected. Selection bias does not occur in prospective cohort and experimental studies because only the exposure has occurred by the time of selection.

It is often easier to understand selection bias if it is described in the context of a specific study design. Selection bias occurs in a case–control study if selection of cases and controls is based on differing criteria that are related to exposure status. In contrast, selection bias occurs in a retrospective cohort study if selection of exposed and unexposed individuals is related to developing the outcome of interest.[3(pp273–274)]

Selection bias can occur in several ways, including selection of an inappropriate control group in case–control studies (control selection bias); refusal, nonresponse, or agreement to participate that is related to the exposure and disease (self-selection bias); selection of the general population as a comparison group in an occupational cohort study ("healthy-worker effect"); and differential surveillance, diagnosis, or referral of study subjects according to their exposure and disease status.[3(pp273–274)] Examples of these types of selection bias in case–control and cohort studies are described in the following sections.

Selection Bias in a Case–Control Study

CONTROL SELECTION BIAS Consider a hypothetical case–control study in which investigators are evaluating the role of Pap smears in the prevention of cervical cancer. Investigators identify newly diagnosed cases of cervical cancer by reviewing medical records from the hospitals where cancer patients are treated. They select population controls from among women who live in the same neighborhoods as cases. Investigators identify controls by canvassing neighborhoods on foot during weekday working

TABLE 10–2 Observed Relationship Between Cervical Cancer and Pap Smears

Pap smear	Cases	Controls
Yes	100	100
No	150	150
Total	250	250

hours. Thus, only controls who are at home during canvassing periods are included in the study. The investigators select and enroll 250 cases and 250 controls. Women are considered "exposed" if they had a Pap smear within 1 year of their diagnosis date (for cases) or an index date (for controls). Comparable index dates are assigned to controls to "match" the cases' diagnosis dates. Let us examine the data that are produced by this study (see Table 10–2).

Exactly 40% of cases and 40% of controls had a Pap smear within the last year. Using the formula for the odds ratio (OR) provided in Chapter 9, we find that there is no association between Pap smears and cervical cancer [OR = (ad/bc) = $(100 \times 150)/(150 \times 100)$ = 1.0].

Unfortunately this study suffers from control selection bias because the researchers included only controls who were home at the time of recruitment. It turns out that women who are at home during the day are less likely to be employed, and so are less likely to have regular medical checkups, including Pap smears. Thus, the selected control group has a lower proportion of women with prior Pap smears than does the source population that produced the cases. The data presented in Table 10–3 depict the true relationship between Pap smears and cervical cancer that would have been produced in the absence of selection bias.

Note that 40% of the cases and 60% of the controls had a Pap smear within the last year. Thus, the true odds ratio is $(100 \times 100)/(150 \times 150)$ or 0.44, which means that there is a 56% reduced risk of cervical cancer among women with recent Pap smears. Thus, the results with control selection bias were biased toward the null.

TABLE 10–3 True Relationship Relationship Between Cervical Cancer and Pap Smears

Pap smear	Cases	Controls
Yes	100	150
No	150	100
Total	250	250

Returning to the description of selection bias in case–control studies, we can conclude that selection bias occurred in this study because investigators did not use the same criteria to select cases and controls (being home during the day was required for controls but not for cases) and these criteria were related to exposure status (recent Pap smear history). Furthermore, because different criteria were used for selecting cases and controls, the control group did not accurately represent the exposure distribution in the source population that produced the cases. Control selection bias can be avoided by remembering the purpose of the control group: to sample the exposure distribution in the base population that gave rise to the cases. Using identical selection criteria will ensure that cases and controls come from the same source population.

SELF-SELECTION BIAS Case–control studies with low and moderate participation rates are susceptible to self-selection bias arising from: (1) refusal or nonresponse by participants that is related to both the exposure and disease, or (2) agreement to participate that is related to both the exposure and disease. A low or moderate participation rate does not necessarily result in selection bias if the reasons and rates of participation are similar for exposed and unexposed cases and controls. However if subjects in a particular exposure-disease category (for example, exposed cases) are more or less likely to participate than subjects in another category, the observed measure of association will be biased. Scenarios with and without self-selection bias are depicted in Table 10–4.

The best way to ensure that self-selection bias does not occur is to obtain high participation rates among both cases and controls. Although there is no magical response rate that guarantees the absence of selection bias (other than 100%), most epidemiologists are satisfied with participation rates greater than 80%. In addition, investigators can assess the pres-

TABLE 10–4   Scenarios With and Without Self-Selection Bias

No Self-Selection Bias: Equal Participation Rates

	Cases*	Controls*
Exposed	60%	60%
Unexposed	60%	60%

Self-Selection Bias: Unequal Participation Rates that Are Associated with the Exposure and Disease

	Cases*	Controls*
Exposed	80%	60%
Unexposed	60%	60%

*Note: The numbers in the cells are participation rates.

ence of self-selection bias in a study by examining the characteristics of participants and nonparticipants.

DIFFERENTIAL SURVEILLANCE, DIAGNOSIS, OR REFERRAL Selection bias can occur in a case–control study as a result of differential surveillance, diagnosis, or referral of cases that is related to the exposure.[3(pp273–274)] For example, investigators conducted a case–control study on the risk of venous thromboembolism among oral contraceptive users.[4] Cases were women aged 20 to 44 years who were hospitalized for a venous thromboembolism. Controls were similarly aged women who were hospitalized for an acute illness or elective surgery at the same hospitals. Of the cases, 72% reported using oral contraceptives and only 20% of controls used them. Based on these findings, investigators calculated a 10.2-fold increased risk of thromboembolism among current oral contraceptive users.

The investigators acknowledged that the high relative risk might be due to "bias in the criteria for hospital admission."[4] Several reports of the association between oral contraceptives and venous thromboembolism had already been published before this study was conducted. As a result of these previously published studies, healthcare providers were more likely to hospitalize women with symptoms of thromboembolism who were currently taking oral contraceptives than symptomatic women who were not taking oral contraceptives. The tendency to hospitalize patients on the basis of their exposure status (selection bias) led to a stronger observed relationship between oral contraceptives and thromboembolism than truly existed. Another study based on cases who were diagnosed before there was widespread knowledge of this association found only a fourfold increased risk.[5]

How could selection bias have been avoided in this study? First, investigators could have conducted a community-based case–control study that included both hospitalized and nonhospitalized subjects. Or, the hospital-based study could have been limited to severe cases of thromboembolism for whom hospitalization was required. Both of these options would have resulted in an unbiased prevalence of oral contraceptive use in the case group. The former option is preferable to the latter one, which restricts the case series by severity and so reduces generalizability.

Selection Bias in a Cohort Study

Selection bias occurs in a cohort study when the choice of exposed and unexposed individuals is related to developing the outcome of interest. Retrospective cohort studies are prone to selection bias because both the exposure and disease have occurred by the time of subject selection.

A real-life example of selection bias occurred in a proportional mortality study among Portsmouth (New Hampshire) Naval Shipyard workers who serviced nuclear-powered submarines.[6] At the time of the study, the shipyard workforce consisted mainly of men who worked as welders, electricians, pipe fitters, and mechanics. Workers who performed "nuclear work" were exposed to radiation during the course of repairing or refueling atomic reactors on the submarines. Concern that radiation exposure was causing leukemia was prompted by a 63-year-old nuclear welder who was diagnosed with the disease. He also reported that several younger fellow workers had died.

The case triggered a proportional mortality ratio (PMR) study that was conducted by an investigative team from a major Boston newspaper. Recall that a PMR study is a special type of cohort study that is commonly used to investigate occupational exposures (see Chapter 8). Based solely on death certificate data, a PMR study compares the observed number of deaths resulting from a specific cause in the exposed group with the expected number of deaths in the general population. Rather than calculating the expected number of deaths using cause-specific mortality *rates*, investigators calculate the expected numbers using cause-specific *proportions* of deaths. The resulting measure of association—the PMR—is interpreted like a relative risk.

The study investigators reviewed more than 100,000 death certificates from New Hampshire, Massachusetts, and Maine from 1959 through 1977, and identified 1722 deaths among former Portsmouth Naval Shipyard workers. Death certificates contain the decedent's name, address, age, occupation, and cause of death, and the name and address of the individual's next of kin or an informant. The investigators used the occupational information noted on the certificate to determine if the decedent was a Portsmouth Naval Shipyard worker. Subsequently, investigators contacted next of kin to determine if the decedent had been exposed to radiation. Relatives were contacted for only 34% of the deceased workers (146 nuclear workers and 379 nonnuclear workers). Then investigators compared the observed number of deaths among the nuclear and nonnuclear workers to the expected number based on the U.S. male population (see Table 10–5).

The investigators reported 56 observed cancer deaths and 31.5 expected cancer deaths among the nuclear workers (PMR = 1.78), and 88 observed cancer deaths and 79.7 expected cancer deaths among nonnuclear workers (PMR = 1.10). For leukemia, investigators found 6 observed deaths and 1.1 expected deaths among the nuclear workers (PMR = 5.6), and 2 observed deaths and 2.8 expected deaths among the nonnuclear workers (PMR = 0.7). Thus, the PMR study suggested a strong association between nuclear shipyard work and cancer deaths, particularly those caused by leukemia.

Although the positive findings were credible because radiation had been established as a cause of leukemia by this time,[7] the authors acknowledged that the results "seem out of proportion to predictions based on prior knowledge of the effects of ionising radiation in man." They also suggested

TABLE 10–5 Results from the Portsmouth Naval Shipyard Proportional Mortality Study: Observed and Expected Deaths Among Nuclear and Nonnuclear Workers

	Nuclear		Nonnuclear	
Cause of death	*Observed*	*Expected*	*Observed*	*Expected*
All deaths	146	146	379	379
All cancer deaths	56	31.5	88	79.7
Leukemia	6	1.1	2	2.8
Other lymphatic and hematopoietic cancers	4	1.8	6	4.3
All other cancer deaths	46	28.6	80	72.6

Source: Data from Najarian T, Colton T. Mortality from leukemia and cancer in shipyard workers. *Lancet.* 1978;1:1019.

that the findings should "prompt more careful and thorough cohort studies of workers in naval yards where nuclear-powered vessels are serviced."[6]

Shortly after these results were published, the National Institute for Occupational Safety and Health (NIOSH) undertook a retrospective cohort study of all 24,545 white male civilian employees of the Portsmouth Naval Shipyard during 1952 to 1977.[8] The study was done at the request of the Subcommittee on Health and the Environment of the U.S. House of Representatives to determine if the PMR study results could be confirmed and to evaluate the dose–response relationship between low-level radiation exposure and cancer.

NIOSH investigators used employment records to identify the workers and examined film badge records to determine their external radiation dose. They traced cohort members through 1977 and found that 76% were still alive, 19% were deceased, and 4% were lost to follow-up. The researchers found 201 cancer deaths among radiation-exposed workers and 726 cancer deaths among unexposed workers. The investigators then compared the observed number of deaths due to a particular cause to the expected number derived from mortality rates (not proportions) based on the U.S. male population (see Table 10–6).

The retrospective cohort study did not find an excess of deaths caused by leukemia, all lymphatic and hematopoietic cancers, or all cancers combined among the radiation-exposed workers. In fact, fewer deaths were observed than were expected for all of the examined causes. For unexposed workers, the number of observed deaths was close to that expected for all cancers, leukemia, and all lymphatic and hematopoietic cancers. Thus, unexposed workers had a higher overall mortality rate and a higher cancer mortality rate than did the exposed workers.

The cohort study investigators thought that the discrepant findings between their study and those of the PMR study "seem to reflect our more

TABLE 10-6   Results from the Portsmouth Naval Shipyard Retrospective Cohort Study: Observed and Expected Number of Deaths Among Radiation-Exposed and Unexposed Workers

Cause of death	Exposed		Unexposed	
	Observed	Expected	Observed	Expected
All deaths	833	1065.3	3733	3801.0
All cancer deaths	201	218.5	726	723.6
Leukemia	7	8.3	31	29.1
All lymphatic and hematopoietic cancers	15	21.1	67	67.7

Source: Data from Rinsky RA, Zumwalde RD, Waxweiler RJ, Murray Jr. WE, Bierbaum PJ, Landrigan PJ, et al. Cancer mortality at a naval nuclear shipyard. *Lancet.* 1981;1:231–235.

complete ascertainment of the PNS [Portsmouth Naval Shipyard] cohort, thus avoiding selection bias, and our more accurate classification of workers as to their radiation dose."[8] In fact, when a third team of investigators conducted a formal comparison of the two studies, they found selection bias as well as observation bias in the PMR study, which apparently biased the results away from the null.[9]

Selection bias occurred in the PMR study because the investigators identified deceased shipyard workers through the death certificate review and, to a lesser extent, because they contacted only about one third of the next of kin. Thus, the PMR study did not identify all deaths, and deaths that were identified were more likely to be leukemia deaths among exposed shipyard workers. Note from comparing the data from Tables 10–5 and 10–6 that the PMR study found 6 of the 7 leukemia deaths among the radiation-exposed workers identified by the retrospective cohort study but found only 2 of 31 leukemia deaths among unexposed workers.[10(p253)] Some disagreements about leukemia as the cause of death also accounted for the different numbers.[9]

The "healthy-worker effect," another form of selection bias, occurred in both studies, but it had a greater impact in the PMR study. The healthy-worker effect means that the rates of death and disease among a working population are typically lower than those of the general population. The lower overall rates can occur even when a noxious substance is present that elevates specific rates of diseases. The healthy-worker effect occurs when the general population, which consists of both healthy and ill people, is selected for comparison to a relatively healthy working population. In the PMR study, the healthy-worker effect was greater among radiation-exposed workers because the health requirements for entry into nuclear work were more stringent than those for nonnuclear work.[8] Workers were required to undergo a special physical examination to be eligible for nuclear work. In addition, nuclear workers were examined every 3 years, and those with abnormal findings were removed from the nuclear program. This difference in health requirements clearly affected the mortality rates: the nuclear workers experienced a 25% lower mortality rate than the general population, and the nonnuclear workers experienced only a 2% lower mortality rate.

The healthy-worker effect influenced the PMR study to a greater extent than it affected the retrospective cohort study because PMR studies suffer from an inherent limitation called the "see-saw effect." In PMR studies the expected numbers are based on proportions rather than rates, and the sum of proportions is, by definition, 1.0. Thus, a deficit in the proportion of one cause of death (such as cardiovascular disease) necessarily results in corresponding increase in the proportion of another cause of death (such as cancer).

Note that the PMR study also suffered from recall bias, a form of observation bias that is described in greater detail later in this chapter. Recall bias arose from inaccurate work exposure histories given by next of kin. Next of kin of nuclear workers were less likely to mention that their relative was a nuclear worker if he did not die of cancer. These inaccurate work exposure histories resulted in an overestimation of the true measure of association between radiation exposure and deaths from cancer. This bias was avoided in the retrospective cohort study because work histories were obtained from employment records.

Unfortunately, once the PMR study was completed, nothing could be done to correct these biases. A valid relationship between shipyard work and the risk of leukemia could only be determined by conducting the more carefully designed retrospective cohort study.

Now let us turn to an example of another form of selection bias—self-selection bias—that occurred in a Centers for Disease Control cohort study on the risk of leukemia among participants in military maneuvers at the 1957 atmospheric nuclear bomb test.[11,12(p119)] This study was prompted by a former paratrooper who thought that his leukemia diagnosis was associated with his presence at the bomb's detonation.

The study included 3224 men who were present at the detonation, which was known as "Smoky." Investigators were able to determine health outcomes for 76% of cohort members—82% of whom were traced by investigators and 18% of whom contacted investigators because of publicity. Given the well-known relationship between radiation and leukemia, it is not unreasonable to think that the 18% who contacted study investigators were more likely to have leukemia. This, in fact, was true. Investigators found a total of 9 leukemia cases in the cohort; 5 cases occurred among the 82% traced by the study investigators and 4 cases occurred among the 18% who self-identified. Thus, there was a much higher proportion of leukemia among self-identified cohort members than among those followed in the

TABLE 10-7 Key Facts about Selection Bias

- Selection bias is an error that arises from systematic differences in selecting the study groups.
- It is more likely to occur in case–control and retrospective cohort studies because both the exposure and disease have occurred by the time of subject selection.
- Specific types include control selection bias in case–control studies; healthy-worker effect in occupational cohort studies; self-selection bias; and differential surveillance, diagnosis, or referral of subjects according to exposure and disease status.
- Little can be done to fix this bias once it has occurred.
- Methods for avoiding it include using the same criteria for selecting cases and controls, obtaining high participation rates, taking diagnostic and referral practices into account when designing a study, and refusing to accept self-referrals into a study.

traditional manner. Although health outcomes were unknown for the 24% of the cohort who were lost to follow-up, it has been estimated that one to three cases of leukemia occurred in this group.[12(p119)] Although self-selection bias in this study was small, the example illustrates why it is unwise to accept self-referrals into a study.

In summary, selection bias can be a serious problem in epidemiologic studies. Because little can be done to correct this bias once it has occurred, epidemiologists must use all available methods to avoid it. The key facts about selection bias are summarized in Table 10–7.

Observation Bias

Observation or information bias is "a flaw in measuring exposure or outcome data that results in different quality (accuracy) of information between comparison groups."[2(p86)] Observation bias arises from a systematic difference in the way that the exposure or outcome is measured between compared groups. For example, observation bias can occur in a case–control study if different techniques are used for interviewing cases and controls. Or, it can occur in a cohort study if different procedures are used to trace and obtain outcome information on exposed and unexposed subjects. Observation bias can be thought of as a measurement error that distorts the true association between an exposure and disease. Key features of this bias are: (1) it occurs after the subjects have entered the study; (2) it pertains to how the data are collected; and (3) it often results in incorrect classification of participants as either exposed or unexposed or as diseased or not diseased.

Like selection bias, observation bias can create either an upward or downward bias. The direction depends on a number of factors, particularly whether the measurement error on one axis (exposure or disease) depends on the other axis (disease or exposure). Unlike selection bias, which is much more likely to occur in retrospective studies, observation bias can occur in both prospective and retrospective studies.

The following section describes and provides examples of the different types of observation bias including recall bias, interviewer bias, loss to follow-up, and differential and nondifferential misclassification. Investigators' decision to use a particular data collection method (such as interviews, preexisting records, biological specimens) is influenced by its potential for observation bias. This bias can be avoided only by carefully designing and conducting the study.

Recall Bias

Recall bias occurs when there is a differential level of accuracy in the information provided by compared groups. Thus, recall bias occurs in a case–control study if cases are more or less likely than controls to recall and report prior exposures, and it occurs in a cohort study if exposed subjects are more or less likely than unexposed subjects to recall and report subsequent diseases. These differences in reporting accuracy are thought to result from subjects' failure to report information rather than a tendency to fabricate information. Differential recall can bias the true measure of association either toward or away from the null. The direction depends on which subjects (cases versus controls or exposed versus unexposed subjects) have less accurate recall.

Although recall bias can occur both in case–control and in retrospective cohort studies, it is typically described in the context of a traditional case–control study with nondiseased controls. For example, consider a hypothetical case–control study of birth defects that includes malformed infants as cases and healthy infants as controls. Exposure data are collected at postpartum interviews with the infants' mothers. In the classical recall bias scenario, the data gathered from case mothers is more accurate than data from control mothers. This is because mothers of malformed case infants have been carefully reviewing every illness that occurred during the affected pregnancy, every medication taken, every alcoholic beverage consumed, and so forth, for a possible reason for their child's defect. In contrast, mothers of healthy control infants have spent less time reviewing their prenatal activities. The results of the hypothetical study are depicted in Table 10–8. Note that 100% of the case mothers (20 of 20) reported their prior exposures, and only 75% of healthy control mothers (15 of 20) did so. Thus the observed odds ratio is biased upward by 40%. If there had been more underreporting among control mothers, the upward bias would have been even larger.

It is also possible to envision a scenario in which the cases' mothers underreport their prior exposures. This is likely to occur with socially sensitive exposures such as drug and alcohol use that mothers may not wish to admit for fear of being blamed for their child's condition. Table 10–9 presents data from a hypothetical study in which all control mothers (20 out of 20) reported their prior exposures and 75% of case mothers (30 out of 40) did so. This differential recall biases the true odds ratio downward by 37% [(2.7 - 1.7)/2.7 x 100% = 37%]. Here, if more underreporting had occurred among case mothers, the downward bias would have been even larger. The two examples presented in Tables 10–8 and 10–9 demonstrate that the direction of the bias is determined by which group has less accurate recall.

Now let us consider a real-life example of recall bias that occurred in a case–control study of drug exposures among children with congenital heart defects.[13] Cases were infants born with congenital heart disease from 1973 through 1975. Controls were randomly selected infants born in the same time period and geographic area. Information on prenatal drug exposure was obtained by self-administered questionnaires. Data on hormonal drug exposures were obtained from closed-ended questions, and data on nonhormonal drug exposures were obtained from an open-ended question ("Did you take any prescription or nonprescription drugs during your pregnancy?").

The study found an 80% increased risk of cardiac malformations among infants of women who recalled using the antinausea medication Benedectin in early pregnancy. Because information about the use of this medication was derived from the open-ended question, the researchers

TABLE 10–8 Recall Bias Scenario: Controls Underreport Exposure

	Truth			Observed study data	
	Case	Control		Case	Control
Exposed	20	20	Exposed	20	15
Unexposed	80	80	Unexposed	80	85
Total	100	100	Total	100	100
	Odds ratio: 1.0			Odds ratio: 1.4	

TABLE 10–9 Recall Bias Scenario: Cases Underreport Exposure

	Truth			Observed study data	
	Case	Control		Case	Control
Exposed	40	20	Exposed	30	20
Unexposed	60	80	Unexposed	70	80
Total	100	100	Total	100	100
	Odds ratio: 2.7			Odds ratio: 1.7	

concluded that it was "likely to be subject to some recall bias." In fact, a later study that was specifically designed to evaluate and remove recall bias found no meaningful increase in the risk of cardiac malformations in association with Benedectin use.[14]

Only a few investigations have been conducted to document the actual occurrence of recall bias. Some of these studies have validated information obtained at postpartum interviews with that in medical records. For example, Werler and colleagues assessed whether recall bias was present in postpartum interviews with mothers of malformed and nonmalformed infants by comparing interview data with that documented during pregnancy in obstetric records.[15] Mothers of malformed infants were more accurate reporters than mothers of nonmalformed infants for some but not all variables. Mothers of malformed infants were more accurate reporters regarding use of birth control after conception and history of urinary tract infections, but the two groups of mothers showed similar reporting accuracy for history of an elective abortion and over-the-counter drug use. These results suggest that recall bias is not widespread and may be exposure-specific.

In another study, investigators evaluated the presence of recall bias by comparing associations with normal controls to those with malformed controls. Investigators analyzed data on 4918 babies with severe defects and 3029 babies without defects from a large population-based case–control study.[16] Odds ratios for 10 specific defect-risk factor associations were compared between normal and malformed controls. For example, the investigators examined associations between advanced maternal age and the risk of Down's syndrome, maternal diabetes, and cardiovascular malformations; and the association between maternal cigarette smoking and the risk of oral clefts. The investigators found that the odds ratios were not appreciably different with either type of control, and they concluded that concern for recall bias was "overrated."

Although we await more research to determine the true extent of recall bias in epidemiologic studies, it is worthwhile to review the steps that epidemiologists take to minimize or avoid its occurrence. The most common method for minimizing recall bias is to select a diseased control group. For example, the study of Benedectin and cardiac malformations compared cases with a specific cardiac malformation to cases with other cardiac malformations.[14] This type of comparison assumes that the exposure is unlikely to cause a general increase in the risk of all types of defects.

Another way to avoid recall bias is to design a structured questionnaire so that exposure ascertainment is complete and accurate. This strategy is important because the opportunity for recall bias *increases* as exposure ascertainment *decreases*. For example, a study was conducted to examine the effect of questionnaire design on the ascertainment of drug use during pregnancy.[17] Investigators obtained information on drug use in the past year from a sequence of three questions. The first question was open ended: "Were any medications prescribed to you during pregnancy?" The second question asked about drug use for selected indications: "Did you take any medication for the following indications: pain, tension, seizures, or nausea and vomiting?" The third question asked about the use of specifically named drugs: "Did you take any of the following medications? Aspirin, Tylenol, Valium, Compazine, Benedectin. . . ." The investigators found that the open-ended question led to vast underreporting of drug use (see Table 10–10). There was much less underreporting in response to questions about drug use for certain indications and use of specifically named drugs. The investigators concluded that a comprehensive series of questions is necessary to obtain as complete information as possible.

Another way to improve the accuracy of questionnaire data, particularly for socially sensitive topics that the study subject is reluctant to reveal to another individual, is to use either a self-administered questionnaire or Audio Computer-Assisted Self-Interviewing (A-CASSI). Self-administered questionnaires are usually scannable to facilitate computer entry. The study subject simply fills out the questionnaire using paper and pencil. A laptop computer with an audio component is used to administer the A-CASSI questionnaire. The computer reads each question to the subject and waits for the subject to enter a response before moving onto the next question.

Both approaches have been useful for obtaining information on sensitive topics such as alcohol drinking, illicit drug use, and sexual behaviors. For example, the HIV (Human Immunodeficiency Virus) Vaccine Preparedness Study, a prospective cohort study of nearly 5000 individuals at high risk for HIV-1 infection, compared A-CASSI to in-person interviews for gathering information on sexual behaviors.[18] Subjects were randomized to receive either personal or computer interviews. The investigators found that men who had sex with men were much more likely to report

TABLE 10–10   Ascertainment of Drug Use According to Type of Question Asked

| | Question asked* | | | | | | | |
| | Open-ended | | Indication | | Specific drug name | | Total users | |
Drug	No.	%	No.	%	No.	%	No.	%
Valium	4	13	18	58	9	29	31	100
Darvon	5	25	8	40	7	35	20	100
Aspirin	2	1	146	77	41	22	189	100
Acetaminophen	0	0	58	61	37	39	95	100

*Asked in sequence
Source: Data from Mitchell AA, Cottler LB, Shapiro S. Effect of questionnaire design on recall of drug exposure in pregnancy. Am J Epidemiol. 1986;123:670–676.

that they had unprotected receptive anal intercourse using the A-CASSI format. Although the true prevalence of unprotected receptive anal intercourse was unknown in this population, the higher proportion reported using A-CASSI is probably more accurate than that reported in personal interviews.

Either self-administered questionnaires or A-CASSI interviewing can be used in clinical and research settings. For example, the subject can fill out the questionnaire in the clinic waiting room. Or, a self-administered questionnaire can be mailed to subjects at home to be filled out at their convenience. Of course, self-administered questionnaires require that subjects have an adequate reading and comprehension level; that they fill out the questionnaire completely; and, if mailed, that they return the completed questionnaire to the investigator. Although a small token of appreciation is often included with mailed questionnaires (such as cash or movie passes), response rates are typically lower than those for other formats. The A-CASSI format avoids many of these problems because little or no reading is required, and the questionnaire can be taken into the field with laptop computers.

Still another way to avoid recall bias is to forgo questionnaires entirely and rely instead on biological measurements and preexisting records for the necessary study data. For example, medical records are often used to provide detailed information on diseases and their treatment. These records are also used to validate information provided at interviews and to provide evidence for or against recall bias. For example, exposure data in the case–control study of Benedectin use and congenital heart disease came from two sources: a postdelivery telephone interview and the prenatal obstetric record.[14] Drug use noted in the prenatal record was assumed to be free of recall bias because it was recorded before the pregnancy outcome was known. Investigators analyzed Benedectin exposure according to the interview alone, the obstetric record alone, and both sources combined. They found virtually identical results, and so provided evidence against differential recall.

Investigators often determine if recall bias is present by asking subjects about their knowledge of the study hypothesis, usually at the end of the interview. The association between the exposure and outcome is analyzed separately among those with and without knowledge of the hypothesis. Those with knowledge are thought to be more prone to recall bias than those without such knowledge.

For example, women were asked the following questions in a study of periconceptional folic acid exposure and the risk of neural tube defects: "Have you heard there are any vitamins, minerals, or anything else, that may cause or reduce the risk of birth defects?" If a participant answered "Yes," she was asked, "What vitamin or mineral?" and "Is this related to any particular birth defect?"[19] About 17% of case mothers and 3% of control mothers reported that folic acid reduced the risk of neural tube defects. Daily use of folic acid was associated with a 20% decreased risk of neural tube defects among women who were familiar with the study hypothesis and a 60% reduction among women who did not have any *knowledge* of the hypothesis. These findings led the investigators to conclude that recall bias was present among women who knew the study hypothesis and to draw their main conclusions from women without knowledge of the hypothesis.

Interviewer Bias

Interviewer bias is a systematic difference in soliciting, recording, or interpreting information that occurs in studies using in-person or telephone interviews. Interviewer bias can occur in every type of epidemiologic study. It can occur in a case–control study when interviewers are aware of the disease status of a subject and question cases and controls differently about their exposures. It can occur in cohort and experimental studies when interviewers are aware of the exposure or treatment status of a subject and query exposed and unexposed subjects differently about their diseases.

Interviewer bias can be avoided by masking interviewers to the subject's disease (in case–control studies) or exposure status (in cohort and experimental studies). However, masking interviewers is often impossible because of the information they learn while talking with the subjects. For example, a case–control study of the risk of spontaneous abortion among women with a prior induced abortion collected data using personal interviews during the subject's hospital stay.[20] It was impossible to mask the interviewers to subjects' disease status because cases who had spontaneous abortions were placed on gynecology floors, and delivery patient controls were placed on obstetric floors and were frequently interviewed in the presence of their newborn infants.

Another way to avoid interviewer bias is to design standardized questionnaires consisting of closed-ended, easy-to-understand questions with appropriate response options. This decreases the likelihood that the interviewer will "interpret" the question for the subject or will need to "probe" the subject for an appropriate response. Understandable questions that are asked in exactly the same manner are key components for reducing interviewer bias.

Writing understandable questions is both an art and a science that falls under the discipline of psychometrics. Epidemiologists should collaborate with psychometricians when designing questionnaires in order to avoid several problems.[21(pp309–336)] First, investigators should avoid the use of ambiguous wording that can be interpreted in various ways. For example, the question "Have you ever smoked?" is ambiguous because it is unclear if cigarettes, cigars, pipes, or a nontobacco product are the intended focus of the question. Second, researchers should avoid using two questions in one such as "Do you get out of breath when you walk up a hill?" This question is problematic because a negative answer might mean that the respondent does not walk up hills or that he or she does not get out of breath doing so. Third, researchers should avoid the use of words such as medical terms or the names of chemicals that the respondent may not understand. Fourth, they should avoid asking about events and activities that the subjects cannot possibly remember, such as "Tell me the names of all the brands of condoms that you have used since you first started having sex." Fifth, investigators should avoid questions that are not self-explanatory, such as "How is heat delivered to your home?" Although the investigator may be interested in responses such as hot air, steam, gas, or oil, the respondent might reply "In a truck!" Finally, researchers should avoid questions that have too many ideas, such as "Have you ever used oral contraceptives, condoms, diaphragms, or intrauterine devices?" A positive response will indicate that one or more of these contraceptives has been used but will not indicate which one(s).

Investigators need to write clear questions in the subject's native language. In addition, given the international nature of epidemiologic research and the populations being studied, epidemiologists often need to translate their questionnaires into several languages. For example, a study of lead exposure among children in Boston conducted interviews in English, Spanish, and Cape Verdean creole.[22] Because accurate translation can be tricky, it is standard practice to have one person translate the questionnaire into the foreign language and have another person translate it back to English and compare the back-translation to the original. Word-for-word translations are often but not always the goal, for it is necessary to take into account cultural differences in the conceptualization of health-related events and exposures.

Another way to avoid interviewer bias is to instruct interviewers on appropriate questioning techniques, such as nondirective probing—a neutral way of searching for a suitable answer. These probes are needed when it is clear from a respondent's response that he has not understood the question. Nondirective probing techniques include simply repeating the question or asking "What do you mean by . . . ?" It is also important to note that the race, gender, age, and sexual orientation of an interviewer will have an impact on data quality. The demographic characteristics of the interviewer are usually matched to those of the subject in order to obtain the most accurate responses.

Loss to Follow-up

A serious concern in both cohort and experimental studies, loss to follow-up arises when subjects can no longer be located or when they no longer want to participate in a study. Loss to follow-up is problematic because it can reduce the power of the study to detect associations that are truly present (because of the smaller sample size available for analysis), and it can bias the study results. A number of epidemiology textbooks classify loss to follow-up as a form of selection bias—specifically, self-selection bias. However, we believe that it is more appropriate to consider it a form of observation bias because loss to follow-up typically occurs long after the subjects have been selected for study. Selection bias, on the other hand, refers to the selective entry of subjects into a study.

Nondifferential loss to follow-up refers to losses on one axis (disease or exposure) that are unrelated to the other axis. An example is the loss of diseased individuals that occurs equally among exposed and unexposed individuals. Differential loss to follow-up refers to losses that are related to both exposure and disease. An example is when these losses are more or less likely to occur among exposed individuals who develop the disease than among unexposed individuals who develop the disease.

Whether or not loss to follow-up biases the results depends on the measure of association being used (that is, absolute or relative) and whether the losses are nondifferential or differential. For example, non-differential loss to follow-up that is associated only with disease (for example, there are equal losses of diseased individuals among exposed and unexposed subjects) results in observed disease incidences that are lower than true incidences. This means that the relative measure of association will not be affected, but the absolute measure will be biased toward the null. On the other hand, differential loss to follow-up can bias relative and absolute measures of association either upward or downward. For example, if loss to follow-up occurs only among exposed subjects who develop the disease, the observed measure of disease frequency in the exposed group will be lower than the truth, and so relative and absolute measures of association will be biased toward the null. On the other hand, if loss to follow-up occurs only among unexposed subjects who develop the disease, the observed measure of disease frequency in the unexposed group will be lower than the truth, and both relative and absolute measures of association will be biased upward.

Unfortunately, it is rarely possible to determine if losses are differential or nondifferential because outcome information is unknown. Thus, it is important to maintain high and similar follow-up rates for compared groups. To achieve this goal, epidemiologists use many methods to maximize retention and trace study subjects including collecting baseline information to help locate study subjects, maintaining regular mail or personal contact with participants, sending additional mailings to nonrespondents, and checking numerous tracing resources. These methods are described in detail in Chapter 8.

It is very difficult to determine if a study with high losses to follow-up is valid. Consider, for example, a randomized experimental study of factory workers in Zimbabwe to determine if a peer-led condom distribution and educational program about HIV and sexually transmitted diseases would reduce HIV-1 incidence more than counseling and testing alone.[23] A total of 2719 HIV-negative individuals were recruited at 40 factories and followed for a 3-year period. Ninety-four individuals became infected during 3731 person-years of follow-up. The incidence rate at the 20 factories that received the intervention was 2.12 per 100 person-years, and the incidence rate at the 20 control factories was 3.20 per 100 person-years. Thus, there was a 34% reduced risk of infection among the intervention factory workers. Although the study suggested that the peer-led condom distribution and education program was highly effective at reducing transmission of HIV-1, the results were difficult to believe given the high losses to follow-up. The clue that high losses occurred is the number of person-years of follow-up (3731 person-years). If no losses had occurred, the population of 2719 individuals would have accrued approximately 8000 person-years of follow-up. (This calculation assumes that the 2625 individuals who remained uninfected each accrued 3 follow-up years, and that the 94 individuals who became infected each accrued 1.5 follow-up years.) The 3731 person-years of follow-up accrued by the study population represent only 46% of the possible total. In fact, the investigators related that 22% of the participants did not have a single follow-up visit. Such high losses make the results difficult to interpret. If these losses were differential (that is, losses were more or less likely among infected intervention factory workers than among infected control factory workers), the results could be biased either toward or away from the null. Thus, the observed benefit of the intervention could be either much greater or much smaller than reported.

As another example, the results of a recent HIV incidence study are difficult to interpret because of high losses to follow-up. This study determined the incidence rate of HIV-1 infection among injecting drug users in New York City from 1992 through 1997, and compared rates during this time period to those seen in prior years.[24] The investigators gathered data from 10 separate incidence studies, each of which included from 96 to 1671 injecting drug users. HIV-1 incidence rates in these 10 populations ranged from 0 to 2.96 per 100 person-years during 1992 to 1997, with a weighted average of 0.7 per 100 person-years. These incidence rates were well below rates observed in studies in New York City from the late 1970s and early 1980s (13 per 100 person-years) and mid-1980s and early 1990s (4.4 per 100 person-years). The authors concluded that "the very large HIV epidemic among injecting drug users appears to have entered a declining phase" and that "very large high-seroprevalence HIV epidemics may be reversed."[24(p352)] These results were widely publicized and ultimately resulted in funding cuts to drug treatment and prevention programs because it appeared that the HIV epidemic had ended among New York

City drug users. Unfortunately, it is difficult to know if the observed decline was real or spurious, because follow-up rates in the 10 cohorts ranged from 36% to 95%. Only two of the cohorts reported follow-up rates greater than 80%—the typical standard of success. A time trend such as this is believable only if all the follow-up rates are above 80%, including those from earlier periods.

Misclassification

Misclassification, also called measurement error, is probably the most common form of bias in epidemiologic research. Misclassification means that there is an error in the classification of the exposure or the disease. For example, misclassification occurs when an exposed individual is classified as unexposed or vice versa. It also occurs when a diseased individual is classified as nondiseased or vice versa.

Misclassification arises in many ways. In case–control and retrospective cohort studies, the relevant exposures may have occurred many years before data collection, and so it is difficult for subjects to recall their exposures accurately. For example, a case–control study of cigarette smoking and the occurrence of breast cancer gathered exposure data from childhood through the present, thereby requiring subjects to recall exposures over a 50-year period.[25] Exposure misclassification also occurs when broad exposure definitions are used. For example, occupational exposure definitions such as job title (for example, individuals who ever worked as a plumber) are misclassified because it is unlikely that all individuals with a particular job title actually sustain the exposure(s) of interest. Characteristics of the work environment such as ventilation and the use of personal protective equipment also influence whether an individual in a particular job is actually exposed.

Like exposure misclassification, disease misclassification can also occur as a result of an overly broad definition. For example, because birth defects are rare, investigators often group together defects into larger organ group categories such as cardiovascular defects, central nervous system defects, and so on. This leads to misclassification when the exposure is related to some but not all defects in the group. For example, if all cardiovascular defects are grouped together, misclassification of disease will occur if the exposure increases the risk of one type of cardiovascular defect but not others.

Like losses to follow-up, there are two types of misclassification— nondifferential and differential. Differential misclassification refers to errors on one axis (exposure or disease) that are related to the other axis (exposure or disease). For example, if there is an error in exposure classification, it is more or less likely to occur for a diseased individual than a nondiseased individual. Depending on who is misclassified, differential misclassification can bias results either upward or downward. Non-differential misclassification refers to errors on one axis that are unrelated to the other axis. For example, if there is an error in exposure classification, it occurs with equal likelihood among diseased and nondiseased individuals. Nondifferential misclassification of dichotomous variables biases results toward the null.

Consider the following hypothetical example illustrating the effect of exposure misclassification in a case–control study. Completely accurate data are described in Table 10–11. The odds ratio based on the completely accurate data is as follows: OR = ad/bc = (200×200)/(100×100) = 4.0.

Table 10–12 presents data with a high degree of differential misclassification. In this scenario, 50% of the exposed controls and 100% of the exposed cases provide accurate exposure information. Note that the different degree of accuracy between the compared groups is a key feature of differential misclassification. The odds ratio for these data is: (200×250)/(100×50) = 10.0. In this scenario, differential misclassification biased results away from the null (from 4.0 to 10.0). If there had been less misclassification (say 75% of the exposed controls gave accurate information), there would have been less bias away from the null.

What happens when the reverse occurs—that is, when exposure information from controls is more accurate than that obtained from cases? A scenario in which 50% of the exposed cases and 100% of the controls provided accurate exposure information is shown in Table 10–13. Now the odds ratio is calculated as follows: (100×200)/(100×200) = 1.0. In this scenario, differential misclassification biased the results toward the null (from 4.0 to 1.0). Again, if there had been less misclassification, the bias would not have been as strong.

TABLE 10–11 Completely Accurate Exposure Data from a Hypothetical Case–Control Study

	Cases	Controls
Exposed	200	100
Unexposed	100	200
Total	300	300

TABLE 10–12 Differential Misclassification of the Exposure in a Hypothetical Case–Control Study: Case Information Is More Accurate Than Control Information

	Cases	Controls
Exposed	200	50
Unexposed	100	250
Total	300	300

What happens if both cases and controls give similarly inaccurate information on their exposure histories? For example, say that 50% of the exposed cases and 50% of the exposed controls do not remember their exposure and are classified as unexposed (see Table 10–14). This scenario is an example of nondifferential misclassification, because there is the same degree of accuracy between the compared groups.

The odds ratio is now $(100 \times 250)/(50 \times 200) = 2.5$. This is lower than the odds ratio based on the completely accurate data (4.0). Again, there would be less bias toward the null if less nondifferential misclassification had occurred.

This hypothetical example illustrates that differential exposure misclassification can lead to either an upward or downward bias, and that the direction depends on which group has more misclassification. It also illustrates that nondifferential misclassification of a dichotomous exposure biases results toward the null. In fact, it can bias the results beyond the null if misclassification is severe. In the most extreme case, it can lead to a completely inverse association (for example, a twofold increased risk becomes a 50% decreased risk). The bias is much less predictable when the misclassified exposure variable has three or more categories. Of course, nondifferential exposure misclassification does not affect truly null associations.

Nondifferential exposure misclassification probably occurred in a 1981 study of vaginal spermicides and congenital disorders.[26] This cohort study was conducted among members of the Group Health Cooperative, a Seattle health maintenance organization that provided medical services as well as most prescription drugs. Spermicides were provided either free of

TABLE 10–13 Differential Misclassification of the Exposure in a Hypothetical Case–Control Study: Control Information Is More Accurate Than Case Information

	Cases	Controls
Exposed	100	100
Unexposed	200	200
Total	300	300

TABLE 10–14 Nondifferential Misclassification of the Exposure in a Hypothetical Case–Control Study

	Cases	Controls
Exposed	100	50
Unexposed	200	250
Total	300	300

charge or at reduced cost to cooperative members. The investigators used the cooperative's computerized health and pharmacy records to compare the prevalence proportions of major congenital anomalies among offspring of women who did and did not fill prescriptions for vaginal spermicides. A woman was considered to be a spermicide user if a prescription for any kind of vaginal spermicide was filled within 600 days before the end of a pregnancy and if no subsequent prescription for any other contraceptive, except for a diaphragm, was filled after the spermicide prescription and before the conclusion of the pregnancy. The investigators found that the prevalence of major malformations was about twice as high among users than nonusers. In particular, the prevalence of limb reduction defects, congenital neoplasms, chromosomal abnormalities, and hypospadias was increased among spermicide users.

This study had three potential sources of exposure misclassification that stemmed from the operational definition of spermicide use. The first arose from grouping all types of vaginal spermicides into one exposure category. About 80% of spermicide use in the health plan involved products containing the chemical octoxynol, and about 20% involved products containing nonoxynol 9. Grouping these two chemicals into one exposure variable may result in misclassification if only one of the chemicals is related to risk of congenital disorders. The second potential source resulted from investigators' use of pharmacy records to ascertain the exposure. It is quite possible that some women who were considered exposed never used the prescribed spermicides, and that some women who were considered unexposed used spermicides obtained from other sources (such as the neighborhood drug store). The third source of exposure misclassification resulted from using a wide exposure window—filling a prescription within 600 days before delivery or abortion. The relevant exposure period for the development of most congenital defects in the study is the first 3 months of pregnancy, the period of organogenesis. Although the long exposure window includes this period, it also includes periods during which exposure to spermicides was irrelevant (for example, after the defect formed). These three potential sources of misclassification were most likely nondifferential. That is, the classification error regarding spermicide use was as likely to occur for a malformed infant as for a normal infant. Thus, the results were likely biased toward the null, and so the true relationship between spermicides and congenital disorders is probably stronger than observed.

What can epidemiologists do to reduce misclassification? The main way is to improve the accuracy of the collected data. Investigators can do this by using multiple measurements of exposure and disease. For example, because blood pressure readings are prone to error, investigators typically rely on several readings to determine if a subject has hypertension. Similarly, because air pollution levels vary widely according to the time of day and location of measurement, investigators often set up continuous monitors in several locations in the study area.

Another method for improving accuracy is through validation—that is, corroborating the collected data using several sources. For example, investigators often review medical records to confirm the occurrence of self-reported diseases. Whenever possible, the corroborating evidence should be objective in nature, such as laboratory test results.

Still another way to improve data accuracy is to switch to a better information source for the exposure or disease. For example, the retrospective cohort study of Portsmouth Naval Shipyard workers improved upon the exposure assessments used in the earlier PMR study by using employment records and film badges to determine external radiation exposure instead of next-of-kin reports.[6,8] Investigators from the study on vaginal spermicides and congenital disorders could have improved the exposure data accuracy either by augmenting or substituting pharmacy data with participant interviews.[26]

A final way to reduce misclassification is to define the exposure and disease using sensitive and specific criteria. Regarding the exposure, criteria should be able to discern those truly exposed and to exclude those who are not. Likewise, criteria for the disease should pick up cases of disease as well as eliminate those without disease. For example, criteria for a myocardial infarction definition should include clinical symptoms, electrocardiogram (ECG) findings, and the results of cardiac enzyme tests. Using only a symptom such as chest pain to define this disease would result in misclas-

---

TABLE 10–15 Key Facts About Observation Bias

- Observation error is an error that arises from systematic differences in the way information on exposure and disease is obtained from study groups.

- This type of bias results in participants who are incorrectly classified as either exposed or unexposed or as diseased or not diseased.

- It occurs after subjects have entered the study.

- It can occur in both retrospective and prospective studies.

- Specific types include recall bias, interviewer bias, loss to follow-up, and differential and nondifferential misclassification.

- Methods for avoiding observation bias include masking interviewers and subjects to the study hypothesis (interviewer and recall bias); using a control group that is composed of diseased individuals (recall bias); carefully designing the study questionnaire (interviewer and recall bias); relying on noninterview data (interviewer and recall bias); using a variety of methods to maximize retention and successfully trace study subjects (loss to follow-up); using multiple measurements, the most accurate information source, and sensitive and specific criteria to define the exposure and disease (misclassification).

sification, because people with other conditions that produce chest pain would be erroneously included and because people with "silent" heart attacks that occur without chest pain would be missed.

The key facts about observation bias are summarized in Table 10–15. A good epidemiologic study incorporates a number of design features to minimize or eliminate this type of bias.

Summary

Bias is a systematic error that results in an incorrect estimate of the measure of association. The two main types of bias are selection and observation bias. When evaluating a study for the presence of bias, it is necessary to identify its source, to assess its strength, and to determine its direction. Bias can pull the estimate of association either toward or away from the null. Although a small amount of bias does not usually have a major impact on the results, a large amount of bias can completely alter the study findings. Little can be done to fix or remove a bias once it has occurred, and so investigators must avoid it by carefully designing and conducting the study.

Selection bias arises from systematic differences in selecting the study groups. This type of bias is more likely in case–control and retrospective cohort studies because the exposure and disease have occurred at the time of subject selection. There are several ways that selection bias can occur, including selection of an inappropriate control group in a case–control study (control selection bias); nonresponse or agreement to participate that is related to exposure and disease (self-selection bias); selection of the general population as a comparison in a cohort study (healthy-worker effect); and differential surveillance, diagnosis, or referral of study subjects according to exposure and disease status. Selection bias can be avoided by using the same criteria to select cases and controls, obtaining high participation rates, taking diagnostic and referral practices into account when designing the study, and excluding self-referrals from a study.

Observation bias is an error that arises from systematic differences in the way that information on exposure and disease is obtained from the study groups. It results in participants whose exposure or disease status is incorrectly classified. There are several ways that observation bias may occur including differential accuracy in the information provided by compared groups (recall bias); systematic differences in the way that interview data are solicited, recorded, or interpreted (interviewer bias); differential and nondifferential loss to follow-up; and measurement errors known as differential and nondifferential misclassification. Differential misclassification occurs when misclassification errors on one axis (disease or exposure) are related to the other axis, and nondifferential misclassification occurs when the errors on one axis are unrelated to the other axis. The methods for avoiding observation bias include masking interviewers and study subjects to the study hypothesis (interviewer and recall bias), using a control group consisting of diseased individuals (recall bias), carefully designing the study questionnaire (interviewer and recall bias), using successful methods to retain and trace study subjects, and obtaining accurate exposure and disease data.

References

1. Pickett JP, exec ed. *The American Heritage Dictionary of the English Language.* 4th ed. Boston, MA: Houghton Mifflin Co; 2000.
2. Last JM. *A Dictionary of Epidemiology.* 3rd ed. New York, NY: Oxford University Press; 1995.
3. Hennekens CH, Buring JE. *Epidemiology in Medicine.* Boston, MA: Little, Brown and Company; 1987.
4. Boston Collaborative Drug Surveillance Programme. Oral contraceptives and venous thromboembolic disease, surgically confirmed gall bladder disease, and breast tumors. *Lancet.* 1973;1:1399–1404.
5. Sartwell PE, Masi AT, Arthes FG, Greene GR, Smith HE. Thromboembolism and oral contraceptives: an epidemiologic case–control study. *Am J Epidemiol.* 1969;90:365–380.
6. Najarian T, Colton T. Mortality from leukemia and cancer in shipyard workers. *Lancet.* 1978;1:1018.
7. Bizzozero OJ Jr, Johnson KG, Ciocco A, Kawasaki S, Toyotda S. Radiation-related leukemia in Hiroshima and Nagasaki, 1946–1964. *Ann Intern Med.* 1967; 66:522–530.
8. Rinsky RA, Zumwalde RD, Waxweiler RJ, Murray WE Jr, Bierbaum PJ, Landrigan PJ, et al. Cancer mortality at a naval nuclear shipyard. *Lancet.* 1981; 1:231–235.
9. Greenberg ER, Rosner B, Hennekens C, Rinsky R, Colton T. An investigation of bias in a study of nuclear shipyard workers. *Am J Epidemiol.* 1985;121: 301–308.
10. Monson RR. *Occupational Epidemiology.* 2nd ed. Boca Raton, FL: CRC Press; 1990.
11. Caldwell GG, Kelley DB, Heath CW Jr. Leukemia among participants in military maneuvers at a nuclear bomb test: a preliminary report. *JAMA.* 1980; 244:1575–1578.
12. Rothman KJ, Greenland S. *Modern Epidemiolgy.* 2nd ed. Philadelphia, PA: Lippincott-Raven; 1998.
13. Rothman KJ, Fyler DC, Goldblatt A, Kreidberg MB. Exogenous hormones and other drug exposures of children with congenital heart disease. *Am J Epidemiol.* 1979;109:433–439.
14. Zierler S, Rothman KJ. Congenital heart disease in relation to maternal use of Benedectin and other drugs in early pregnancy. *N Engl J Med.* 1985;313: 347–352.

15. Werler MM, Pober BR, Nelson K, Holmes LB. Reporting accuracy among mothers of malformed and non-malformed infants. *Am J Epidemiol.* 1989;129: 415–421.

16. Khoury MJ, James LM, Erikson JD. On the use of affected controls to address recall bias in case–control studies of birth defects. *Teratology.* 1994;49:273–281.

17. Mitchell AA, Cottler LB, Shapiro S. Effect of questionnaire design on recall of drug exposure in pregnancy. *Am J Epidemiol.* 1986;123:670–676.

18. Metzger DS, Koblin B, Turner C, Navaline H, Valenti F, Holte S, et al. Randomized controlled trial of audio computer-assisted self-interviewing: utility and acceptability in longitudinal studies. *Am J Epidemiol.* 2000;152:99–107.

19. Werler MM, Shapiro S, Mitchell AA. Peri-conceptional folic acid exposure and risk of occurrent neural tube defects. *JAMA.* 1993;269:1257–1261.

20. Levin AA, Schoenbaum, SC, Monson RR, Stubblefield PG, Ryan PG. The association of inducted abortion with subsequent pregnancy loss. *JAMA.* 1980;243: 2495–2499.

21. Kelsey JL, Thompson WD, Evans AS. *Methods in Observational Epidemiology.* New York, NY: Oxford University Press; 1986.

22. Aschengrau A, Hardy S, Mackey P, Pultinas D. The impact of low technology lead hazard reduction activities among children with mildly elevated blood lead levels. *Environ Res.* 1998;79:41–50.

23. Mzezewa V, Basset M, Machekano R, McFarland W, Katzenstein D. *Challenges in implementing a workplace-based peer-led AIDS education program in Harare: the Zimzabwe AIDS Prevention Project (ZAPP) experience.* Paper presented at: 12th World AIDS Conference; 1998; Geneva, Switzerland.

24. DesJarlais DC, Marmor M, Friedman P, et al. HIV incidence among injection drug users in New York City, 1992–1997: evidence for a declining epidemic. *Am J Public Health.* 2000;90:352–359.

25. Lash TL, Aschengrau A. Active and passive cigarette smoking and the occurrence of breast cancer. *Am J Epidemiol.* 1999;149:5–12.

26. Jick H, Walker AM, Rothman KJ, et al. Vaginal spermicides and congenital disorder. *JAMA.* 1981;245:1329–1332.

EXERCISES

1. Briefly define each of the following terms:
    A. Recall bias
    B. Healthy-worker effect
    C. Control selection bias

2. State the main difference between differential and nondifferential mis-classification, and state which direction(s) each type of error can bias the study results.

3. A case–control study was conducted to determine if using antihista-mines around the time of conception increased the risk of birth defects in the offspring. No personal interviews were conducted regarding the subjects' antihistamine use. Instead, women were considered exposed if computerized pharmacy records from their health maintenance organization indicated that they had filled at least one prescription for antihistamines within 500 days before the birth of the child.
    A. Which type of observation bias is this data collection method most susceptible to?
    B. Which type of observation bias is this data collection method least susceptible to?

4. A prospective cohort study was conducted to determine the risk of heart attack among men with varying levels of baldness. Third-year residents in dermatology conducted visual baldness assessments at the start of the study (which was before any heart attacks had occurred). Four levels of baldness were coded: none, minimal, moder-ate, and severe. Which of the following types of bias were surely avoided in this study?
    A. Recall bias of the exposure information
    B. Differential misclassification of the exposure
    C. Nondifferential misclassification of the exposure
    D. Selection bias

5. State the different ways that each of the following biases can be minimized:
    A. Interviewer bias
    B. Recall bias
    C. Selection bias
    D. Misclassification

11

Confounding

LEARNING OBJECTIVES

By the end of this chapter, the reader will be able to:

- Define and provide examples of confounding.
- Describe the methods for assessing the presence of confounding.
- Describe the methods for controlling confounding including restriction, randomization, matching, and stratified and multivariate analyses.

Introduction

Epidemiologists evaluate whether a study result is valid by assessing the presence of random error, bias, and confounding. These three phenomena are considered *alternative explanations* for the observed association between an exposure and disease. Random error is the probability that the observed result is due to "chance." Bias is a systematic error committed by the investigator during the course of a study. In contrast, confounding is not the fault of the investigator. It simply reflects the fact that epidemiologic research is conducted among free-living humans with unevenly distributed characteristics. As a result, epidemiologic studies of the relationship between an exposure and disease are susceptible to the disturbing influences of extraneous factors called confounders. This chapter provides several definitions of confounding and describes the main methods to control for confounding in the design and analysis of a study.

Definition and Examples of Confounding

Confounding is most simply defined as the *mixing of effects* between an exposure, an outcome, and a third extraneous variable known as a confounder.[1(p120)] In fact, confounding can be considered the "third variable problem." When it is present, the association between the exposure and outcome is distorted because of the relationships between the confounder and the exposure, and between the confounder and the disease.

Confounding can also be considered in terms of the counterfactual ideal.[1(pp137–138)] As described in Chapter 8, the ideal comparison group in a cohort study consists of exactly the same individuals in the exposed group had they not been exposed. Because it is impossible for the same person to be exposed and unexposed simultaneously, epidemiologists select different sets of individuals for the exposed and comparison groups. Even though different people form each group, the investigator chooses groups that are as similar as possible on characteristics that influence getting the disease. Accordingly, the rate of disease in the exposed and comparison groups will be identical if the exposure has no effect on disease occurrence.

Confounding can be thought of as a failure of the comparison group to reflect the counterfactual experience of the exposed group. Thus, even if the exposure has no effect on disease occurrence, the exposed and comparison groups will have different disease rates because they differ on other risk factors for the disease. In other words, risk factors apart from the exposure are distributed differently between the exposed and unexposed groups when confounding is present.

For example, consider a hypothetical cohort study on the risk of dementia among adults with diabetes. The investigators enrolled a group of newly diagnosed diabetic adults (the exposed group) and a group of adults without diabetes (the unexposed group), and followed them to determine the cumulative incidence of dementia. They found that participants with diabetes were four times more likely to develop dementia than those without diabetes over a 10-year follow-up period (see Table 11–1).

TABLE 11–1   Hypothetical Data on the Association Between Diabetes and Dementia

| | Dementia | | |
Diabetes	Yes	No	Total
Yes	400	600	1000
No	100	900	1000
Total	500	1500	2000
	Relative risk = 4.0		

Although the results imply that there was a strong association between diabetes and the subsequent occurrence of dementia, the findings may be invalid because of the distorting influence of confounding factors. For example, a close inspection of the study population revealed that subjects with diabetes were, on average, older than subjects without diabetes. Thus, perhaps the reason or part of the reason for the increased incidence of dementia among subjects with diabetes was their older age. This is a plausible explanation because the risk of dementia is influenced by age. When confounding by age was "controlled," the subjects with diabetes were twice as likely to develop dementia than those without diabetes. Thus, the initial results were exaggerated by confounding by age. Confounding occurred because age was associated with diabetes and with dementia. More specifically, the subjects with diabetes were older than those without diabetes, and the risk of dementia increased with age.

A variable must meet several criteria in order to be a confounder. First, the variable must be associated with the exposure in the population that produced the cases. That is, the confounding variable must be more or less common in the exposed group than in the comparison group. Second, the variable must be an independent cause or predictor of the disease, which means that the association between the confounder and the disease is present among both exposed and unexposed individuals. For example, the association between age and dementia is present for both diabetics and nondiabetics. Third, a confounding variable cannot be an intermediate step in the causal pathway between the exposure and disease. We identify intermediate steps by evaluating the biological mechanism by which the exposure is thought to cause the disease. For example, consider the inverse association between modest alcohol consumption and the risk of heart disease.[2] Modest alcohol consumption is thought to lower the risk of heart disease by increasing the level of high-density lipoproteins (HDL). In other words, modest alcohol consumption increases a person's HDL level which, in turn, decreases his risk of heart disease. HDL level is a step in the causal chain between modest alcohol consumption and a lowered risk of heart disease, and thus is not a confounder. Figure 11–1 depicts the relationship between the confounder, the exposure, and the disease; Figure 11–2 depicts a variable that is a step in the causal pathway between an exposure and a disease.

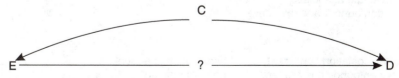

FIGURE 11–1. The Confounder (C) is Associated Both With the Exposure (E) and the Disease (D)

E ⎯⎯⎯⎯⎯⎯⎯⎯⎯⎯⎯⎯→ S ⎯⎯⎯⎯⎯⎯⎯⎯⎯⎯⎯→ D

FIGURE 11–2. The Variable (S) is a Step in the Causal Pathway Between the Exposure (E) and the Disease (D) and, Thus, is Not a Confounder of This Relationship.

How do epidemiologists determine if a variable is a confounder? One way is to evaluate the strength of the associations between the confounder, the exposure, and the disease. First, the strength of the association between the confounder and the disease is evaluated (C and D in Figure 11–1). If there is no association, we can conclude that the variable is not a confounder. If there is an association, we next determine if this association is present among both exposed and unexposed individuals. If not, we can conclude that the variable is not a confounder. If yes, we determine if there is an association between the confounder and the exposure (C and E in Figure 11–1). If there is no association, we can conclude that the variable is not a confounder. In summary, epidemiologists conclude that confounding is present if there is an association between the confounder and the disease among the exposed and unexposed groups, and between the confounder and the exposure. The decision tree for determining if a variable is a confounder is depicted in Figure 11–3.

Consider again the hypothetical cohort study on the risk of dementia among people with diabetes. Data on the relationship between age, diabetes, and the risk of dementia are described in Tables 11–2 and 11–3. Recall that subjects with diabetes had a fourfold increased risk of dementia, but that the risk was reduced to a twofold increase after controlling for

Evaluate association between confounder and disease
(overall and separately among exposed and unexposed).

If association is present,
confounding is possible.

If association is absent,
no confounding.

Evaluate association between
confounder and exposure.

If association is present,
confounding is present.

If association is absent,
no confounding.

FIGURE 11–3. Decision Tree for Determining if a Variable is a Confounder

TABLE 11–2   Hypothetical Data on the Association Between Age and Dementia among Diabetics and Nondiabetics

Age	Dementia among participants with diabetes			Age	Dementia among participants without diabetes		
	Yes	*No*	*Total*		*Yes*	*No*	*Total*
80–99 years	360	540	900	80–99 years	20	80	100
45–79 years	20	80	100	45–79 years	90	810	900
Total	380	620	1000	Total	110	890	1000
	Relative risk = 2.0				Relative risk = 2.0		

TABLE 11–3   Hypothetical Data on the Association Between Age and Diabetes

	Diabetes		
Age	*Yes*	*No*	*Total*
80–99 years	900	100	1000
45–79 years	100	900	1000
Total	1000	1000	2000
	Relative risk = 9.0		

age. The mixing of effects between age, diabetes, and dementia caused confounding. Note from the data in Table 11–2 that there was a twofold increased risk of dementia among subjects aged 80 to 99 years as compared to subjects aged 45 to 79 years that was present for both diabetics and non-diabetics. Thus, there was a positive association between the confounder and the disease among both exposed and unexposed individuals. There was a ninefold increased risk of diabetes with older age (Table 11–3), and so there was also an association between the exposure and the confounder. Confounding occurred when these complex associations were ignored in the crude analysis.

Confounding is not an all or none condition described merely by its presence or absence. Rather, confounding is a quantitative issue. Thus, it is vital to ask the following questions about the presence of confounding in a particular study. First, what is the magnitude or extent of confounding? Second, what is the direction of confounding? The question regarding the magnitude of confounding can be answered by using the following formula:

Magnitude of confounding = (RR crude − RR adjusted)/RR adjusted,

where RR is the relative risk. Note that the crude measure of association (RR crude) has not been adjusted for confounding, and the adjusted measure (RR adjusted) has been corrected for confounding. In this example, the crude relative risk of dementia among participants with diabetes was

4.0 while the age-adjusted relative risk was 2.0. Thus, the magnitude of confounding was [(4.0 − 2.0)/2.0] x 100 or 100%, indicating that a large amount of confounding was present.

Regarding the direction of confounding, confounding pulls the observed association away from the true association. Thus, it can either exaggerate the true association (positive confounding) or hide it (negative confounding). An example of positive confounding is when the true relative risk is 1.0 and the confounded relative risk is 2.0; an example of negative confounding is when the true relative risk is 2.0 and the confounded relative risk is 1.0. In the hypothetical study of the association between diabetes and dementia, age was a positive confounder of the relationship.

Confounding occurs in all types of epidemiologic studies. An interesting example of confounding occurred in a study of the relationship between myopia or near-sightedness and light exposure.[3] In particular, the investigators hypothesized that night-time ambient light exposure increased the risk of myopia among children. The cross-sectional study included 479 outpatients aged 2 to 16 years from a university pediatric opthalmology clinic. Children who slept with room lights and night lights before the age of 2 years had an increased risk of myopia as compared to children who slept in darkness during these years. In particular, the investigators observed a 5.5-fold increased risk of myopia associated with full room lights and a 3.4-fold increased risk with night lights. Although the investigators acknowledged that the study was limited by the lack of information on confounders, they concluded, "It seems prudent that infants and young children sleep at night without artificial lighting in the bedroom."[3]

In retrospect, this conclusion was incorrect given the lack of information on crucial confounding factors. That is, no data were collected on independent risk factors for myopia that were also associated with the use of lighting. A subsequent study of this relationship found that family history of myopia was an important confounder.[4] In particular, the study found that families with two myopic parents were much more likely to employ night-time lighting aids for their children, and were much more likely to have myopic children. The investigators hypothesized that the parents' own poor visual acuity necessitated the lighting.

Confounding by Indication and Severity

Two special types of confounding occur in observational studies of the intended effects of treatments: confounding by indication and confounding by severity. Confounding by indication reflects the fact that treatments are given to individuals with a particular disease, and so there is a mixing of effects between the treatment, the disease for which the treatment is given, and the outcome under study.[5] For example, studies of the association between antidepressant drug use and infertility need to consider depression, the indication for the drug treatment, as a confounder. This is because antidepressant drug use is associated with depression (patients are not given the drug unless they have the condition), and because depression itself is a known risk factor for infertility.[6] Confounding by indication occurs when individuals who are treated for their condition are compared to individuals who have neither the condition nor the treatment. Thus, a common way to control for this type of confounding is to compare different treatments for the same condition. For example, investigators could compare one antidepressant drug to another drug among women who have a diagnosis of depression.

Confounding by severity is a type of confounding "in which not only the disease that forms the indication but also its severity is the potential confounder. . . . Here, the stage of the disease and its corresponding severity and complications are important."[7(p982)] For example, a recent study found that the initiation of antiretroviral therapy for HIV disease was associated with more severe disease.[8] In particular, individuals who initiated antiretroviral therapy had more compromised immune systems and higher plasma viral loads than did individuals who did not initiate such therapy. Confounding by severity in observational studies usually makes the therapy appear less effective than it appeared in experimental studies. For example, because antiretroviral therapy is more likely to be given to patients with more severe disease and hence worse prognoses, this treatment is associated with higher crude mortality rates than other treatments. Experimental studies do not suffer from this problem, mainly because randomization balances the severity distribution of the compared groups.

Controlling for Confounding: General Considerations

Epidemiologists control or adjust for confounding variables because they consider confounders nuisance variables that distort the true association between an exposure and disease. Confounding can be controlled either in the design phase, the analysis phase, or a combination of the two. In order to control for confounding, the investigator must have information on all variables that are potential confounders. Except for randomization, it is impossible to control for a confounder without data.

Epidemiologists typically determine which variables are potential confounders by conducting a literature review to ascertain all currently known risk factors for the disease under study. Note that risk factors include variables that either increase or decreases a person's risk of disease. For example, potential confounders in a study of the relationship between tetrachloroethylene-contaminated drinking water and the risk of breast cancer included age at diagnosis of breast cancer, race, religion, age at first live- or stillbirth, prior history of breast cancer, prior history of benign breast disease, family history of breast cancer, and prior history of medical treatment with radiation. In particular, the risk of breast cancer is increased among women with a positive family history, who are Jewish, and whose first birth occurs at a later age (older than 30 years).[9]

After determining which variables are potential confounders and collecting data on them, epidemiologists determine if the variable is an actual confounder. This is typically accomplished by comparing the crude and adjusted estimates of the measure of association. If the crude and adjusted measures differ appreciably, then the variable that has been controlled is considered an actual confounder. The definition of an "appreciable" difference is arbitrary. Epidemiologists commonly use a 10 to 20% difference. Age clearly met this criterion in the diabetes–dementia relationship.

Controlling for Confounding in the Design

There are three main ways to control for confounding in the design stage of a study: randomization, restriction, and matching (see Table 11–4). Randomization is the "act of assigning or ordering that results from a random process."[10(p220)] Random methods include flipping a coin, using a random number table, or using a computerized random number generator. Randomization ensures that the treatment assignment occurs in an unbiased fashion and will, on average, result in a balanced distribution of both known and unknown confounders, if the sample size is large enough. Recall, for example, the CAPRIE (Clopidogrel versus Aspirin in Patients at Risk of Ischemic Events) study described in Chapter 7. This study enrolled about 19,000 patients with atherosclerotic vascular disease and randomly assigned them to receive either clopidogrel or aspirin.[11] As shown in Table 7–2, randomization achieved baseline comparability of the patients in the two arms of the CAPRIE study because the size of the study was so large.

A unique advantage of randomization is that it will control for variables that study investigators are unable to measure. Although there is no absolute guarantee that randomization will control for unknown confounders (it may not work just by chance), known and unknown confounders are considered unlikely if the sample size is sufficient. Randomization is one of the few aspects of epidemiologic research for which there are numerous advantages and no disadvantages. Unfortunately, it can be used only in experimental studies.

Restriction, another method investigators use to control for confounding in the design phase, means that admissibility criteria for study subjects are limited. In other words, entrance into the study is confined to individuals who fall within a specified category of the confounder. For example, confounding by age can be reduced by restricting a study to individuals within a narrow age range, say from 25 to 35 years. Other examples of restriction include limiting the study population to one gender or only one

TABLE 11–4 Methods to Control for Confounding in the Design and Analysis

Design stage
- Randomization
- Restriction
- Matching

Analysis stage
- Standardization
- Stratified analysis
- Matched analysis (needed for case–control studies but not for cohort or experimental studies)
- Multivariate analysis

race. The goal of restriction (and all other methods to control for confounding) is to eliminate or reduce the variability of the confounder. It is important to remember that a variable is a confounder only if its distribution differs between compared groups. Thus, when a study is restricted to one confounder category, the compared groups are identical on that variable. For example, a study restricted to men cannot be confounded by gender.

The advantages of restriction include its simplicity, convenience, low expense, and effectiveness. Confounding can be completely eliminated if a categorical variable such as gender is restricted. In addition, confounding can be greatly reduced if a continuous variable such as age is restricted. How much confounding is reduced depends on the narrowness of the range. For example, for most exposure–disease relationships, restricting to ages 25 to 30 years will control for confounding by age better than restricting to ages 25 to 45 years.

Restriction also has a few drawbacks. First, it makes it difficult to find enough study subjects, and so it is usually applied to only a few variables. Second, it limits the generalizability of the study. For example, when investigators restrict a study to men, its results may not be generalizable to women because of biological, social, and other differences between the sexes.

Another way to control for confounding in the design stage is to match on one or more confounders. Matching is defined as "the process of making a study group and a comparison group comparable with respect to extraneous factors."[12(p101)] Matching means that investigators select the study subjects so that potential confounders are distributed in an identical manner. Thus, there will be identical confounder distributions among exposed and unexposed groups in a cohort study, and among cases and controls in a case–control study.

The most common forms of matching are individual matching and frequency matching. Both types of matching are used more often in case–control than cohort studies. Individual matching involves "identifying individual subjects for comparisons, each resembling a study subject on the matched variable."[12(p101)] For example, consider a cohort study on the relationship between exercise and the risk of colon cancer. A literature review reveals that potential confounders of this association include age, gender, and obesity. Thus, when an exposed subject (an exerciser) is enrolled who is a 55-year-old male with a normal body mass index, an unexposed subject (a nonexerciser) would be enrolled who is a 55-year-old male with a normal body mass index. (Body mass index is a measure of obesity.) If it is difficult to find an exact match on a continuous variable such as age, a looser match may be acceptable, say 55 years plus or minus a few years.

Frequency matching is a type of category matching that balances the proportion of people with a confounding factor in the compared groups. For example, consider a cohort study in which exposed subjects had the following age distribution: 20% were aged 40 to 49 years, 40% were 50 to 59 years, 20% were 60 to 69 years, and 20% were 70 years and older. Frequency matching would ensure that 20% of the unexposed subjects were aged 40 to 49 years, 40% were aged 50 to 59 years, and so on. Once investigators filled a particular age category, they would select no more unexposed individuals in that category. Frequency matching is less exact than individual matching, which makes it easier to find matches.

When matching is conducted in a cohort study, exposed and unexposed groups have the same distribution of the matched confounder, and so the crude measure of association is not confounded by the matched variable(s). However, matching in the design of a case–control study does not control confounding by itself. The investigator must perform a special matched analysis. The reason for matching in the design phase of a case–control study is to ensure sufficient numbers of subjects in each category of the matched variable in order to conduct the matched analysis efficiently. In fact, the crude odds ratio from a matched case–control study will be biased toward the null because matching makes the cases' and controls' exposure histories more similar because the matching variable is associated with the exposure.

Matching has several disadvantages. First, it is not possible for investigators to study the relationship between the matching factor and outcome. Second, it is difficult and expensive to find subjects who are appropriate matches. Third, it is possible to "overmatch" on a confounder in a case–control study. This can occur when investigators match on a potential confounder that is strongly associated with the exposure but either weakly associated or not associated with the disease. Overmatching is problematic because it makes the matched analysis very inefficient. This occurs because information on the large number of matched sets with concordant exposure histories is lost.

Despite these disadvantages, matching is desirable and even necessary in a number of situations. First, matching is advantageous when the cases series in a case–control study is very small, and so other options for controlling confounding do not work well. Second, matching is needed when the confounder is a complex nominal variable such as occupation, neighborhood, or familial characteristic such as sibship. Each of these variables represents a complex web of environmental and, occasionally, genetic factors that are difficult to measure and to control in other ways.

Controlling for Confounding in the Analysis

Even when the study design does not feature randomization, restriction, and matching, it is still possible to achieve excellent control for confounding using methods available during the analysis phase. The three main ways to control for confounding in the analysis of a study are standardization, stratification, and multivariate methods (see Table 11–4). Epidemiologists commonly use standardization to control for demographic variables such as age, race, gender, and calendar time. Chapter 3 contains an example of age standardization, which allows us to make a fair comparison between the mortality rates in Alaska and Florida, despite very different age distributions in these two states.

Stratification, which is used both to evaluate and to control for confounding, is defined as "the process of or result of separating a sample into several subsamples according to specified criteria such as age groups, socioeconomic status, and so forth. The effect of confounding variables may be controlled by stratifying the analysis of results."[12(p161)] With stratification, the investigator evaluates the association within homogeneous categories of the confounder. The homogeneous categories are called strata, and each stratum should be free of confounding by the stratification variable. For example, consider a hypothetical case–control study of DDE exposure (DDE is the metabolic byproduct of the pesticide DDT) and the risk of breast cancer in which age is a confounder. Table 11–5 describes the crude results without stratification by age. Overall, there is a 1.9-fold increased risk of breast cancer among women who were exposed to high DDE levels (odds ratio = $[500 \times 3400]/[600 \times 1500] = 1.9$).

TABLE 11–5   Crude Data from a Hypothetical Case–Control Study of DDE Exposure and Breast Cancer

DDE level	Cases	Controls
High	500	600
Low	1500	3400
Total	2000	4000
	Odds ratio = 1.9	

TABLE 11–6 Age-Stratified Data from a Hypothetical Case–Control Study of DDE Exposure and Breast Cancer

	Age less than 50 years		*Age 50 years and older*	
DDE levels	*Cases*	*Controls*	*Cases*	*Controls*
High	50	300	450	300
Low	450	2700	1050	700
Total	500	3000	1500	1000
Stratum-specific odds ratio = 1.0			Stratum-specific odds ratio = 1.0	

Now let us examine these results stratified into two age groups: women less than 50 years of age and women 50 years and older (see Table 11–6). Note that all of the numbers in the cells of two stratified tables add up to the numbers in the cells of the crude data table (see Table 11–5). Each stratum can be considered a restricted analysis. That is, each stratum restricts the analysis to a narrow range of the confounder. When we stratify the data, we see that there is no association between DDE and breast cancer among women who are less than 50 years of age and among those who are 50 years and older. The odds ratio is $(50 \times 2700)/(300 \times 450)$ or 1.0 among women less than 50 years of age, and it is $(450 \times 700)/(300 \times 1050)$ or 1.0 among women aged 50 years and older. The magnitude of the association does not differ across the strata, but the stratum-specific odds ratios (1.0) are different from the crude odds ratio (1.9). The appreciable difference between the crude and stratum-specific odds ratios indicates that confounding by age is present.

When epidemiologists conduct stratified analyses, they have the option of reporting either the stratum-specific results or calculating a summary measure using standardization or pooling. Standardization involves taking weighted averages of the relevant measures of disease frequency. The weights typically come from the exposed group in the study population. Pooling involves calculating a weighted average of the relative risks instead of the measures of disease frequency. A commonly used method for calculating a pooled estimate of association was first proposed by Mantel and Haenszel.[13] Table 11–7 gives the formulas for the Mantel-Haenszel pooled estimates of relative risk for case–control studies, and cohort and experimental studies with count and person-time denominators. In the example above, the Mantel-Haenszel pooled odds ratio is $[(50 \times 2700/3500) + (450 \times 700/2500)] / [(300 \times 450/3500) + (300 \times 1050/2500)] = 1.0$.

Pooling should only be conducted if the stratum-specific estimates are similar to one another. Pooling should not be undertaken if the estimates are appreciably different because this means that effect modification is present. Briefly, effect modification indicates that the strength of the asso-

TABLE 11–7 Formulas for Calculating Mantel-Haenszel Pooled Relative Risks

Type of study	Formula	
Case–control study	$$\dfrac{\sum a_i d_i / T_i}{\sum b_i c_i / T_i}$$	where a_i, b_i, c_i, and d_i are the cells of each stratified two-by-two table and T_i is the total number of subjects in each stratum.
Cohort or experimental study with count denominators	$$\dfrac{\sum a_i (c_i + d_i) / T_i}{\sum c_i (a_i + b_i) / T_i}$$	where a_i, b_i, c_i, and d_i are the cells in each stratified two-by-two table and T_i is the total number of subjects in each stratum.
Cohort or experimental study with person-time denominators	$$\dfrac{\sum a_i (PT_{0i}) / PT_i}{\sum c_i (PT_{1i}) / PT_i}$$	where a_i is the number of exposed cases, c_i is the number of unexposed cases in each stratified two-by-two table, PT_{0i} is amount of person-time among the unexposed in each stratum, PT_{1i} is the amount of person-time among the exposed in each stratum, and PT_i is the total amount of person-time in each stratum.

ciation is modified or differs according to the level of another variable. For example, the relationship between body mass index and breast cancer varies according to menopausal status. Higher body mass index decreases the risk of breast cancer among premenopausal women, and it either increases or does not affect risk among postmenopausal women.[14] For more about effect modification, see Chapter 13.

It is unusual for stratum-specific measures of association to be exactly the same, even when no effect modification is present. Epidemiologists determine when stratum-specific results are different enough to suggest effect modification either by visually inspecting the results or by performing a statistical test such as the chi-square test for homogeneity. Chapter 12 contains more details about this statistical test.

Stratified analyses have several advantages. They are straightforward and easy to carry out. Even more important, they allow epidemiologists to view the raw data underlying the complex relationships under study. Their chief disadvantage is that they do not allow investigators to control simultaneously for many variables. This is because they generate a large number of strata relative to the number of study subjects. For example, if investigators wanted to control for four variables simultaneously—gender (two categories: male and female), age (five categories: less than 50 years, 50–59, 60–69, 70–79 and 80 years and older), and race/ethnicity (three categories: white, black, and Hispanic), and cigarette smoking status (three categories: current smoker, past smoker, and never smoked), they would need 90 strata (2 x 5 x 3 x 3 = 90) to describe all the possible combinations of these four variables. Even if the study size were relatively large, the number of subjects in the cells of some strata would be small or even zero, making the analysis questionable.

Consequently, epidemiologists rely on multivariate analysis when it is necessary to control for many confounding variables. Multivariate analysis involves the construction of a mathematical model that describes the association between exposure, disease, and confounders. Numerous multivariate models have been developed for this purpose, each with a certain set of assumptions. The choice of a particular model depends on the relationships among the relevant variables and the study design. For example, multiple linear regression models are used when the dependent variable is continuous, logistic regression models are used when the outcome is dichotomous as in a case–control study, and Cox proportional hazard and Poisson models are used when rates from a cohort or experimental study are being compared. A disadvantage of multivariate models is that the study data must comport with the model's assumptions. If not, the results of the multivariate analysis produce incorrect results. For example, if the model incorrectly assumes that there is a linear relationship between the independent and dependent variables, the results of the multivariate analysis will be skewed. An additional disadvantage is that investigators lose sight of the data when conducting these types of analyses.

Multivariate analyses should never be performed without first conducting a stratified analysis. The stratified analysis should be used to determine which variables are actual confounders that need to be controlled in the multivariate model. Any variable that changes the crude measure of association by an appreciable amount in the stratified analysis should be retained for the multivariate model. For example, investigators conducted a stratified analysis to identify confounders of the association between first- and second-degree family history of breast cancer and the risk of breast cancer.[15] The crude data were stratified by each of the following confounders, one at a time: race, age at diagnosis, age at first birth, religion, body mass index, prior history of benign breast disease, and prior history of ionizing radiation. The investigators planned to control simultaneously in a logistic regression analysis all variables that changed the crude measure of association by 10% or more. However, comparison of the crude and stratified estimates of association indicated little or no confounding by these variables.

Residual Confounding

Residual confounding is a term for the confounding that remains even after many confounding variables have been controlled. Residual confounding arises from several sources. The first source consists of confounders for which data were not collected. For example, a study of the relationship between tetrachloroethylene (PCE)-contaminated drinking water and the risk of bladder cancer, kidney cancer, and leukemia found that the risks of bladder cancer and leukemia were moderately increased among subjects with high PCE exposure levels (the odds ratio for leukemia was 5.8 among subjects with high levels of exposure).[16] Data on other drinking water contaminants such as disinfection byproducts could not be gathered because of the historical nature of the exposure–disease relation, and so residual confounding by these variables was possible. However, the investigators stated: "Residual confounding by uncontrolled factors . . . remains a possible but unlikely explanation for the results. These risk factors would need to be related strongly to risk, tightly correlated with PCE exposure, and sufficiently common to have produced the large odds ratios observed in our study."[16(p951)] Thus, the residual confounding could not have been large enough to account for the strong associations seen in the study. In contrast, residual confounding from missing information on family history of myopia was the likely reason for the positive association between myopia and early childhood light exposure.[4]

The second source of residual confounding arises from persistent differences in risk within a category of a confounder. It usually occurs when the confounder is classified in very broad categories. For example, if investigators used frequency matching to control for age in 10-year categories, residual confounding might be present if the risk of disease varied within the 10-year age group. The solution for this problem is to categorize the confounder into smaller groups—for example, 5-year age groups.

Third, residual confounding can occur when the confounder is mismeasured—that is when there is confounder misclassification. Misclassification is the "erroneous classification of an individual, a value, or an attribute into a category other than that to which it should be assigned."[12(p106)] Any kind of variable can be mismeasured, including confounders. Misclassification of confounders makes it more difficult to control for that confounder. Greater misclassification leads to greater residual confounding.

Summary

Confounding may be defined as a mixing of effects between an exposure, an outcome, and a third extraneous variable known as a confounder. Epidemiologists consider confounding a nuisance because it distorts the true association between an exposure and disease. A study may have a small, moderate, or large amount of confounding. A small degree of confounding may not significantly affect the study results, but a large degree may completely distort the findings. The distortion can either exaggerate or minimize the true association. The former is known as positive confounding, and the latter is known as negative confounding.

A confounding variable has three key features. (1) It is associated with the exposure in the population that produced the cases. (2) It is an independent cause or predictor of disease. (3) It is *not* an intermediate step in the causal pathway between the exposure and disease. Special types of confounding include confounding by indication, which is confounding between a treatment and the disease for which the treatment is given, and confounding by severity, which is confounding between a treatment and the seriousness of a disease. Both varieties occur in observational but not experimental studies.

Confounding can be controlled in the design, the analysis, or a combination of the two. Unless investigators conduct a study for which randomization is appropriate, they cannot control for confounders without collecting information on them. Crude and adjusted measures of association are compared to determine if confounding is present. The crude measure is calculated without controlling for confounding, and the adjusted measure is corrected for confounding. If crude and adjusted measures differ appreciably, then the variable is considered a confounder.

Three ways to control for confounding in the design phase are randomization, restriction, and matching. Randomization means that subjects are assigned to the study groups through a random process. It generally ensures that compared groups are balanced on both known and unknown confounders, if the sample size is sufficient. Although randomization is an excellent method for controlling confounding, its use is limited to experimental studies. Restriction means that admissibility criteria for enrollment are limited. It is a simple and excellent means to control for confounding, but it limits the generalizability of study results. Matching means that study subjects with identical or nearly identical characteristics are selected. The process is often expensive because it can be difficult to find appropriate matches, particularly when several variables are involved. Thus, matching is typically used to control for complex characteristics (such as neighborhood) that are difficult to control using other methods.

Techniques for controlling for confounding in the analysis include stratified and multivariate analyses. Stratification involves separating the study population into homogeneous categories of a confounder. A meaningful difference between the stratum-specific and crude measures of association indicates the presence of confounding. Stratum-specific or summary measures of association, such as the Mantel-Haenszel pooled estimate, should be used to present results in this situation. Stratified analyses are popular because they are straightforward and easy to carry out; however, they are inefficient for controlling for many confounders simultaneously. Thus, multivariate analysis, which involves specification of a mathematical model, is used in this setting. Although they are powerful, multivariate analyses are conducted in a "black-box," and so the investigator loses sight of the data.

Residual or persistent confounding may be present even after many confounding variables have been controlled. This occurs when data on certain confounders are unavailable, when confounders are controlled in overly broad categories, and when confounders are collected with measurement error.

References

1. Rothman KJ, Greenland S. *Modern Epidemiolgy*. 2nd ed. Philadelphia, PA: Lippincott-Raven; 1998.
2. Klatsky AL. Moderate drinking and reduced risk of heart disease. *Alcohol Alcohol*. 1999;23:15–23.
3. Quinn GE, Shin CH, Maguire MG, Stone RA. Myopia and ambient lighting at night. *Nature*. 1999;399:113–114.
4. Gwiazda J, Ong E, Held R, Thorn F. Myopia and ambient night-time lighting. *Nature*. 2000;404:144.
5. Greenland S, Neutra R. Control of confounding in the assessment of medical technology. *Int J Epidemiol*. 1980;9:361–367.
6. Lapane KL, Zierler S, Lasater TM, et al. Is a history of depressive symptoms associated with an increased risk of infertility in women? *Psychosom Med*. 1995; 57:509–513.
7. Salas M, Hofman A, Stricker BH. Confounding by indication: an example of variation in the use of epidemiologic terminology. *Am J Epidemiol*. 1999;149: 981–983.
8. Ahdieh L, Gange S, Greenblatt R, et al. Selection by indication of potent antiretroviral therapy usage in a large cohort of HIV-infected women. *Am J Epidemiol*. 2000;152:923–933.
9. Aschengrau A, Paulu C, Ozonoff D. Tetrachloroethylene-contaminated drinking water and the risk of breast cancer. *Environ Health Perspect*. 1998;106: 947–953.
10. Meinert CL. *Clinical trials dictionary, terminology and usage recommendations*. Baltimore, MD: The Johns Hopkins Center for Clinical Trials; 1996.
11. CAPRIE Steering Committee. A randomized, blinded trial of clopidogrel versus aspirin in patients at risk of ischemic events (CAPRIE). *Lancet*. 1996;348: 1329–1339.
12. Last JM. *A Dictionary of Epidemiology*. 3rd ed. New York, NY: Oxford University Press; 1995.
13. Mantel N, Haenszel WH. Statistical aspects of the analysis of data from retrospective studies of disease. *J Natl Cancer Inst*. 1959;22:719–748.
14. van den Brandt PA, Spiegelman D, Yaun S-S, Adami H-O, Beeson L, Folsom AR, et al. Pooled analysis of prospective cohort studies on height, weight, and breast cancer risk. *Am J Epidemiol*. 2000;152:514–527.
15. Bradbury B, Aschengrau A. *First and second degree family history of breast cancer and the risk of breast cancer* (unpublished manuscript).
16. Aschengrau A, Ozonoff D, Paulu C, Coogan P, Vezina R, Heeren T, et al. Cancer risk and tetrachloroethylene-contaminated drinking water in Massachusetts. *Arch Environ Health*. 1993;48:284–292.

ESSENTIALS OF EPIDEMIOLOGY IN PUBLIC HEALTH

EXERCISES

1. Briefly define each of the following terms:
   A. Confounding
   B. Residual confounding
   C. Positive and negative confounding

2. What are the key characteristics of a confounding variable?

3. Consider each of the following scenarios and state whether the variable in question is a confounder:
   A. A study of the relationship between contact lens use and the risk of eye ulcers. The crude relative risk is 3.0 and the age-adjusted relative risk is 1.5. Is age a confounder in this study?
   B. A case–control study of the relationship between cigarette smoking and pancreatic cancer. In this study, coffee drinking is associated with smoking and is a risk factor for pancreatic cancer among both smokers and nonsmokers. Is coffee drinking a confounder in this study?
   C. A study of the relationship between exercise and heart attacks that is conducted among men who do not smoke. Is gender a confounder in this study?
   D. A cohort study of the risk of liver cirrhosis among female alcoholics. Incidence rates of cirrhosis among alcoholic women are compared to those among nonalcoholic women. Nonalcoholics are individually matched to alcoholics on month and year of birth. Is age a confounder in this study?

4. Describe three methods for controlling confounding in the study design, and give one advantage and one disadvantage for each method.

5. Describe two methods for controlling confounding during the analysis, and give one advantage and one disadvantage for each method.

6. How do you determine if a variable confounds an association?

7. State which method to control for confounding is being used in the following scenarios. In each scenario, exercise is the exposure, myocardial infarction is the disease, and gender is the confounder.
   A. A study of exercise and myocardial infarction that is limited to men.
   B. A case–control study of exercise and myocardial infarction that includes men and women. Controls are selected so that the proportions of male and female subjects groups are identical.
   C. A study of exercise and myocardial infarction that includes men and women. The study determines the relative risk separately for men and for women and compares these to the crude relative risk.

12

Random Error

LEARNING OBJECTIVES

By the end of the chapter, the reader will be able to:

- Discuss the key phases in the history of biostatistics.
- Define chance, precision, and random error.
- Describe the process of hypothesis testing, calculate hypothesis testing statistics, and interpret a P value.
- Describe the process of confidence interval estimation and interpret 95% confidence intervals.
- Calculate measures of central tendency and dispersion for data with normal, binomial, and Poisson distributions.
- Calculate 95% confidence intervals for measures of disease frequency and association.
- Explain the elements of sample size and power calculations.

Introduction

Epidemiologists evaluate whether study results are valid by assessing the presence of three alternative explanations: bias, confounding, and random error. Bias is an error committed by the investigator either in the design or conduct of a study that leads to a false association between the exposure and disease. Confounding stems from the natural mixing of effects between the exposure and disease and a third variable called the confounder. Both bias and confounding are considered systematic errors because they arise from a discernible process.

In contrast, random error leads to a false association between the exposure and disease that arises from "chance," an uncontrollable force that seems to have no assignable cause.[1(p309)] Unlike bias and confounding, random errors are considered unsystematic because they arise from an unforeseeable and unpredictable process. Random errors in epidemiologic research originate from two sources. First, they can result from measurement errors—that is, mistakes in assessing the exposure and disease. For example, when investigators measure an incidence rate in a particular population, random errors may occur during the process of identifying cases of disease or calculating person-time of follow-up. Second, random errors arise from sampling variability when selecting particular subjects for a study. Sampling variability may cause an unrepresentative sample of the population to be selected "just by chance."

This chapter describes a variety of topics related to random error including the history of biostatistics in public health, the definition of precision (which is the lack of random error) and factors that influence precision, sampling, hypothesis testing and P values, confidence interval estimation, random variable probability distributions, statistical tests for hypothesis testing, and sample size and power calculations.

History of Biostatistics in Public Health

The evaluation of random error in epidemiologic research involves the use of statistics. The field of statistics was first developed in the 19th century as "a science concerned with information that was important to the state."[2(p1932)] Following the industrial revolution, various governments supported the collection of a wide variety of "statistics" on the social, economic, and health conditions of the populace, such as the number and causes of deaths and the number and characteristics of births.

Biostatistics, the branch of statistics that applies statistical methods to medical and biological phenomena, has been used by epidemiologists and other public health practitioners for more than 200 years. Its history, which is inextricably entwined with the history of epidemiology, can be divided into four distinct phases.[2(p1931)] During the first phase in the 19th century, biostatisticians and epidemiologists showed that the patterns of disease followed "law-like" characteristics. These discoveries could not have been made without the pioneering work of individuals such as William Farr, who developed and used statistics to summarize public health information on births and deaths during his 40-year tenure as the compiler of statistical abstracts for the General Registry Office in Great Britain (see Chapter 1 for more details). One of the chief epidemiologic discoveries of the mid-19th century, John Snow's demonstration that cholera was caused by drinking water contamination, relied on mortality statistics.[2(p1932)]

Although 19th-century pioneers such as Farr and Snow made important discoveries by using descriptive statistics, they placed little emphasis on mathematical reasoning.[2(p1933)] Karl Pearson changed this practice during the second phase of biostatistics in the early 20th century, when he developed a philosophy of statistical reasoning asserting that all scientific reasoning is fundamentally statistical. Pearson became one of the chief architects of the modern theory of mathematical statistics.

During the third phase of biostatistical history, between World Wars I and II, researchers took methods for testing hypotheses used in agricultural research and applied them to medicine and public health.[2(p1934)] During this period, R.A. Fisher developed theoretical methods for statistical inference, a method for generalizing results from a sample to a population. Fisher also made important contributions to the theory of experimental study design while working as a statistician at an agricultural research station in the United Kingdom. As he discovered the inadequacies of experimental studies of grain productivity, Fisher formulated the principles of randomization, adequate replication, and confounding. These principles, particularly those involving randomization, were later extended to medical research by Sir Austin Bradford Hill in one of the first modern experimental studies of streptomycin treatment of pulmonary tuberculosis.[3]

During the fourth phase, following World War II, researchers extended the statistical techniques developed by Fisher and others to nonexperimental studies including cohort and case–control designs.[2(pp1934–1935)] During this period, epidemiologists shifted their focus from infectious to noninfectious diseases. This new focus provided the impetus for biostatisticians to solve difficult statistical issues, such as developing appropriate methods for assessing and controlling confounding and for dealing with repeated measurements over time.

Today, biostatisticians and epidemiologists receive professional training in one another's field, and the two groups continue to collaborate closely in the design, conduct, and analysis of epidemiologic studies. The emphasis upon random error has recently been questioned. Although many epidemiologists and biostatisticians emphasize the role of random error as an explanation for study findings, others believe that it is overemphasized to the point of misinterpreting study results. This misinterpretation typically occurs when investigators mistakenly use statistical significance, a topic covered later in this chapter, as a stringent criterion for judging the presence of an association.

Precision

Precision can be thought of as the lack of random error. It is formally defined as "the state or quality of being precise or exact."[1(p1381)] However, most measurements in epidemiologic research are not exact, and epidemiologists use the term *measurement error* to describe these problems. Consider, for example, a study that uses interviews to measure women's use of vaginal spermicide over the past decade. Although most women would be able to recall whether they ever used spermicides during this period, many would be unable to recall exactly the brand, time, frequency, and duration of use. Inexact recall is a form of measurement error that leads to imprecise data.

There are two schools of thought on the nature of random error.[4(p116)] Epidemiologists known as probabilists believe that random error or chance is an important, even chief, explanation for events. Probabilists believe that it is impossible to predict the outcome of a coin toss (assuming the coin is fair) because chance rules its unpredictable occurrence. Epidemiologists known as determinists think that every event, act, or decision is the inevitable consequence of prior events, acts, or decisions.[1(p495)] They believe that all events are "predestined to unravel in a theoretically predictable way that follows inexorably from the previous pattern of actions."[4(p116)] Therefore, determinists believe that it would be possible to predict the outcome of a fair coin toss if one could measure accurately all of the antecedent variables that determine its outcome, including the weight of the coin, the force and torque of the throw, the presence of wind, and so forth.

Even determinists acknowledge that it is impossible to measure accurately all variables needed to predict events, even simple ones such as the outcome of a coin toss. This makes it impossible to distinguish determined outcomes from random occurrences, and so determinists regard random variation as the equivalent of ignorance about determinants for it is the "part of our experience that we cannot predict."[4(p116)]

In epidemiologic research there are three principal ways to increase precision and reduce random error in a study: (1) increase the sample size of the study, (2) repeat a measurement within a study or repeat the entire study, and (3) use an efficient study design that maximizes the amount of information obtained for a given sample size.[4(pp116–118)]

The absence or reduction of random errors does not guarantee the absence or reduction of systematic errors. In other words, it is possible to have precise but inaccurate findings. Consider, for example, a scale that is used to weigh a particular individual. The scale is precise and so, whenever the individual steps onto the scale, the digital read-out is "125.225 pounds." The scale is also consistent, giving the same read-out (125.225 pounds) every time the individual is weighed. However, because the scale was calibrated incorrectly, it always overestimates the individual's true weight of 123.000 pounds. Thus, improper calibration has led to a systematic error, even in a precise measuring instrument.

Sampling

Random error arises from measurement error and sampling variability. Measurement errors stem from inaccuracies in assessing the exposure and disease occurrence, and sampling variability stems from the selection of specific study subjects. Errors in subject selection may lead to an unrepresentative sample of a parent population just by the "luck of the draw." This is another way of saying that the uncontrollable force known as "chance" caused the sample selection problem.

Samples can be drawn from a parent population either randomly or nonrandomly. A random sample is one that has a probabilistic element in the selection process. In other words, each person has "a fixed and determinate probability of selection."[5(p140)] In order to select a random sample, investigators first must make a list of individuals in the parent population and then assign a sequential number to each individual. Next, they select a predetermined number of individuals (say 100 or 1000) using a random number table or another similar process. Tables of random sampling numbers are lists of randomly generated numbers. These tables and more details on the mechanics of their use can be found in most biostatistics textbooks.

There are two main types of random samples: simple and stratified random samples.[5(p151)] In a simple random sample, each person has an equal chance of being selected out of the entire parent population. In a stratified random sample, the parent population is first divided into subgroups or strata, and then a random sample is selected from each stratum. The proportion of the sample drawn from each stratum is weighted according to the population distribution of the stratification variable. For example, if 60% of the parent population consists of men, then 60% of the stratified random sample will also consist of men.

In contrast to a random sample, a nonrandom sample has no probabilistic element in the selection process. For instance, a sample of individuals who volunteer for a study or a sample of individuals who happen to use a medical care facility on a particular day are examples of nonrandom samples. Even selecting subjects according to a systematic process (such as all persons whose names begin with a particular letter or who are born on certain dates) is considered nonrandom because there is no random element in the selection process.

Although not all epidemiologic studies involve any sampling, particularly random sampling, it is standard practice to consider participants selected samples. "In this view, the subjects in a study, whether literally sampled or not, are viewed as a figurative sample of possible people who could have been included in the study or of the different possible experiences the study subjects have had. . . . Conceptually, the actual subjects are always considered a sample of a broader experience of interest."[4(p117)]

Statistical inference is the process of making generalizations from a sample to the source or parent population. The basis for making statistical inferences is the mathematical theory of probability. The probability of an event may be defined as "the event's long-run relative frequency in repeated trials under similar conditions."[6(p63)] Thus, the probability of heads on the toss of a fair coin is 0.5 or 50%. This means that, if one conducts a large number of coin tosses (say 1000) in exactly the same manner, heads will come up in about half of the tosses.

Probability-based statistics were developed in order to make inferences beyond actual data. Two commonly used statistics—P values and confidence intervals—are covered in detail in the following sections. Note that these statistics presume that a random sample was taken from the population under study. Because random samples are uncommon in epidemiologic research, many epidemiologists question the use of these statistics, particularly P values, in observational studies. At the very least, they encourage cautious interpretation of these statistics.

Hypothesis Testing and P Values

Epidemiologists commonly use hypothesis testing to assess the role of random error in their research. Hypothesis testing is considered a "uniform decision-making criterion" for evaluating random error that is superior to subjective impressions of the data.[7(p211)] The hypothesis testing framework has three main steps. First, investigators specify null and alternative hypotheses. Second, the investigators determine the compatibility of the study results with the null hypothesis using probabilistic methods. Third, they decide whether to reject or not to reject the null hypothesis according to the degree of compatibility with the null hypothesis.

The null hypothesis (H_O) states that there is no association between the exposure and disease. Thus, a null hypothesis in an epidemiologic study might be that the ratio measure of association is equal to one, or the difference measure of association is equal to zero. The alternative hypothesis (H_A) states that there is an association between the exposure and disease. Sometimes the direction of the alternative hypothesis is specified—for example, there is a positive association between the exposure and disease. Note that the alternative hypothesis contradicts the null hypothesis.

Next, the compatibility of the study data with the null hypothesis is evaluated using a statistical test. The particular test depends on the study design and type of measurement. For example, the chi-square test, which is covered later in this chapter, is used to assess random errors in categorical count data. The computation of the test statistic yields a P value, which quantifies the compatibility of the study data with the null hypothesis. It is important to note that hypothesis testing assumes that the null hypothesis is true. Accordingly, the P value is defined as the probability of obtaining the observed result and more extreme results by chance alone, given that the null hypothesis is true.

P values can be either one-sided or two-sided. A one-sided P value refers to the probability of observing a result at least as extreme as the observed result in one direction or another, but not both. An upper one-sided P value corresponds to the probability of obtaining the observed result or a greater one (see Figure 12–1). For example, if the observed relative risk is 2.0, the upper one-sided *P* value refers to the probability of observing relative risks greater than or equal to 2.0. A lower one-sided *P* value is the probability of obtaining the observed result or a lesser one. For example, if the observed relative risk is 0.5, the one-sided *P* value refers to the probability of observing relative risks less than or equal to 0.5. In contrast, a two-sided *P* value corresponds to a probability of seeing either a greater or lesser result. Thus, two-sided *P* values can be calculated by summing the upper and lower probabilities (areas A and B in Figure 12–1). Two-sided *P* values are more conservative than one-sided *P* values and suggest that the true population parameter may be either above or below the null hypothesis value.

Note that the *P* value is a continuous statistic ranging from 0.0 to 1.0. A small *P* value indicates a low degree of compatibility between the observed data and null hypothesis because there is only a small chance that a result at least as extreme would have been generated if the null hypothesis were true. Thus, a small *P* value means that the alternative hypothesis is a better explanation for the results than the null hypothesis. A large *P* value indicates a high degree of compatibility between the observed data and null hypothesis. Thus, a large *P* value means that the null hypothesis is a better explanation for the results than the alternative hypothesis. However, no *P* value—no matter how small—excludes chance, and no *P* value—no matter how large—mandates chance.

Epidemiologists commonly use a cutoff point of 0.05 to determine if the null hypothesis should or should not be rejected. This cutoff is known as the *alpha* or *significance level*. Thus, when a *P* value is less than or equal to 0.05, we reject the null hypothesis in favor of the alternative because random error is an unlikely explanation of the discrepancy between the results and the null hypothesis. When the *P* value is greater than 0.05, we do not reject the null hypothesis because random error is a likely explanation for the discrepancy. Results are considered statistically significant when the *P* value is less than or equal to 0.05 and are considered not statistically significant when the *P* value is greater than 0.05.

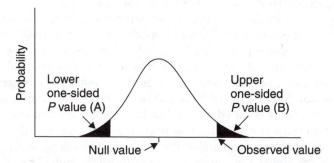

FIGURE 12–1. Representation of Lower and Upper One-Sided *P* Values

Consider, for example, a hypothetical study on the risk of breast cancer among women who are long-term users of oral contraceptives. Assume that the study measured a 1.8-fold increased risk of breast cancer among long-term pill users, and that the P value associated with this relative risk was 0.04. This means that, if the null hypothesis is true, there is a 4% probability of obtaining the observed result or one more extreme (that is, a relative risk of 1.8 or greater) by chance alone. Because the P value is less than 0.05, we may conclude that the results are statistically significant and we may reject the null hypothesis.

As another example, consider a hypothetical study on the risk of breast cancer among women who are long-term users of spermicidal creams. Assume that this study found a 1.4-fold increased risk of breast cancer among long-term spermicide users, and that the P value associated with this relative risk was 0.15. This means that, if the null hypothesis is true, there is a 15% probability of obtaining the observed result or one more extreme by chance alone. Because the P value is greater than 0.05, we can conclude that the results are not statistically significant and we do not reject the null hypothesis.

The statements "statistically significant" and "not statistically significant" do not indicate the probability that the null hypothesis is true. It does not mean that the null hypothesis has been proven when results are not statistically significant. In fact, it is impossible to prove that the null hypothesis (or any other hypothesis) is true. The most that can be said about results that are not statistically significant is that the data fail to provide sufficient evidence to doubt the null hypothesis. This means that the null hypothesis remains viable until evidence to the contrary is obtained.

This line of reasoning comports with the hypothetico-deductive philosophy of causal inference proposed by Karl Popper in the 1930s[8] (see Chapter 15 for more details). According to Popper's philosophy, hypotheses are formed using creativity and imagination. Predictions are made on the basis of these hypotheses, and observations are collected and compared with predictions. If the observations are incompatible with the predictions, the hypothesis is falsified. Otherwise, the hypothesis remains a reasonable explanation until a better one comes along.

Because the significance level is an arbitrary cutoff, it is possible to incorrectly reject or not reject the null hypothesis. When a significance level of 0.05 is used, there is a 5% chance of erroneously rejecting the null hypothesis when, in fact, it is true. The incorrect rejection of a null hypothesis is known as a *type I* or *alpha error*. It is also possible to erroneously fail to reject the null hypothesis when it is false. The incorrect failure to reject a false null hypothesis is called a *type II* or *beta error*. The complement of the type II or beta error (1 minus beta) is known as the power of the statistical test. Thus, *statistical power* measures the ability of a test to correctly reject the null hypothesis when the alternative hypothesis is true. The differences between the two types of errors are summarized in Table 12–1. Alpha and

TABLE 12–1 Possible Outcome of Hypothesis Testing

	Truth	
Conclusion of significance test	Null hypothesis (H_o) is true	Alternative hypothesis (H_A) is true
Do not reject H_o (not statistically significant)	Correct conclusion: H_o is true, and we do not reject H_o	Type II or beta error: H_A is true, but we do not reject H_o
Reject H_o (statistically significant)	Type I or alpha error: H_o is true, but we reject H_o	Correct conclusion: H_A is true and we reject H_o

beta errors are taken into account when investigators plan the appropriate sample size for a study. This topic is addressed later in this chapter.

In recent years, hypothesis testing, particularly significance testing, has come under criticism for numerous limitations and misuses. The chief limitation of significance testing is the use of a purely arbitrary cutoff for deciding whether to reject the null hypothesis. For example, it is difficult to argue that there is a meaningful difference between two sets of results whose associated P values are 0.04 and 0.06. Yet, significance testing would require that the null hypothesis be rejected on the basis of the former but not the latter. Significance testing has been criticized as a simplistic strategy for studying the complex biological and social phenomena being investigated in epidemiologic studies.

Hypothesis testing was originally developed in order to facilitate decision making in agricultural experiments. Although making decisions is an integral part of public health practice, decisions are rarely based on the results of a single epidemiologic study. Furthermore, making decisions on the basis of several studies that have been degraded to either being "statistically significant" or "not statistically significant" can give misleading impressions. Consider, for example, five hypothetical studies on the risk of breast cancer among women who lived with smokers during their childhood. Assume that the five studies represent the worldwide literature on the topic, and that all of the studies are free from bias and confounding. The results of these hypothetical studies are shown in Table 12–2. Note that the relative risks are fairly consistent, ranging from 1.4 to 1.8. Thus, on the

TABLE 12–2 Results of Five Hypothetical Studies on the Risk of Breast Cancer Following Childhood Exposure to Tobacco Smoke

Study (No. subjects)	Relative risk	P value	Statistically significant
A (n = 2500)	1.4	0.02	Yes
B (n = 500)	1.7	0.10	No
C (n = 2000)	1.6	0.04	Yes
D (n = 250)	1.8	0.30	No
E (n = 1000)	1.7	0.06	No

basis of the measure of association, the studies suggest a modest increase in breast cancer risk among tobacco-exposed women. However, the five studies appear to be inconsistent on the basis of statistical significance: two studies have statistically significant results, and three have statistically nonsignificant results.

Which assessment is correct? We believe that the measure of association (in this case, the relative risk) gives the most accurate picture of the strength of the relationship between tobacco exposure and breast cancer risk. The *P* value, on the other hand, gives a sense of the "stability" of the measure of association. Some studies produce more stable results than others, mainly because their size is larger. For example, studies A and C produced more stable results than studies B, D, and E because of larger numbers.

The following analogy about a horse race may help to illustrate the relative importance of the measure of association (e.g., relative risk) and the measure of statistical stability (*P* value). A person must answer two questions when betting on the outcome of a horse race: "Which horse should I bet on?" and "How much money should I wager?" In epidemiologic studies, investigators should examine the measure of association when deciding on the winning horse. The best choice for the *true* measure of association is the one that is obtained in a particular study. For example, the results of Study A suggest that the best choice for the true relative risk is 1.4.

Epidemiologists should examine the *P* value when deciding how much money to bet. A large amount of money should be wagered when the *P* value is small because this indicates that the results are statistically stable. Thus, one would wager a large bet on the results of study A (relative risk of 1.4). In contrast, one would wager less money when the *P* value is large because this indicates that the results are statistically unstable. Note that this process does not degrade the *P* value into the dichotomous statistically significant or not statistically significant. Instead epidemiologists examine the numerical *P* value to determine the size of the wager.

The measure of statistical stability may also be used to help decide on the winning horse—that is, the best estimate for the true relative risk among the five studies, assuming they are all valid. Because studies A, C, and E (which have larger study populations) have more stable results than studies B and D (which have smaller study population), the best estimate for the true risk lies between 1.4 and 1.7 (the range of results from studies A, C, and E) rather than between 1.7 and 1.8 (the range of results from studies B and D).

Another reason why *P* values have been criticized is that they mix together two pieces of information: the size of the association and the precision of the association.[9] In other words, *P* values are confounded statistics because they simultaneously reflect the magnitude of the association and the study size. When study results are summarized only with *P* values, it is impossible to determine whether a *P* value is small because the measure of association is strong or the sample size is large. In fact, it is possible to have a trivial increase in the measure of association (say a relative risk of 1.1) but a highly significant *P* value (say 0.001) just because the study size is large. In addition, it is impossible to determine whether a *P* value is large because the measure of association is weak or the sample size is small. For example, it is possible to have a study with a large increase in relative risk (say 5.0) but a large *P* value (say 0.15) because the study size is small.

Statistical testing has led to the dubious practice of "adjusting for multiple comparisons" when examining many hypotheses in a large body of data.[10] The line of reasoning to support this practice is as follows. Under the null hypothesis that there is no association between an exposure and a disease and that any observed association is due to chance, a statistically significant association will be observed with a probability of alpha, the significance level. Thus, if alpha is set at the traditional level of 0.05, there is a 5% probability of rejecting a correct null hypothesis.

The theoretical basis for adjusting for multiple comparisons is the "universal null hypothesis," which states that all associations seen in a given body of data reflect only random variation.[10] Thus, when many independent associations are examined for statistical significance, the probability that at least one will be found significant increases in proportion to the number of associations examined, even if all null hypotheses are true. For example, if we test 10 hypotheses within a body of data with an alpha level of 0.05, there is a 40% probability that at least 1 finding will be statistically significant, assuming that all 10 null hypotheses are true. Thus, in order to protect against false detection of significant differences that arise when making too many comparisons, statisticians have developed "multiple comparison procedures" that make the criterion for statistical significance more stringent.

However, the assumption of the universal null hypothesis is incorrect because it "undermines the basic premises of empirical research, which hold that nature follows regular laws that may be studied through observations."[10] Making adjustments for multiple comparisons also implies that investigators should not follow up "chance" or unusual associations with further investigation. However, potentially important findings will be missed if scientists do not follow all possible leads, even those that turn out to be wrong.

Still another reason why significance testing has been criticized is that investigators often misinterpret *P* values. One common misinterpretation is to equate the *P* value with the probability that the null hypothesis is true. As stated earlier, the *P* value assumes that the null hypothesis is true and tests the compatibility of the data with the null. Another misinterpretation is to equate a statistically significant association with a causal association. As is discussed in Chapter 15, statistical significance is not one of the suggested guidelines for discriminating between causal and noncausal associations.

Furthermore, statistical significance does not mean that bias or confounding have been ruled out as alternative explanations for study findings. Thus, it is entirely possible to have a statistically significant association that is invalid. Finally, statistical significance does not imply medical, biological, or public health significance. Thus, it is quite possible to have statistically significant findings that are unimportant by all other meaningful criteria.

Confidence Interval Estimation

Another method for quantifying random error in epidemiological studies is confidence interval estimation. A confidence interval is typically calculated around a point estimate, which is either a measure of disease frequency or measure of association. The confidence interval quantifies the variability around the point estimate. Several formulas for calculating confidence intervals around measures of disease frequency and association are presented later in this chapter. Note that the width of the confidence interval is determined by: (1) random error stemming from measurement error and sampling variability and (2) an arbitrary certainty factor, which is usually set at 95%. Thus, a wider confidence interval indicates a larger amount of random error, and a narrower interval indicates a smaller amount of random error. Given a similar degree of measurement error, a narrow confidence interval also indicates that a large sample generated the results and a wide confidence interval indicates that a small sample produced the results. For example, consider again the five hypothetical studies on the risk of breast cancer among women who lived with smokers during their childhood (see Table 12–3). Assume that the measurement error involved in assessing smoke exposure was similar across studies. Note that the 95% confidence intervals from the larger studies (A, C) are narrower than those from the smaller studies (B, D, E).

Most epidemiologists use 95% confidence intervals, although some use 90% or 99%. The strict statistical definition of a 95% confidence inter-

TABLE 12–3   Results of Five Hypothetical Studies on the Risk of Breast Cancer Following Childhood Exposure to Tobacco Smoke: Confidence Intervals

Study (No. subjects)	Relative risk	95% confidence interval	Statistically significant
A (n = 2500)	1.4	1.2–1.7	Yes
B (n = 500)	1.7	0.7–3.1	No
C (n = 2000)	1.6	1.2–2.1	Yes
D (n = 250)	1.8	0.6–3.9	No
E (n = 1000)	1.7	0.9–2.5	No

val is as follows: If a study were repeated 100 times and 100 point estimates and 100 confidence intervals were calculated, 95 out of 100 confidence intervals would contain the *true* measure of association. The remaining 5% will exclude the true measure of association.

There are two other useful ways to interpret confidence intervals. First, a confidence interval can be considered the range of possible values within which the true magnitude of effect lies with a stated level of certainty. For example, the 95% confidence interval for Study A ranges from 1.2 to 1.7 (see Figure 12–2). Thus, we may state that we have 95% confidence that the true measure of association lies somewhere inside the interval from 1.2 to 1.7. Second, a confidence interval can be considered the range of hypotheses that are compatible with the observed data. Thus, we may state that the results from Study A are consistent with hypotheses that the strength of the association lies between 1.2 and 1.7. Although these two interpretations are incorrect from a strict statistical viewpoint, they are useful alternative explanations.

Confidence intervals may also be used to determine if results are statistically significant. For example, if the 95% confidence interval does not include the null value (a relative risk of 1.0), the results are considered statistically significant. If the 95% confidence interval does include the null value, the results are not statistically significant. For example, the 95% confidence intervals for studies A and C indicate that these study results are statistically significant, whereas the 95% confidence intervals for studies B, D, and E indicate that these results are not statistically significant (see Table 12–3). However, we strongly discourage the degradation of the confidence interval into the dichotomous designations of statistically significant and not statistically significant because this practice can result in misleading conclusions. Even a cursory examination of the point estimates

FIGURE 12–2. Point Estimates and 95% Confidence Intervals from Five Hypothetical Studies on the Risk of Breast Cancer Following Childhood Exposure to Tobacco Smoke

and confidence intervals in Figure 12–2 reveals that the results of the five hypothetical studies on the risk of breast cancer following childhood exposure to tobacco smoke are quite consistent. Not only are the point estimates close together but the confidence intervals are overlapping.

Many epidemiologists prefer confidence intervals to P values for evaluating the role of random error. The main reason is that, unlike P values, confidence intervals are not confounded statistics. In other words, confidence intervals do a better job separating the magnitude of the association from the sample size. First, the width of the confidence interval is mainly influenced by the sample size. For studies with a similar amount of measurement error, a wider interval reflects a smaller sample size and a narrower interval reflects a larger sample size. Note from the data in Table 12–3 and Figure 12–2, the confidence intervals for studies A and C are much narrower than those of studies B and D because the former are based on many more study subjects than the latter. (Of course, we must assume that the level of measurement error is similar across studies.)

A second reason that confidence intervals are preferable to P values is that the general position of the confidence interval reflects the magnitude of the association. When a confidence interval is high on the relative risk scale, it means that the point estimate (the measure of association) is large. When the confidence interval is low on the relative risk scale, it indicates that the point estimate is small. This characteristic stems from the construction of the interval around the point estimate. As can be seen from Figure 12–3, the point estimate anchors the interval.

Still another reason why most epidemiologists prefer confidence intervals to P values is that they are in the same units as the measure of association. Thus, one can "guesstimate" the point estimate by examining the confidence interval. Depending on the measure around which the interval is constructed, the point estimate will be either in the center or very close to the center of the interval. In contrast, one cannot "guesstimate" the point estimate by examining a P value.

FIGURE 12–3. Point Estimates and 95% Confidence Intervals for Associations of Different Magnitude (The numbers in parentheses indicate the point estimates and the parentheses indicate the ends of the confidence intervals.)

However, confidence intervals have some of the same limitations as *P* values. For example, they do not provide information on other explanations for the results such as bias and confounding, and they do not indicate that the observed association is causal.

P-Value Function

The *P* value measures the consistency between the observed data and the null hypothesis. This is why the traditional *P* value is often described as the "null *P* value." However, it is possible to determine the consistency between the data and other hypotheses by graphing a "*P*-value function."[11(pp42–45)] For example, the *P*-value function shown in Figure 12–4 gives the *P* values for all possible values of a relative risk. The peak of the *P* value function corresponds to the point estimate of the relative risk, and the width of the function indicates the precision of the data. A narrow function indicates a high degree of precision, and a wide function indicates a low degree of precision.

The *P*-value function can be used to determine which values of the relative risk are most likely in light of the study results. For example, the *P*-value function in Figure 12–4 shows that positive relative risks are most compatible with the study results because the area under the function is mainly associated with relative risks greater than 1.0. The *P*-value function also shows the null *P* value—the *P* value for the relative risk of 1.0 and all possible confidence intervals. Figure 12–4 also shows the null *P* value and 90% and 95% confidence intervals.

FIGURE 12–4. *P*-value Function Depicting the Point Estimate and 90% and 95% Confidence Intervals

Probability Distributions

Mathematical probability theory is the basis for making statistical inferences from a sample to a parent population. In order to calculate P values and confidence intervals, it is necessary to postulate a particular probability distribution for the data under the null hypothesis. The normal, binomial, and Poisson probability distributions are commonly used in epidemiologic research. The normal distribution is used for continuous variables, and the binomial and Poisson distributions are used for discrete events with two mutually exclusive outcomes. These probability distributions are described in the following sections.

Normal Distribution

The normal distribution, also known as the Gaussian or "bell-shaped" distribution, is the cornerstone of hypothesis testing and confidence interval estimation for continuous biomedical variables such as height, blood pressure, and weight. Although many biological variables follow approximately this distribution, variables can be normalized by transforming the data onto a different scale. For example, log transformations of serum triglyceride measurements usually follow a normal distribution.[7(p121)] In addition, an important statistical principle known as the central limit theorem allows us to assume a normal distribution for variables whose underlying distribution of individual observations is not normal. (This principle is discussed later in this chapter.)

Consider, for example, the distribution of heights among the adult residents of Wayland, Massachusetts, a suburban town about 20 miles west of Boston. According to recent data, 13,840 adult men and women live in the town.[12] Let us assume that we visit every home in Wayland and measure the heights of all resident adults. The distribution of heights among these individuals is bell-shaped or normally distributed. Every distribution, including the normal distribution, is typically described by a measure of location or central tendency and a measure of dispersion or spread. The measure of central tendency summarizes the center or middle of the distribution and the measure of dispersion describes the spread of the distribution (see Figure 12–5).

The mean, median, and mode are popular measures for describing central tendency. The formula for calculating the population *mean* is as follows:

$$\mu = \frac{\sum_{i=1}^{N} X_i}{N}$$

where μ is the population mean, X_i is each individual's measurement (height), and N is the number of people in the population. The *median* is the middlemost observation of the distribution—that is, the observation

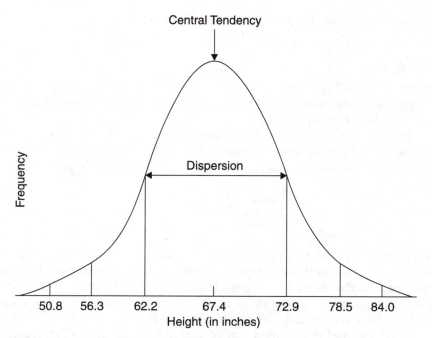

FIGURE 12–5. Normal Distribution of Heights Among Adult Residents of Wayland, Massachusetts

where 50% of the observations fall above it and 50% of the observations fall below it. In particular, if N is the number of observations in a population, the median will be the $(N+1)/2^{th}$ largest observation if N is odd; the median will be the average of $(N/2)$ and $(N/2 + 1)^{th}$ largest observation if N is even.[7(p10)] The *mode* is the most commonly occurring observation, and distributions with one mode are termed unimodal.

The mean, median, and mode of heights among adults in Wayland are identical at 67.4 inches because the distribution is perfectly symmetrical (see Figure 12–5). If the distribution were skewed or asymmetrical, the three measures would be different. For example, in 1999, the mean annual income among U.S. households was much higher ($54,842) than the median annual income ($40,816) because the distribution is skewed with a tail to the right.[13] The mean is more sensitive to extreme values (in this case, individuals with extraordinarily high incomes) than the median.

Commonly used measures of dispersion are the range, variance, and standard deviation. The *range* is defined as the difference between the highest and lowest values in the distribution. Although range is the simplest measure to calculate, it has a tendency to increase with the number of observations. For this reason, the more stable variance and standard deviation are generally preferred measures of dispersion.

The formula for the *population variance* is as follows:

$$\sigma^2 = \frac{\sum_{i=1}^{N}(X_i - \mu)^2}{N}$$

where σ^2 is the population variance, X_i is each individual's measurement (height), μ is the mean value for the population, and N is the number of individuals in the population.

Because the variance is the square of the original observations, the square root of the variance, known as the *population standard deviation*, is more commonly used to describe the degree of dispersion. Its formula is as follows:

$$\sigma = \sqrt{\sigma^2} = \sqrt{\frac{\sum_{i=1}^{N}(X_i - \mu)^2}{N}}$$

where σ is the standard deviation, σ^2 is the population variance, X_i is each individual's measurement (height), μ is the population mean, and N is the number of individuals in the population. The population variance and population standard deviation of heights among adult residents in Wayland are 30.58 inches and 5.53 inches, respectively.

Every normal distribution can be completely described by its mean and standard deviation. For a normal distribution, about 68% of observations in the distribution fall within one standard deviation of the mean, about 95% fall within two standard deviations of the mean, and about 99% fall within three standard deviations of the mean. This is another way of saying that the normal distribution falls off rapidly and has few values in its tails (see Figure 12–5).

Because it is usually impossible or impractical to gather data on an entire parent population in order to calculate the population mean and variance, investigators commonly collect data from a sample of the population in order to estimate the population mean and standard deviation. For example, instead of measuring the heights of the entire adult population of Wayland, Massachusetts, we could select a simple random sample of 20 individuals from the population in order to approximate the population mean and variance. The heights of the 20 individuals selected for this hypothetical sample are listed in Table 12–4.

The *sample mean* is calculated using the following formula:

$$\bar{x} = \frac{\sum_{i=1}^{n} x_i}{n}$$

where x is the sample mean, x_i is the measurement for each individual in the sample, and n is the number of individuals in the sample. The mean height in the simple random sample of 20 Wayland adults is: (59.0 + 60.6 + 60.8 + 61.0 + 62.5 + 63.5 + 64.1 + 64.4 + 64.8+ 65.4 + 66.0 + 66.4 + 67.6 + 67.7 + 67.7 + 69.2 + 72.2 + 75.0 + 76.6 + 77.0) ÷ 20 or 66.6 inches.

TABLE 12-4   Height (in Inches) for a Simple Random Sample of Adult Residents of Wayland, Massachusetts

59.0	60.6
60.8	61.0
62.5	63.5
64.1	64.4
64.8	65.4
66.0	66.4
67.6	67.7
67.7	69.2
72.2	75.0
76.6	77.0

The *sample standard deviation* is calculated using the following formula:

$$SD = \sqrt{\frac{\sum_{i=1}^{n}(x_i - \bar{x})^2}{n-1}}$$

where SD is the standard deviation, x_i is each individual's measurement, $\bar{x}$ is the sample mean, and n is the number of individuals in the sample. Thus, the standard deviation in the Wayland sample is 5.24 inches as calculated from:

$$\sqrt{\frac{(59.0-66.6)^2 + (60.6-66.6)^2 + (60.8-66.6)\ldots}{20-1}}$$

When the sample mean and standard deviation are computed from a random sample, such as described above, these figures should be good estimates of the mean and standard deviation of the population from which the sample was drawn. However, sampling variability predicts that different random samples will yield slightly different estimates of the population mean and standard deviation.

Another statistic called the *standard error* is used to quantify the accuracy of these estimates. For example, the standard error of the mean quantifies the degree to which the sample mean estimates the population mean. Its formula is as follows:

$$SEM(\bar{x}) = \frac{SD(\bar{x})}{\sqrt{n}}$$

where SEM is the standard error of the sample mean which is denoted by $\bar{x}$, SD is the standard deviation of the sample mean, and n is the size of the sample.

The standard error and standard deviation are commonly confused. To illustrate the difference between the two, let us suppose that we draw 50 random samples of 20 Wayland residents each and measure the height of all 1000 participants. Although each sample mean provides a good estimate of the population mean, *the mean of the means* gives a more accurate estimate than any particular sample mean. According to the statistical principle known as the central limit theorem, when a large number of random samples is drawn, the distribution of sample means will be approximately normal, regardless of the distribution of the original variables.[6(pp101–102)] The standard error expresses the variation of sample means around the parent population mean, while the standard deviation expresses the variation of individual values around a sample mean. The standard error of height measurements from 50 random samples of 20 Wayland residents is 1.17, and the previously calculated standard deviation from one sample of 20 Wayland residents is 5.24.

Binomial Distribution

The binomial distribution is another commonly used theoretical probability distribution that describes random variables with two possible discrete outcomes.[7(pp91–97)] In epidemiologic settings, it is used to describe dichotomous health outcomes such as diseased versus not diseased or dead versus alive. One outcome is considered the "success," and the other is considered the "failure." Note that these terms are used arbitrarily; for example, the occurrence of disease might be considered the success, and its nonoccurrence might be considered the failure.

The binomial distribution assumes that the frequency of success and failure occur with certain probabilities. The probability of success is designated by p, and the probability of failure is designated by 1 − p or q. The probabilities of success and failure are evaluated within the context of a Bernoulli trial, which is formally defined as a random variable that takes on the value of 1 with probability of p and a value of 0 with a probability of 1 − p.[7(p140)] For example, a coin toss can be considered a Bernoulli trial that takes on the value of heads with a probability of 0.5 and the value of tails with a probability of (1 − 0.5) or 0.5. Similarly, each person in an epidemiologic study can be considered a Bernoulli trial. For example, each subject in a cohort study can be considered a Bernoulli trial for the occurrence or nonoccurrence of disease. The probability that an individual will develop the disease is p, and the probability that he will not develop the disease is q. Likewise, each subject in a case–control study can be considered a Bernoulli trial for the presence or absence of exposure. The probability that the individual is exposed is p, and the probability that he is unexposed is q.

Bernoulli trials are based upon several assumptions. First, the probabilities of success and failure are assumed to be the same for each trial. Second, the trials are assumed to be independent of one another. This means that the outcome of one trial does not affect the outcome of any other trial. Third, the trials are assumed to be conducted in an identical manner.

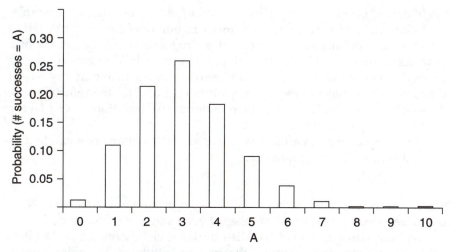

FIGURE 12–6. Binomial Distribution With the Probability of Success (p) = 0.3 and the Number of Bernoulli Trials (n) = 10

The binomial distribution describes the probability of k successes in n independent trials, where p is the probability of success in each trial, k is the number of successes, and n is the number of trials. The mean of the binomial distribution is estimated as follows:

$$\mu = np,$$

where μ is the mean, n is the number of Bernoulli trials, and p is the probability of success in each trial. The variance is estimated by:

$$\sigma^2 = np(1 - p),$$

where σ^2 is the variance, n is the number of independent Bernoulli trials, and p is the probability of success in a trial. The shape of a binomial distribution for 10 Bernoulli trials when p equals 0.3 is shown in Figure 12–6. Note that the distribution has a tail to the right. If p were nearer to zero or one, the distribution would be more severely skewed.

Because the binomial distribution is very cumbersome to use when the number of trials or sample size is large, the normal distribution is typically used to approximate the binomial in this setting. In fact, the normal distribution is a good approximation of the binomial distribution when n is moderately large and p is not extreme (too near zero or one).[7(p139)]

Poisson Distribution

The Poisson distribution is a discrete distribution commonly used to describe rare events.[7(p98)] It is frequently used in epidemiologic research because many diseases are uncommon, particularly if one considers the likelihood of occurrence in a short period of time. Consider, for example, the occurrence of new cases of human immunodeficiency virus (HIV) infection in a population of intravenous drug users over the course of a year. Assuming that (1) the probability of a new HIV infection on any given day is very small, (2) the number of cases occurring on any day is independent of that number on any other day, and (3) the infection rate does not change over time, then the number of HIV infections over a 1-year period follows a Poisson distribution.

Both the mean and variance of a Poisson distribution are equal to μ as defined by the following formula:

$$\mu = \lambda\tau,$$

where λ is the expected number of events per unit time and τ is time. Note that μ describes the expected number of events over the time period t.

Not surprisingly, the Poisson distribution is closely related to the binomial distribution. For example, the two distributions are quite similar when the number of Bernoulli trials is large and the probability of success is small. The normal distribution is also used to approximate the Poisson distribution when μ is very large because the Poisson distribution is too unwieldy in this situation.

Hypothesis-Testing Statistics

Many statistical tests are used for hypothesis testing. Commonly used tests in epidemiological research include the Student t test and the chi-square test. A third type of test is the Z test, which is not described in this chapter. The decision to use a particular statistical test depends on the nature of the data under investigation. For example, the Student t test is used to test hypotheses about continuous variables when the variance is unknown or sample size is small, and the chi-square test is used for discrete data.

The Student t statistic can be used to test a hypothesis about the heights of adult residents in Wayland, Massachusetts (a continuous variable). For example, let us test the null hypothesis that the average height of males is equal to the average height of females by selecting two simple random samples of 20 men and 20 women each. Suppose that we find that the mean height and variance for the male sample are 69.1 and 34.8, respectively, and the mean height and variance for the female sample are 63.7 and 31.4, respectively. The following formula for the two-sample t test can be used to compare these two independent samples:

$$t_{df} = \frac{\overline{x}_1 - \overline{x}_2}{\sqrt{s_p^2 \frac{1}{n_1} + \frac{1}{n_2}}}$$

where t is the test statistic, $\bar{x}_1$ is the mean of the first sample and $\bar{x}_2$ is the mean of the second sample, s_p is the pooled estimate of the common variance, and n_1 and n_2 are the number of individuals in each sample. The degrees of freedom (df), the number of independent comparisons that can be made among members of a sample, equals $n_1 + n_2 - 2$. This equals the total number of quantities in a series ($n_1 + n_2$) minus the number of restrictions placed on the series (two, in this case because two means have been estimated).[6(p32)]

The pooled estimate of the common variance (s^2) estimates the variance of the entire study population (20 males and 20 females), and is calculated as follows:

$$s_p^2 = \frac{(n_1 - 1)s_1^2 + (n_2 - 1)s_2^2}{n_1 + n_2 - 2}$$

where s_p^2 is the pooled variance, n_1 is the number of individuals in the first sample, n_2 is the number of individuals in the second sample, s_1 is the variance of the first sample, and s_2 is the variance of the second sample. Using the data from the samples of men and women, we find that:

$$t_{20+20-2} = \frac{69.1 - 63.7}{\sqrt{33.1\left(\dfrac{1}{20} + \dfrac{1}{20}\right)}}$$

Thus, the t statistic equals 2.97 and has 38 degrees of freedom. This statistic can be converted into a probability statement or P value by looking up its value in a t table (which can be found in most biostatistics textbooks). The t value of 2.97 with 38 degrees of freedom corresponds to a P value of approximately 0.01. Thus, there is about a 1% probability of obtaining the observed result and more extreme results by chance alone, given that the null hypothesis is true.

Now let us use the chi-square statistic to test a hypothesis about the political affiliations of men and women in Wayland, (a discrete variable). In particular, let us test the null hypothesis that the proportion of registered Democrats is identical for men and women by selecting two new simple random samples of 20 men and 20 women each. Suppose that we find that the proportion of Democrats in the male sample is 40%, and the proportion of Democrats in the female sample is 50%. The following chi-square formula can be used to compare these two independent samples:

$$\chi_{df}^2 = \sum \frac{(O_i - E_i)^2}{E_i}$$

where χ^2 is the chi-square statistic, O_i is the observed count in a category, and E_i is the expected count in the category under the null hypothesis. Again, df stands for the number of degrees of freedom associated with the

TABLE 12–5 Observed and Expected Numbers of Democrats and Republicans among Men and Women in Wayland

Gender	Democrats	Republicans
Men		
Observed	8	12
Expected	9	11
Women		
Observed	10	10
Expected	9	11

statistic. Table 12–5 gives the observed counts and the expected values according to the null hypothesis. Note that we expect to see an equal proportion of Democrats among men and women.

Using these data, we calculate the chi-square statistic as follows: $(8 - 9)^2/9 + (12 - 11)^2/11 + (10 - 9)^2/9 + (10 - 11)^2/11 = 0.40$. The number of degrees of freedom is equal to the product of the number of categories in each variable minus one. Here, there are two categories of each variable (men and women, Democrats and Republicans), and so the number of degrees of freedom is $(2 - 1)(2 - 1)$ or 1. The chi-square statistic can be converted to a P value by looking up its value in a chi-square table. A chi-square value of 0.40 with 1 degree of freedom corresponds to a P value of approximately 0.50. Thus, there is a 50% probability of obtaining the observed result and more extreme result, by chance alone, given that the null hypothesis is true.

Confidence Intervals for Measures of Disease Frequency and Association

Many epidemiologists prefer to quantify random error by estimating confidence intervals. Either approximate or exact methods may be used to calculate confidence intervals. Approximate confidence intervals are easy to calculate because they assume that the point estimate is normally distributed. Exact confidence intervals, which are based on the binomial or Poisson distributions, are difficult to calculate because many values must be tested successively before one arrives at the correct interval value. Thus, epidemiologists primarily use exact intervals when normality cannot be assumed.

This section describes commonly used formulas for calculating approximate 95% confidence intervals around several measures of disease frequency—cumulative incidence, prevalence, incidence rate—and several absolute and relative measures of comparison.

Cumulative Incidence

The cumulative incidence is defined as the proportion of a candidate population that becomes diseased over a specified period of time (see Chapter 2). Mathematically, it is expressed as follows:

number of new cases of disease
number in candidate population over a specified time period

Let us use data presented in Chapter 3 to illustrate the calculation of a 95% confidence interval for cumulative incidence. Recall that the "Six Cities Study" was a prospective cohort study that investigated the association between air pollution and mortality. Investigators followed a sample of adults from six locations around the United States in order to measure the cumulative incidence of mortality.[14] The six locations provided a wide range of pollution levels from the highly polluted city of Steubenville, Ohio, to the relatively unpolluted city of Portage, Wisconsin.

The investigators observed an increased risk of death in the polluted areas. In particular, the cumulative incidence of mortality was 291/1351 (or 21.5%) among subjects from Steubenville and 232 per 1631 (or 14.2%) among subjects from Portage. Exact confidence intervals for cumulative incidence are calculated using the binomial distribution. However, when the sample size is large, the following normal distribution approximation formula can be used to quantify random error around these measurements:

$$CI_{L,U} = \frac{A}{N} \pm 1.96\sqrt{\frac{\frac{A}{N}\left(1-\frac{A}{N}\right)}{N}}$$

where $CI_{L,U}$ are the lower and upper bounds of the confidence interval, A is the number of cases of disease (the numerator of the cumulative incidence), and N is the number of individuals in the group (the denominator of the cumulative incidence denominator). This formula works best when the sample size is large and the outcome frequency is fairly high. Because these conditions are met in the Six Cities Study, we can calculate the approximate 95% confidence interval for the cumulative incidence of mortality in Steubenville as follows:

$$CI_{L,U} = \frac{291}{1351} \pm 1.96\sqrt{\frac{\frac{291}{1351}\left(1-\frac{291}{1351}\right)}{1351}}$$

Thus, the 95% confidence interval ranges from 20.4% to 22.6%. This means that our best estimate for the true mortality rate in Steubenville is 21.5%; however, we are 95% confident that the true mortality rate lies between 20.4% and 22.6%.

Prevalence

Prevalence is defined as the proportion of the total population that is diseased at a point or during a period of time (see Chapter 2). Mathematically, it is expressed as follows:

$$\frac{\text{number of existing cases of disease}}{\text{number in total population}}$$

The confidence interval formula for cumulative incidence is also appropriate for prevalence measures. For example, let us assume that we measure a prevalence of diabetes among a random sample of adults in Steubenville, Ohio, at 25 per 1000 people. We calculate the approximate 95% confidence interval for the diabetes prevalence as follows:

$$CI_{L,U} = \frac{25}{1000} \pm 1.96\sqrt{\frac{\frac{25}{1000}\left(1 - \frac{25}{1000}\right)}{1000}}$$

Thus, the 95% confidence interval ranges from 15.3 per 1000 to 34.7 per 1000. This means that our best estimate for the true prevalence of diabetes among adults in Steubenville is 25 per 1000, but we are 95% confident that the true prevalence lies between 15.3 and 34.7 per 1000.

Incidence Rate

The incidence rate is defined as the occurrence of new cases of disease arising during at-risk person-time of observation (see Chapter 2). Mathematically, it is expressed as follows:

$$\frac{\text{number of new cases of disease}}{\text{person-time of observation}}$$

Let us use incidence rate data from the Six Cities Study to illustrate calculation of the approximate 95% confidence interval for this measure of disease frequency. The incidence rate of death was 291 per 17,914 person-years (or 16.24/1000 person-years) in Steubenville, Ohio.[14] Exact confidence intervals for incidence rates are calculated using the Poisson distribution. However, when the sample size is large, the following normal distribution approximation formula can be used to quantify the random error around this type of measurement:

$$CI_{L,U} = \frac{A}{R} \pm 1.96\sqrt{\frac{A}{R^2}}$$

where $CI_{L,U}$ are the lower and upper bounds of the confidence interval, A is the number of cases, and R is the time at risk in the study population.

Thus, we calculate the 95% confidence interval for the incidence rate of mortality in Steubenville as follows:

$$\text{CI}_{L,U} = \frac{291}{17{,}914} \pm 1.96 \sqrt{\frac{291}{17{,}914^2}}$$

Thus, we are 95% confident that the true mortality rate in among adults in Steubenville lies in the range from 14.37 to 18.11 per 1000 person-years.

Absolute Measures of Comparison

Now, let us calculate an approximate 95% confidence interval for an absolute measure of comparison. Absolute comparisons are calculated either for exposed individuals or for the total population. When exposed individuals are the focus, the absolute difference measure is as follows:

$$\text{RD} = R_e - R_u$$

where RD = rate or risk difference (incidence rate difference, cumulative incidence difference, or prevalence difference), R_e = rate or risk (incidence rate, cumulative incidence, or prevalence) in the exposed group, and R_u = rate or risk (incidence rate, cumulative incidence, or prevalence) in the unexposed group. The particular formula for the 95% confidence intervals for risk or rate differences depends on the underlying measure of disease frequency and sample size. The following formula for an approximate 95% confidence interval may be used to quantify the random error around an incidence rate difference when the sample size is large:

$$\text{CI}_{L,U} = \text{RD} \pm 1.96 \sqrt{\frac{A_1}{R_1^2} + \frac{A_0}{R_0^2}}$$

where $\text{CI}_{L,U}$ are the lower and upper bounds of the confidence interval, RD is the rate or risk difference, A_1 is the number of exposed cases, A_0 is the number of unexposed cases, R_1 is the time at risk in the exposed group, and R_0 is the time at risk in the unexposed group.

Let us use results from the Six Cities Study to illustrate calculation of a 95% confidence interval for an incidence rate difference between Steubenville (the most polluted city) and Portage (the least polluted city). The incidence rates of mortality among subjects in these cities were 291 per 17,914 person-years (or 16.2 per 1000 person-years) and 232 per 21,618 person-years (or 10.7 per 1000 person-years), respectively.[14] Thus, the incidence rate difference is equal to 5.5 per 1000 person-years, and we calculate the corresponding 95% confidence interval as follows:

$$\text{RD} \pm 1.96 \sqrt{\frac{291}{17{,}914^2} + \frac{232}{21{,}618^2}}$$

Thus, we are 95% confident that the true incidence rate difference among adults from the two cities ranges from 3.2 to 7.8 per 1000 person-years.

Relative Measures of Comparison

The relative measure of comparison is based on the ratio of two measures of disease frequency. Mathematically, the relative measure is expressed as follows:

$$RR = R_e/R_u$$

where RR = rate or risk ratio; R_e = incidence rate, cumulative incidence, or prevalence in the exposed group; and R_u = incidence rate, cumulative incidence, or prevalence in the unexposed group. The following normal approximation formula may be used for a 95% confidence interval for a relative risk based on incidence rates when the sample size is large:

$$\ln RR_{L,U} = \ln RR \pm 1.96 \sqrt{\frac{1}{A_1} + \frac{1}{A_0}}$$

where L and U are the lower and upper bounds of the confidence interval, ln RR is the natural log of the rate ratio, A_1 is the number of cases in the exposed group, and A_0 is the number of cases in the unexposed group. Because this formula gives the confidence interval for the natural log of the rate ratio, it is necessary to take the antilog of the two bounds to obtain the confidence interval for the rate ratio itself. Using the incidence rate data from the Six Cities Study, we measure the incidence rate ratio at 16.24 per 1000 person-years/10.73 per 1000 person years or 1.51,[14] and we calculate the approximate 95% confidence interval as follows:

$$\ln RR_{L,U} = \ln 1.51 \pm 1.96 \sqrt{\frac{1}{291} + \frac{1}{232}}$$

Thus, taking the antilog of the two bounds, we are 95% confident that the true relative risk comparing adults from the two cities lies between 1.27 and 1.79.

It is usually impossible to calculate the rate or risk of disease in exposed and unexposed groups in a case–control study, and so the odds ratio must be used as the relative measure of comparison in this setting. Recall from Chapter 9 that either the disease odds ratio (the odds of being a case [a/b] among the exposed versus the odds of being a case among the unexposed [c/d]), or the exposure odds ratio (the odds of being exposed among cases [a/c] versus the odds of being exposed among controls [b/d]) may be calculated.

Consider the following hypothetical case–control study of DDE exposure and the risk of breast cancer presented in Chapter 11 (see Table 12–6).

TABLE 12–6 Crude Data from a Hypothetical Case–Control Study of DDE Exposure and Breast Cancer

	Breast Cancer	
DDE levels	Cases	Controls
High	500	600
Low	1500	3400
Total	2000	4000

According to these data, women with high serum DDE levels have a 1.9-fold increased risk of breast cancer as compared to women with low serum DDE levels (odds ratio = (500×3400)/(600×1500) = 1.9). The following formula for an approximate 95% confidence interval may be used to quantify the random error around an odds ratio:

$$\ln OR_{L,U} = \ln OR \pm 1.96\sqrt{\frac{1}{a}+\frac{1}{b}+\frac{1}{c}+\frac{1}{d}}$$

where ln OR is the natural log of the odds ratio, and a, b, c, and d are the cells of the two-by-two table that refer to the number of exposed cases (a), the number of exposed controls (b), and so forth. Using this formula, we calculate the 95% confidence interval as follows:

$$\ln OR_{L,U} = \ln 1.9 \pm 1.96\sqrt{\frac{1}{500}+\frac{1}{600}+\frac{1}{1500}+\frac{1}{3400}}$$

Thus, after taking the antilog of the calculated numbers, we can say that we are 95% confident that the true odds ratio ranges from 1.7 to 2.2. The formulas for approximate 95% confidence intervals are summarized in Table 12–7.

Sample Size and Power Calculations

Epidemiologists often use sample size calculations to plan the appropriate size of a study because they believe that correct inferences about the parent population can only be made with a sufficient sample size. But exactly what constitutes a "sufficient" sample size? To answer this question, investigators often turn to sample size formulas. These formulas, which can be found in most biostatistics textbooks, take into account the following factors: (1) the expected magnitude of the association, (2) the outcome rate in the comparison group (if a cohort or experimental study is being planned) or the exposure prevalence in the control group (if a case–control study is being planned), (3) the probability of rejecting the null hypothesis when it is true (known as the *type I* or *alpha error*, (4) the probability of missing a true association (known as the *type II* or *beta error*), and (5) the relative size of the compared groups.[15(p79)] In general, a large sample size is needed

TABLE 12-7 Approximate 95% Confidence Intervals for Measures of Disease Frequency and Comparison

Point estimate	Definition	95% confidence interval formula
Prevalence (P)	Number of existing cases (A)/number in total population (N)	$\dfrac{A}{N} \pm 1.96\sqrt{\dfrac{\dfrac{A}{N}\left(1-\dfrac{A}{N}\right)}{N}}$
Cumulative incidence (CI)	Number of new cases (A)/number in candidate population (N)	$\dfrac{A}{N} \pm 1.96\sqrt{\dfrac{\dfrac{A}{N}\left(1-\dfrac{A}{N}\right)}{N}}$
Incidence rate (IR)	Number of new cases (A)/person-time at-risk (R)	$\dfrac{A}{R} \pm 1.96\sqrt{\dfrac{A}{R^2}}$
Incidence rate difference (IRD)	Incidence rate$_\text{exp}$ (A_1/R_1) – incidence rate$_\text{unexp}$ (A_0/R_0)	$\text{IRD} \pm 1.96\sqrt{\dfrac{A_1}{R_1^2} + \dfrac{A_0}{R_0^2}}$
Incidence rate ratio (IRR)	Incidence rate$_\text{exp}$ (A_1/R_1)/incidence rate$_\text{unexp}$ (A_0/R_0)	$\ln \text{IRR} \pm 1.96\sqrt{\dfrac{1}{A_1} + \dfrac{1}{A_0}}$
Odds ratio (OR)	Exposure odds among cases (a/c)/exposure odds among controls (b/d), or disease odds among exposed (a/b)/disease odds among unexposed (c/d)	$\ln \text{OR} \pm 1.96\sqrt{\dfrac{1}{a} + \dfrac{1}{b} + \dfrac{1}{c} + \dfrac{1}{d}}$

when alpha and beta errors are small, when the expected magnitude of the association is small, and when the outcome rate in the comparison group of a cohort or experimental study or exposure prevalence in the control group of a case–control study is either very small or very large.

The information needed for the formula is gathered from several sources. The expected magnitude of the association comes from prior research. A scientifically important association is used, say a relative risk of 1.5 or 2.0, when prior studies are absent or ambiguous. The outcome rate in the comparison group (in a cohort or experimental study) or the exposure prevalence in the control group (in a case–control study) comes from pilot data from the actual study population or other populations. For example, a cohort study was designed to investigate the relationship between drinking water contaminants and reproductive and developmental abnormalities in the Cape Cod area of Massachusetts.[16] Outcome rates for the power calculations were gathered from national statistics on low birthweight, prematurity, and birth defects among demographically similar individuals during the years under study. The alpha and beta errors are assigned arbitrarily; usually the alpha error is set at 0.05 and the beta error is set at 0.20 or less. The latter implies that investigators aim for a sample size with at least 80% power (power is equal to 1 minus beta) to detect an association, if one truly exists.

Although sample size formulas are helpful, the information that goes into their calculations are either arbitrary (for example, alpha and beta errors) or educated guesses (such as expected magnitude of association). Furthermore, sample size calculations fail to account for numerous other factors including the value of the information gained from a study; the balance between precision and cost; and many unquantifiable social, political, and biological factors.[4(p117)] Thus, these estimates should not be cast in stone but rather should be considered "ballpark" figures of a sufficient sample size.

Some epidemiologists believe that power curves are more informative than sample size calculations for determining the needed study size.[15(pp79–80)] Power refers to the ability of a test to correctly reject the null hypothesis when the alternative hypothesis is true. When an association is present, the power of a study will increase as the study size increases. Power curves can be constructed that plot power against sample size for various estimates of an association. As displayed in Figure 12–7, power curves show the degree to which the study size must increase in order to attain greater power at differing estimates of an association.[15(p80)] These curves share some of the same drawbacks as sample size calculations. However, because they illustrate the informativeness of a particular sample size, they are more valuable for planning a study than sample size calculations. In the end, however, "the question of the most appropriate study size is not a technical decision . . . but a judgment to be determined by experience, intuition, and insight."[15(pp81–82)]

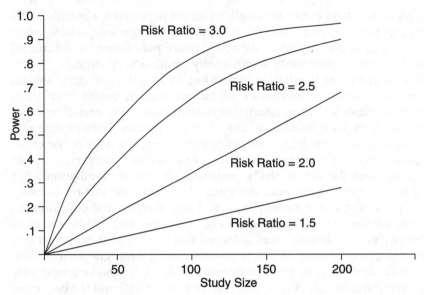

FIGURE 12-7. Power Curves for a Cohort Study with an Equal Number of Exposed and Unexposed Subjects (alpha error is 0.05; outcome frequency is 0.10)

Summary

Random error is considered an unsystematic error because it arises from an unforeseeable and unpredictable process known as chance. Precision is a term for the lack of random error. Two sources of random error are measurement error and sampling variability. Measurement error stems from inaccuracies in assessing the exposure and disease, and sampling variability stems from the selection of specific study subjects. Errors in subject selection lead to an unrepresentative sample of a parent population just by the "luck of the draw." This is another way of saying the uncontrollable force known as chance caused the sample selection problem.

Epidemiologists commonly use hypothesis testing to assess the role of random error and to make statistical inferences—that is, generalizations from a study sample to the parent population. In hypothesis testing, investigators specify the null and alternative hypotheses, evaluate the compatibility of the study results with the null hypothesis using statistical tests and P values, and decide whether to reject or not reject the null hypothesis. Commonly used statistical tests include the chi-square test and Student t test. The decision to use a particular test depends on the nature of the data under investigation (for example, continuous or discrete).

An integral part of hypothesis testing is the calculation of a P value, which is defined as the probability of obtaining the observed result (or a more extreme result) by chance alone when the null hypothesis is true. Although the P value is a continuous statistic, epidemiologists commonly use a cutoff of 0.05 (known as the alpha or significance level) to determine if the null hypothesis should be rejected. In recent years, hypothesis testing, particularly the use of P values, has come under criticism. Critics argue that the significance level of 0.05 is a purely arbitrary cutoff that can lead to incorrect interpretations of study results, and that the P value is confounded (that is, it mixes together the impact of the magnitude of the association with the impact of the sample size).

Today many epidemiologists prefer to use confidence intervals for quantifying random error. A confidence interval is calculated around a point estimate, which is typically a measure of disease frequency or association. Typically, 95% confidence intervals are calculated, and particular formulas for calculating them vary according to the point estimate. Epidemiologists prefer confidence intervals mainly because they are not confounded like P values, which means they can separate better the magnitude of the association from the sample size. The width of the confidence interval is influenced by the sample size, and the general position of the interval reflects the magnitude of the association. The strict statistical definition of a 95% confidence interval is as follows: If a study were repeated 100 times and 100 point estimates and confidence intervals were obtained, 95% of the intervals would contain the true measure of association. Although incorrect from a statistical viewpoint, two other ways to interpret confidence intervals are: (1) the range of possible values within which the true magnitude of effect lies with a certain level of certainty, and (2) the range of possible hypotheses that are compatible with the observed data with a certain level of certainty.

Mathematical probability theory is the basis for making statistical inferences from a study sample to a parent population. In fact, it is necessary to postulate a particular probability distribution for the data under the null hypothesis in order to calculate a P value and confidence interval. The normal, binomial, and Poisson distributions are commonly employed in epidemiologic research. The normal distribution is used for continuous variables, and the binomial and Poisson distributions are used for discrete events with two mutually exclusive outcomes. Each probability distribution is described by measures of central tendency and dispersion. The mean, median, and mode are commonly used central tendency measures; range, variance, standard deviation, and standard error of the mean are measures of spread. Formulas to calculate these measures vary according to the probability distribution.

Because correct inferences about the parent population can be made only with a sufficient sample size, epidemiologists use sample size calculations, power curves, experience, and intuition to plan the appropriate size for a study. Sample size formulas take into account the expected magnitude of the association, the outcome rate in the comparison group, and the alpha and beta levels. Power curves plot statistical power against sample size for various estimates of association.

References

1. Pickett JP, ed. *The American Heritage Dictionary of the English Language.* 4th ed. Boston, MA: Houghton Mifflin Company; 2000.
2. Armitage P, Colton T, ed-in-chief. *Encyclopedia of Biostatistics.* Vol 3. Chichester, England: John Wiley and Sons; 1998.
3. Medical Research Council. Streptomycin in Tuberculosis Trials Committee. Streptomycin treatment of pulmonary tuberculosis. *Br Med J.* 1948;2:769–782.
4. Rothman KJ, Greenland S. *Modern Epidemiology.* 2nd ed. Philadelphia, PA: Lippincott-Raven; 1998.
5. Last JM, ed. *A Dictionary of Epidemiology.* 3rd ed. New York, NY: Oxford University Press; 1995.
6. Colton T. *Statistics in Medicine.* Boston, MA: Little, Brown and Company; 1974.
7. Rosner, B. *Fundamentals of Biostatistics.* 5th ed. Pacific Grove, CA: Duxbury Thompson Learning; 2000.
8. Popper KR. *The Logic of Scientific Discovery.* New York, NY: Basic Books; 1959 (reprint of 1935 ed).
9. Lang JM, Rothman KJ, and Cann CI. That confounded P value. *Epidemiology.* 1998;9:7–8.
10. Rothman KJ. No adjustments are needed for multiple comparisons. *Epidemiology.* 1990;1:43–46.
11. Ahlbom A. *Biostatistics for Epidemiologists.* Boca Raton, FL: Lewis Publishers; 1993.
12. Wayland, Massachusetts Home Page. Available at: www.wayland.ma.us/aboutwayland.html. Accessed June 2001.
13. U.S. Census Bureau. Type of household—Households (all races) by median and mean income: 1980 to 1999, Table H–9. Available at: http://www.census.gov/hhes/income/histinc/h09.html.
14. Dockery DW, Pope CA, Xu X, Spengler JD, Ware JH, Fay ME, Ferris BG, et al. An association between air pollution and mortality in six U.S. cities. *N Engl J Med.* 1993;329:1753–1759.
15. Rothman KJ. *Modern Epidemiology.* 1st ed. Boston, MA: Little, Brown and Co; 1986.
16. Aschengrau A, Rogers S, Ozonoff D. Tetrachloroethylene-contaminated drinking water and the risk of reproductive and developmental disorders (Unpublished Manuscript).

EXERCISES

1. Define each of the following terms:
   A. Chance
   B. Precision
   C. Statistical inference

2. What is the main assumption involved in hypothesis testing and the calculation of P values?

3. What is the main limitation of significance testing?

4. Why are P values considered confounded statistics?

5. A case–control study was conducted in Europe to determine the association between dietary factors and coronary heart disease. The investigators found an odds ratio of 1.8 for coronary heart disease among subjects who cooked with margarine (the exposed group) compared to those who cooked with olive oil (the reference group). The 95% confidence interval for this odds ratio was 0.8 to 4.3, and the upper one-sided P value was 0.10.
   A. State in words your interpretation of the odds ratio.
   B. State in words your interpretation of the 95% confidence interval.
   C. Do you think that this confidence interval is relatively wide or narrow?
   D. State in words your interpretation of the P value.

6. Give one reason why many epidemiologists prefer to use confidence intervals instead of P values to assess the role of random error.

7. State the probability distributions that are commonly used in epidemiologic research and describe the settings in which they are used.

13

Effect Measure Modification

LEARNING OBJECTIVES

By the end of this chapter, the reader will be able to:

- Define and provide examples of effect measure modification including synergy and antagonism.
- Distinguish between confounding and effect measure modification.
- Describe the methods for evaluating effect measure modification.
- State the relationship between the measure of association and effect measure modification.

Introduction

As described in Chapters 10 through 12, epidemiologists evaluate whether a study result is valid by assessing the presence of bias, confounding, and random error. Confounding is a mixing of effects between an exposure, an outcome, and a third variable known as the confounder.[1(p120)] Epidemiologists control for confounding using a variety of methods in the design and analysis of a study. While assessing and controlling for confounding during the analysis, investigators also determine if the magnitude of the association between an exposure and disease is changed or modified by a third variable. If the size of the association changes according to the level of a third variable, then effect measure modification is present. Unlike bias and confounding, which are problems that the investigator needs to eliminate, effect modification is a natural phenomenon of scientific interest that the investigator aims to describe and understand. This chapter defines and describes effect measure modification, explains how it differs from confounding, and describes the principal ways to evaluate its presence.

Definitions and Terms for Effect Measure Modification

Effect measure modification, also known as *heterogeneity of effect*, means that the strength of the association between an exposure and disease differs according to the level of another variable. This other variable is called the effect modifier. For example, age is a modifier of the relationship between race and breast cancer incidence. There is no difference in breast cancer incidence rates between black and white women under the age of 50 years.[2] However, the breast cancer incidence rate is about 16% higher among white women aged 50 years and older than among black women of the same age.

The term *homogeneity of effect* is used when effect modification is absent. An example of homogeneity of effect is the relationship between religion, age, and breast cancer. Jewish women have a higher risk of breast cancer than do women who belong to other religious groups at both young and old ages.[3] Furthermore, older women have a higher risk of breast cancer than younger women, regardless of their religious affiliation.

Epidemiologists often use the term "effect modification" instead of effect measure modification to describe the change in an association according to the level of the third variable. However, this simplification leads to ambiguity, because effect measure modification depends on the particular measure of association describing the relationship between the exposure and disease.[1(p254)] That is, it depends on whether a ratio measure or a difference measure is being used. When effect modification is present using a ratio measure of association, it will be necessarily absent when a difference measure of association is used, and vice versa. (This concept is discussed later in the chapter.) Consequently, it is important to describe the presence of effect measure modification as specifically as possible, for example, by stating "heterogeneity of the risk ratio was observed." The expression "statistical interaction" is also commonly used to describe effect measure modification. It, too, should be avoided because the term is too vague.

Effect measure modification should not be considered merely an arbitrary statistical phenomenon, but rather it should be regarded as a causal framework for gaining insight into a natural phenomenon.[1(p329-342)] For example, age modifies the relationship between a woman's weight and her risk of breast cancer.[4] Thinness increases a woman's relative risk of breast cancer before 50 years of age, and obesity increases her relative risk at older ages. These different associations likely reflect biological differences such as differences in circulating hormone levels between pre- and postmenopausal women, and so provide important clues to the pathological mechanism whereby a normal breast cell is transformed into a cancerous one.

The epidemiologic literature contains many well-known examples of effect measure modification that have both helped epidemiologists to understand the biology of a particular disease and have led to important medical and public health policy recommendations. One example is the modification of the relationship between cigarette smoking and bronchogenic cancer (cancer of the lung, bronchus, and trachea) by asbestos exposure.[5] In a landmark study, Selikoff and colleagues found that asbestos insulation workers in general had a 10-fold increased risk of dying from bronchogenic cancer but that asbestos insulation workers who smoked had 92 times the risk of dying from bronchogenic cancer as compared to men who did not smoke and were not exposed to asbestos. This tremendous increased risk among individuals with both exposures reflects the pathological process whereby the carcinogens in cigarette smoke and asbestos fibers exacerbate one another to transform normal cells into malignant ones. These data have also been used to guide occupational and safety health recommendations to reduce workplace exposure to chemical and physical agents such as asbestos and to initiate smoking-cessation campaigns among working groups, especially those exposed to asbestos.[6]

Another well-known example of effect measure modification is the modification of the relationship between oral contraceptives and myocardial infarction by the presence of other factors such as cigarette smoking and obesity.[7] For example, Mann and colleagues found that women who had recently used oral contraceptives had about a threefold increased risk of myocardial infarction as compared to women who did not use oral contraceptives. However, women who had at least two additional risk factors for myocardial infarction (such as high lipid levels, cigarette smoking, and obesity) had a 78-fold increased risk of myocardial infarction compared to women who did not have any of these risk factors. Again, the heterogeneity of the risk ratio has helped us understand the biological basis of myocardial infarction and has provided a rational basis for physicians' recommendation that certain women avoid using oral contraceptives.[8] In addition, it may have prompted manufacturers to produce safer formulations of oral contraceptives.

Effect Measure Modification Versus Confounding

Confounding and effect measure modification are sometimes confused. This is because effect measure modification, like confounding, involves a third variable in addition to the exposure and disease and is evaluated by conducting stratified analyses. However, one has nothing to do with the other. In fact, a particular variable may be: (1) a confounder but not an effect modifier, (2) an effect modifier but not a confounder, (3) both a confounder and an effect modifier, or (4) neither a confounder nor an effect modifier. The key difference is that confounding is a problem that epidemiologists aim to eliminate and effect measure modification is an interesting occurrence that epidemiologists aim to describe. The occurrence of interest is the change in the relation of an exposure and disease according to the level of another variable. Thus, we pose two different questions when we consider confounding and effect measure modification in stratified analyses. For confounding, we are asking whether the crude measure of association is distorted and whether the stratum-specific and adjusted summary estimates are different from the crude estimate. For effect modification, we are asking if the association differs according to the level of a third variable—that is, whether the stratum-specific estimates are different from one another.

Evaluation of Effect Measure Modification

To explain effect measure modification, it is helpful to return to the crude and stratified analyses from Chapter 11 that examined the hypothetical relationship between DDE exposure and the risk of breast cancer. Let us first reexamine the crude data (see Table 13–1). There is a 1.9-fold increased risk of breast cancer among women who were exposed to high DDE levels (odds ratio = (500×3400)/(600×1500) = 1.9).

Now let us reexamine these results stratified into two age groups— women less than 50 years of age and women aged 50 years and older (see Table 13–2). Note that there is no association between DDE and breast cancer among women who are less than 50 years or among those who are 50 years and older. Each stratum-specific odds ratio is 1.0. Thus, the magnitude of the odds ratio does not differ across the strata but the stratum-specific odds ratios (1.0) are different from the crude odds ratio (1.9). As discussed in Chapter 11, the noticeable difference between the crude and

TABLE 13–1 Crude Data from a Hypothetical Case–Control Study of DDE Exposure and Breast Cancer

	Breast Cancer	
DDE levels	Cases	Controls
High	500	600
Low	1500	3400
Total	2000	4000
	Odds ratio: 1.9	

stratum-specific odds ratios indicates that confounding by age is present. On the other hand, the lack of a difference between the two stratum-specific odds ratios indicates that effect measure modification (in this case, heterogeneity of the odds ratio) is absent.

Now let us consider the impact of lactation history on the relationship between DDE levels and breast cancer risk (see Table 13–3). The women are divided into two groups: those who never breast fed and those who breast fed at least one child before their diagnosis or index year. (The index year is a cutoff date for controls that is comparable to the diagnosis year for cases. Only exposures and effect measure modifiers that occur before the index or diagnosis year are etiologically relevant.)

Here, the association varies according to a woman's lactation history. The odds ratio among women who never breast fed is 2.2, and the odds ratio among those who breast fed at least one child is 1.0. In other words, women who have high DDE exposure levels and never breast fed have a 2.2-fold increased risk of breast cancer, and women who have high DDE levels but did breast feed have no elevation in risk. The heterogeneity of the stratum-specific odds ratio indicates that lactation history is an effect modifier of the relationship between DDE exposure level and breast cancer. These data support two possible underlying physiological mechanisms: (1) breastfeeding may reduce the susceptibility of the breast tissue to environmental carcinogens through tissue differentiation[9] or (2) breastfeeding may reduce breast tissue exposure to environmental carcinogens through excretion.[10]

TABLE 13–2 Age-Stratified Data from a Hypothetical Case–Control Study of DDE Exposure and Breast Cancer

	Age less than 50 years			*Age 50 years and older*	
DDE levels	*Cases*	*Controls*	*DDE levels*	*Cases*	*Controls*
High	50	300	High	450	300
Low	450	2700	Low	1050	700
Total	500	3000	Total	1500	1000
Stratum-specific odds ratio = 1.0			Stratum-specific odds ratio = 1.0		

TABLE 13–3 Data from a Hypothetical Case–Control Study of DDE Exposure and Breast Cancer Stratified According to Lactation History

	Never breast fed			*Breast fed*	
DDE levels	*Cases*	*Controls*	*DDE levels*	*Cases*	*Controls*
High	140	300	High	360	300
Low	550	2600	Low	950	800
Total	690	2900	Total	1310	1100
Stratum-specific odds ratio = 2.2			Stratum-specific odds ratio = 1.0		

Epidemiologists generally use two methods to determine if the stratum-specific results are different from one another: visual inspection or a statistical test. In the example above, simple visual inspection indicates clearly that the two odds ratios are different. If a more formal assessment is desired, numerous statistical tests are available to test the null hypothesis that the differences in the stratum-specific measures of association reflect merely random variation. In this example it is appropriate to use the chi-square test for homogeneity of the odds ratios over different strata with the Woolf method.[11(pp603–604)] This analysis tests the null hypothesis (H_O) that the stratum-specific odds ratios are equal versus the alternative hypothesis (H_A) that at least two of the stratum-specific odds ratios are different. The number of stratum-specific odds ratios depends on the number of strata. There are only two strata in the example above, but there can be more.

The test is based on the following chi-square test statistic:

$$\chi^2_{HOM} = \sum^{I=1 \text{ to } k} w_i \left(\ln OR_i - \ln OR\right)^2$$

where $\ln OR_i$ is the log odds ratio relating disease to exposure in the ith stratum of the potential effect modifier, $\ln OR$ = the weighted average log odds ratio over all strata, and w_i is the weight that is inversely proportional to the variance of $\ln OR_i$.

More specifically, $\ln OR_i$ = log odds ratio in the ith stratum = $\ln [(a_i d_i)/(b_i c_i)]$, where a_i, b_i, c_i, d_i are the cells of the two-by-two table relating disease to exposure in the ith stratum; weight=$w_i = [1/a_i + 1/b_i + 1/c_i + 1/d_i]^{-1}$, and $\ln OR = \sum^{I=1 \text{ to } k} w_i \ln OR_i / \sum^{I=1 \text{ to } k} w_i$.

Note that the purpose of the weighting is to weight strata with lower variances more than strata with higher variances. This is done because low variance strata have more subjects than high variance strata. The weighted differences between $\ln OR_i$ and $\ln OR$ are summed over all of the strata (1 to k). Once the chi-square statistic is calculated, a P value may be obtained from a table of chi-square values, as described in Chapter 12. This chi-square test has $k - 1$ degrees of freedom, where k is the total number of strata.

The null hypothesis (H_0) in the hypothetical example described above is as follows: the odds ratio among women who never breast fed is equal to the odds ratio among women who breast fed at least one child. In addition, the alternative hypothesis (H_A) is: the odds ratio among women who never breast fed is different from the odds ratio among women who did breast feed. Using the formula given above, we perform the following calculations:

$$\chi^2_{HOM} = \sum^{I=1 \text{ to } k} w_i \left(\ln OR_i - \ln OR\right)^2, \text{ where}$$

$\ln OR_1$ among women who never breast fed = $\ln [(140 \times 2600/300 \times 550)]$ = 0.79

w_1 among women who never breast fed = $[1/140 + 1/2600 + 1/300 + 1/550]^{-1}$ = 62.15

ln OR_2 for a positive breastfeeding history = ln $[(360 \times 800/300 \times 950)]$ = 0.0
w_2 for a positive history of breast feeding = $[1/360 + 1/800 + 1/300 + 1/950]$ = 118.91
ln OR = $[(0.79) \times (62.15) + (0) \times (118.91)]/(62.15 + 118.91)$ = 0.2715

Thus, the test statistic is given as follows:

χ^2_{HOM} = 62.15 $(0.791 - 0.2715)^2$ + 118.906 $(0 - 0.2715)^2$ = 25.54 with one degree of freedom

Referring to a chi-square table, we note that the corresponding P value is less than 0.001. This indicates that we can reject the null hypothesis that the odds ratios are the same across breastfeeding history strata, and we can conclude that effect measure modification of the odds ratio is present. Thus, the visual inspection and statistical test lead us to the same conclusion.

Now let us turn to a real-life example of effect measure modification from the Boston Partners Study, a cohort study of biologic and behavioral risk factors for transmission of the human immunodeficiency virus (HIV) among infected men and their partners. Investigators conducted this analysis to clarify the risk of HIV infection from unprotected receptive anal intercourse with and without the use of the drug amyl nitrite.[12] This example illustrates another method for assessing the presence of effect measure modification: comparison of the excess relative risk.

The investigators hypothesized that amyl nitrite inhalation relaxed the smooth muscles and dilated the blood vessels around the anal sphincter, thereby allowing for more traumatic sexual activity and facilitating entry of HIV into the bloodstream during anal intercourse. Thus, they compared the odds ratios for the four possible exposure categories: (1) a history of nitrite use and a history of unprotected receptive anal intercourse, (2) no history of nitrite use and a history of unprotected receptive anal intercourse, (3) a history of nitrite use and no history of unprotected receptive anal intercourse and, (4) no history of nitrite use and no history of unprotected receptive anal intercourse. The last exposure category—a negative history of both exposures—served as the referent category for all the comparisons. The results are provided in Table 13–4.

Note that, compared to men with a negative history of both unprotected receptive anal intercourse and nitrite use, the risk of HIV infection was higher among men with a positive history of unprotected receptive anal intercourse and nitrite use (RR = 10.1), than among men with a positive history of unprotected receptive anal intercourse and a negative history of nitrite use (RR = 4.1), and among men with a positive history of nitrite use and a negative history of unprotected anal intercourse (RR = 2.7).

Now let us compare the excess relative risks to determine if effect measure modification is present. The excess relative risk is defined as the

TABLE 13–4   Risk Ratios for HIV Infection According to History of Nitrite Use and Unprotected Receptive Anal Intercourse

Exposure category	Number of persons	Risk ratio
Nitrite use/unprotected receptive anal intercourse	317	10.1
No nitrite use/unprotected receptive anal intercourse	102	4.1
Nitrite use/no unprotected receptive anal intercourse	31	2.7
No nitrite use/no unprotected receptive anal intercourse	31	1.0

Source: Data from Seage GR III, Mayer KH, Horsburgh CR, Holmberg SD, Moon MW, Lamb GA. The relation between nitrite inhalants, unprotected receptive anal intercourse, and the risk of human immunodeficiency virus infection. *Am J Epidemiol.* 1992;135:1–11.

relative measure of association minus one (e.g., risk ratio minus one). Thus, the excess relative risk associated with having both factors is 9.1 (10.1 – 1.0), the excess relative risk associated with only unprotected receptive anal intercourse is 3.1 (4.1 – 1.0), and the excess relative risk associated with only nitrite use is 1.7 (2.7 – 1.0). Because the excess relative risk associated with having both factors together (9.1) is larger than the sum of the excess relative risk associated with each factor alone (3.1 + 1.7 = 4.8), we may conclude that there is effect measure modification known as "the departure from additivity."

It is possible to have a stronger level of effect measure modification known as "the departure from multiplicity." This occurs when the excess relative risk associated with having both factors together is larger than the product of the excess relative risk associated with each factor alone. In fact, supplemental data from the Boston Partners Study found that men who always used nitrite inhalants when participating in unprotected receptive anal intercourse had a 33.8-fold increased risk of HIV infection as compared to men who never used inhalants and never engaged in unprotected receptive anal intercourse. The excess relative risk associated with such frequent nitrite use (32.8) represents a departure from multiplicity, because it is greater than the product of the excess relative risks associated with each factor alone (3.1 × 1.7 = 5.3). Note that departure from additivity represents a low to moderate level of effect measure modification, and departure from multiplicity represents a high level.

Synergy and Antagonism

The terms synergy and antagonism are used to describe effect measure modification. *Synergy,* which is also known as positive interaction, is said to occur when the excess relative risk among individuals with both factors

TABLE 13–5 Hypothetical Risk Ratios for Gastroenteritis According to Consumption of Contaminated Fish and Alcoholic Beverages

Exposure category	Risk ratio
Ate contaminated fish/drank alcoholic beverage	1.5
Ate contaminated fish/did not drink alcoholic beverage	5.0
Did not eat contaminated fish/drank alcoholic beverage	1.0
Did not eat contaminated fish/did not drink alcoholic beverage	1.0

is greater than the sum of the excess relative risks of each factor considered alone. Thus, synergy occurs when two factors work in concert to produce more disease than one would expect based on the action of either factor working alone. Synergy is a more general term for "departure from additivity or multiplicity." Several examples of synergy have been given in this chapter including the relationship between nitrite use, unprotected anal intercourse, and the risk of HIV infection; the relationship between smoking, asbestos exposure, and lung cancer; and the relationship between oral contraceptives, smoking and other risk factors, and myocardial infarction.

Antagonism, which is also known as negative interaction, is said to occur when the excess relative risk among individuals with both factors is less than the sum of the excess relative risks of each factor considered alone. It means that one factor reduces the impact or even cancels out the effect of the other factor. Consider, for example, a hypothetical study of the risk of gastroenteritis following the ingestion of contaminated shellfish. Individuals who ate the shellfish were three times as likely to develop gastroenteritis during the 24-hour follow-up period than those who did not eat the shellfish. However, when the consumption of other food items was taken into account, the investigators found that individuals who consumed an alcoholic beverage along with the contaminated shellfish had only a 1.5-fold increased risk of gastroenteritis, and those who did not consume any alcoholic beverages with the contaminated fish had a 5-fold increased risk of gastroenteritis (see Table 13–5). Of course, there was no increased risk of gastroenteritis among individuals who did not eat contaminated shellfish, regardless of their alcohol consumption. Thus, the excess relative risk for individuals with both exposures (1.5 – 1.0 = 0.5) was less than the sum of the excess relative risks for individuals with only one of the exposures [(5.0 – 1.0) + (1.0 – 1.0) = 4.0]. A plausible explanation for these results is that the alcoholic beverage killed the pathogenic bacteria in the subject's gastrointestinal tract.

Choice of Measure

Effect measure modification depends on the measure of association that is being used—that is, whether a ratio measure (rate, risk, or odds ratio) or

TABLE 13–6 Hypothetical Incidence Rates, Rate Ratios, and Rate Differences of Breast Cancer Following Radiation Exposure According to the Age at Which the Exposure Occurred

Constant incidence rate ratios/changing incidence rate differences

Age of exposure (years)	Incidence rate (per 100,000 person-years)	Rate ratio	Rate difference
20	125 among exposed/75 among unexposed	2.5	50
30	300 among exposed/120 among unexposed	2.5	180
40	450 among exposed/180 among unexposed	2.5	270

Constant incidence rate differences/changing incidence rate ratios

Age of exposure (years)	Incidence rates (per 100,000 person-years)	Rate ratio	Rate difference
20	210 among exposed/70 among unexposed	3.0	140
30	310 among exposed/170 among unexposed	1.8	140
40	420 among exposed/280 among unexposed	1.5	140

difference measure (risk or rate difference) is being used. Thus, when effect modification is present using a ratio measure, it will necessarily be absent when a difference measure is used, and vice versa.

Consider a hypothetical example of the risk of breast cancer following exposure to radiation according to the age at which the radiation exposure occurred (see Table 13–6). When the incidence rate ratio is constant at 2.5, the incidence rate difference changes according to the age at exposure. In this hypothetical example, the incidence rate difference increases because the incidence rate increases with age more dramatically among exposed women. In addition, when the incidence rate difference is constant at 140 cases per 100,000 person-years, the incidence rate ratio decreases with age. The higher rate ratios at younger ages may reflect the lower baseline rate of breast cancer at younger ages. In fact, effect measure modification seen on the ratio scale may represent nothing more than different levels of baseline risk.

Evaluating Effect Measure Modification and Confounding in Stratified Analyses

Epidemiologists conduct stratified analyses to evaluate simultaneously the presence of effect measure modification and confounding. Figure 13–1 contains a decision tree for evaluating data for both of these issues and provides information on the proper presentation of the results.

First, investigators conduct a crude analysis of the relationship between the exposure and disease. Next, they conduct a stratified analysis that

Conduct crude analysis.
↓
Conduct stratified analysis.
↓
Evaluate effect measure modification by examining stratum-specific estimates visually or by performing statistical tests.

Effect measure modification is present if estimates are different from one another.
↓
Give stratum-specific results.
↓
Proceed with evaluation of confounding.
↓
If present, give standardized estimates. If not present, give crude estimates.

Effect measure modification is not present if estimates are not different from one another.
↓
Proceed with evaluation of confounding.
↓
If present, give pooled or standardized estimates. If not present, give crude estimates.

FIGURE 13–1 Decision Tree for Evaluating and Presenting Data with Effect Measure Modification and Confounding

separates the crude data according to levels of the potential confounder/ effect modifier. Effect measure modification is evaluated either by examining the stratum-specific estimates visually or by performing a statistical test. Effect measure modification is considered present if the stratum-specific estimates are sufficiently different from one another, and absent if the stratum-specific estimates are not different enough. The results of the visual inspection and statistical test may differ, and so investigators must judge which results are more likely to be correct. Next, investigators evaluate confounding by comparing the stratum-specific estimates with the crude estimate. If both confounding and effect measure modification are present, stratum-specific and standardized estimates should be presented. If effect measure modification is present but confounding is absent, crude and stratum-specific estimates should be presented. If effect measure modification is absent but confounding is present, the pooled or standardized results should be presented; if neither confounding nor effect measure modification are present, the crude results alone are sufficient.

Summary

Effect measure modification is defined as a change in the strength of an association between an exposure and disease according to the level of a third variable. Other commonly used terms for this phenomenon include heterogeneity of effect and (less preferable) statistical interaction. Unlike confounding, which is considered a nuisance that epidemiologists aim to eliminate, effect measure modification is an interesting scientific phenomenon that epidemiologists aim to describe. Because its presence depends on the particular measure of association, effect measure modification should be described using terms that specify the measure (for example, heterogeneity of the risk ratio). Furthermore, when effect measure modification is present using a ratio measure, it will necessarily be absent when a difference measure is used. Departure from additivity represents a low to moderate degree of modification, and departure from multiplicity represents a high degree. Synergy occurs when two factors work together to produce more disease than one would expect based on the action of either factor alone. In contrast, antagonism occurs when one factor reduces the impact or even cancels out the effect of another factor. Effect measure modification is evaluated in stratified analyses through visual inspection, statistical tests, or evaluation of excess relative risks.

References

1. Rothman KJ, Greenland S. *Modern Epidemiology*. 2nd ed. Philadelphia, PA: Lippincott-Raven Publishers; 1998.
2. Ries LAG, Eisner MP, Kosary Cl, Hankey BF, Miller BA, Clegg L, et al, eds. *SEER Cancer Statistics Review, 1973–1998*. Bethesda, MD: National Cancer Institute; 2001.
3. Egan KM, Newcomb PA, Longnecker MP, Trentham-Diaz A, Baron JA, Trichopolous D, et al. Jewish religion and risk of breast cancer. *Lancet*. 1996;347: 1645–1646.
4. Kelsey JL. Breast cancer epidemiology. *Epidemiol Rev*. 1993;15:256–263.
5. Selikoff IJ, Hammond EC, Churg J. Asbestos exposures, smoking, and neoplasia. *JAMA*. 1968;204:104–110.
6. Robbins A. *Adverse Health Effects of Smoking and the Occupational Environment*. NIOSH pub. no. 79–122. Cincinnati, OH: National Institute for Occupational Safety and Health; 1979.
7. Mann JI, Vessey MP, Thorogood M, Doll R. Myocardial infarction in young women with special reference to oral contraceptive practice. *Br Med J*. 1975;2: 241–245.
8. U.S. Department of Health and Human Services. *Facts about oral contraceptives*. Available at: http://www.nih.gov/health/chip/nichd/oralcnt. Accessed October 2000.
9. Russo J, Russo IH. Toward a physiological approach to breast cancer prevention. *Cancer Epidemiol Biomarkers Prev*. 1994;3:353–364.
10. Murrell TG. Epidemiological and biochemical support for a theory on the cause and prevention of breast cancer. *Med Hypotheses*. 1991;36:389–396.
11. Rosner B. *Fundamentals of Biostatistics*. 5th ed. Pacific Grove, CA: Duxbury Thompson Learning; 2000.

12. Seage GR III, Mayer KH, Horsburgh CR, Holmberg SD, Moon MW, Lamb GA. The relation between nitrite inhalants, unprotected receptive anal intercourse, and the risk of human immunodeficiency virus infection. *Am J Epidemiol.* 1992; 135:1–11.

EXERCISES

1. Define each of the following terms:
   A. Effect measure modification
   B. Heterogeneity and homogeneity of effect
   C. Synergy
   D. Antagonism

2. Briefly describe the key difference between confounding and effect measure modification.

3. Briefly describe how epidemiolgists determine if a variable is an effect modifier.

4. A case–control study was conducted to determine if the relationship between cigarette smoking and lung cancer is modified by the presence of asbestos exposure. The following results were obtained:

Exposed to:	Odds ratio for lung cancer
Both smoking and asbestos	50.0
Only smoking	10.0
Only asbestos	5.0
Neither	1.0

   A. Is asbestos an effect measure modifier of the relation between smoking and lung cancer?
   B. State the reason for your answer.

5. The association between heavy alcohol consumption and the risk of oral cancer was investigated in a case–control study with 475 cases and 400 controls. The following results were seen:

Heavy Alcohol Consumption	Cases	Controls
Yes	350	200
No	125	200
Total	475	400

A. Calculate the crude odds ratio based on these data.
B. Gender was considered a potential confounder and/or effect measure modifier in this study. The data were stratified into males and females in order to assess these issues. Calculate the stratum-specific odds ratios among males and females using the following data:

Heavy alcohol consumption	Males		Females	
	Cases	Controls	Cases	Controls
Yes	300	150	50	50
No	50	50	75	150

C. Is gender a confounder in this study?
D. Is gender an effect measure modifier in this study?
E. Briefly justify your answers to parts C and D.

14

Critical Review of Epidemiologic Studies

LEARNING OBJECTIVES

By the end of this chapter, the reader will be able to:

- Describe a method for critically evaluating the published literature.
- Apply the critique outline to published articles.

Introduction

One of the most useful outcomes of studying epidemiology is learning how to evaluate critically the scientific literature. Critical assessment of this literature is an important skill for public health professionals because the findings of epidemiologic research inform so many activities. For example, the application of epidemiologic research methods have helped determine the impact of laws requiring motorcycle helmet use in reducing head injuries,[1] the effectiveness of taking an aspirin every other day in reducing cardiovascular mortality,[2] the interaction between nitrite inhalants and unprotected receptive anal intercourse on the risk of HIV-1 (human immunodeficiency virus, type 1) infection,[3] the scientific basis for setting permissible pollutant levels,[4] ways to reduce cesarean section rates,[5] the effectiveness of niacin fortification of the U.S. food supply in reducing the nutritional deficiency disease pellagra,[6] and methods for improving doctor–patient communication.[7] Epidemiologic research has helped us understand the pattern of occurrence and etiology of diseases throughout the world, including acquired immune deficiency syndrome, (AIDS), tuberculosis, Lyme disease, *Chlamydia* infection, cardiovascular disease, stroke, cancer, diabetes, Alzheimer's disease, osteoarthritis, and depression.

Publishing in scientific journals is a major avenue for communicating the results of epidemiologic studies. The major public health and epidemiology journals include *American Journal of Public Health, American Journal of Epidemiology, Epidemiology, Annals of Epidemiology,* and *International Journal of Epidemiology.* Medical and subspecialty journals also publish the results of epidemiologic studies. Some of the best known are *New England Journal of Medicine, Journal of the American Medical Association,* and *Lancet.*

Journal articles are typically organized in the following format: abstract, introduction, materials and methods, results, discussion, conclusions, and references. The purpose of the abstract is to provide a short summary of the goals, methods, main findings, and conclusions of the study. The introduction describes the context and motivation for the study. The materials and methods section reports on the setting, design, data collection procedures, and analysis of the study. In our opinion, this section is the most important part of the article because it provides critical information about the study's validity. The results section describes the characteristics of the study population and the study findings. It typically includes text, several tables, and figures. The findings of epidemiologic studies are quantitative in nature and usually include the measures of disease frequency and association described in Chapters 2 and 3. The discussion section provides the scientific interpretation of the findings, places the findings in the context of other research, and acknowledges the study's limitations. The conclusions, which are either part of the discussion or in a separate section, briefly summarize the findings and their implications. The conclusions often include recommendations for future research and public health policy; however, the latter practice has been discouraged.[8] The article concludes with references for all cited scientific facts.

The critique outline shown in Exhibit 14–1 has been adapted from an outline originally developed by Richard Monson of Harvard School of Public Health.[9(p94)] We believe that it is a useful guide for learning how to evaluate a study and have used it extensively in our teaching. The outline helps "disentangle the skeins of serendipity, bias, and intent that run throughout epidemiologic research."[10(p556)] In other words, it provides a framework to help epidemiologists assess: (1) whether the methods used to select the study subjects and collect and analyze the data were comparable across groups; (2) whether any errors were committed in the design, conduct, or interpretation of the study; and (3) what impact these errors had on the reported findings.[9(p94)]

The critique outline is organized into three sections: data collection, analysis, and interpretation. All well-written articles published in reputable journals should contain the information needed to answer the critique questions. If an article does not contain most of this information, one can assume that the study quality is poor. If an article is silent on a particular issue, it is usually safe to assume that the issue was not addressed. For

EXHIBIT 14–1

OUTLINE FOR CRITIQUING EPIDEMIOLOGIC STUDIES

A. Collection of data

1. What was the context of the study?

2. What were the objectives of the study?

3. What was the primary exposure of interest? Was this accurately measured?

4. What was the primary outcome of interest? Was this accurately measured?

5. What type of study was conducted?

6. Describe the source of the study population, process of subject selection, sample size, and ratio of propositi to comparison subjects. (Propositi are exposed subjects in an experimental or cohort study and cases in a case–control study.)

7. Could there have been bias in the selection of the study subjects? How likely was this bias?

8. Could there have been bias in the collection of information? How likely was this bias?

9. What provisions were made to minimize the influence of confounding factors prior to the analysis of the data? Were these provisions sufficient?

B. Analysis of data

1. What methods were used to control confounding bias during data analysis? Were these methods sufficient?

2. What measures of association were reported in this study?

3. What measures of statistical stability were reported in this study?

C. Interpretation of data

1. What were the major results of this study?

2. How is the interpretation of these results affected by information bias, selection bias, and confounding? Discuss both the direction and magnitude of any bias.

3. How is the interpretation of these results affected by nondifferential misclassification? Discuss both the direction and magnitude of this misclassification.

4. Did the discussion section adequately address the limitations of the study?

5. What were the authors' main conclusions? Were they justified by the findings?

6. To what larger population can the results of this study be generalized?

Source: Adapted from Monson RR. *Occupational Epidemiology.* 2nd ed, p 94. Boca Raton, FL: CRC Press; 1990.

example, if an article does not mention that the interviewers were masked to the subject's disease status, one can assume that no masking occurred.

Guide to Answering the Critique Questions

The following section provides guidelines for answering the critique questions. We advise students to read an article twice before attempting to answer the questions. The purpose of the first reading is to become familiar with the article. The second reading should be done with the critique questions in mind. Note that the answers to many of these questions can be found in the introduction and materials and methods sections of an article. One last piece of advice—a critique should be brief. A long critique defeats an important benefit of the review process—the production of a brief, easy-to-read summary that makes future readings of the article unnecessary.

Collection of Data

WHAT WAS THE CONTEXT OF THE STUDY? This question deals with the investigators' motivation for the study. For example, the observations that stimulated the study may have come from laboratory research, clinical reports, or other epidemiologic studies. The answer to this question gives the reader a sense of the particular contribution made by the study at hand. For example, the study may be the first of its kind or it may be replicating results of an earlier study in a different population, with larger numbers, or by using more refined methods. For example, Zierler and Rothman conducted a case–control study of congenital heart disease and maternal use of Benedectin in early pregnancy because a study that they had conducted earlier found an association that they suspected was the result of recall bias.[11] The new study was designed "expressly to evaluate and remove any bias that might have arisen when exposure histories obtained from mothers of affected offspring were compared with exposure histories obtained from mothers of healthy controls."[(p347)]

WHAT WERE THE OBJECTIVES OF THE STUDY? This question deals with the purpose of the study—that is, the hypothesis being tested. Hypotheses are suppositions about an exposure–disease relationship that lead to refutable predictions.[12(p80)] Examples of hypotheses are as follows:

- Following American Cancer Society cancer screening guidelines reduces the incidence of colon cancer.
- Unprotected receptive anal intercourse increases the risk of HIV-1 transmission among homosexual men.
- Removal of lead-contaminated soil accessible to children decreases their blood lead levels.

mortality. It is important to consider whether the outcome was accurately defined and measured because loose definitions and inaccurate measurement can result in misclassification. Thus, when evaluating the accuracy of an outcome variable, one should compare its conceptual and operational definitions. For example, the conceptual outcome definition in the study on the cancer risk associated with tetrachloroethylene-contaminated drinking water was breast cancer, which is defined as a malignant neoplasm of the breast tissue.[14] However, as required by the operational definition, all cases of breast cancer were reported to the state cancer registry, were pathologically confirmed, and were diagnosed at stage 1 through 4. These requirements helped ensure that all of the cases in the study truly had breast cancer.

When reviewing an article, the reader should look for measures taken to improve the accuracy of the outcome data such as use of a combination of signs and symptoms, examinations, and tests to define cases of disease; verification of information from one source with another; use of sensitive and specific biomarkers of disease or its precursors as outcome measures; use of the likely causal mechanism to define and group cases of disease; and use of reputable registries (such as cancer registries) to identify or corroborate disease reports.

WHAT TYPE OF STUDY WAS CONDUCTED? The main epidemiologic study designs are experimental, cohort (prospective and retrospective), case–control, cross-sectional, and ecologic studies. It is important to know which design was used because certain designs are more prone to bias than others. The following paragraph briefly reviews the key features of each design.

Experimental studies examine preventions and treatments for disease. Their hallmark is the investigator's assignment of participants to compared groups. Random assignment is recommended but not required. Observational (cohort, case–control, cross-sectional, and ecologic) studies investigate causes, preventions, and treatments for disease. Observational study participants become exposed without the investigator's intervention. Subjects in a cohort study are defined according to their exposure level and are followed for disease occurrence. In contrast, subjects in a case–control study are defined as either cases or controls and their exposure histories are examined. Cross-sectional studies examine the relationship between an exposure and a disease in a well-defined population at a single point in time. Their main limitation is that they do not allow investigators to infer the temporal sequence between exposure and disease if the exposure is a changeable characteristic. Ecologic studies examine rates of disease in relation to a population-level factor and use groups—not individuals—as units of analysis. Their main limitation is known as the ecological fallacy, an inability to apply the group-level relationship to the individual level.

DESCRIBE THE SOURCE OF THE STUDY POPULATION, PROCESS OF SUB-JECT SELECTION, SAMPLE SIZE, AND RATIO OF PROPOSITI TO COMPARISON SUBJECTS. This information allows the reader to evaluate many important topics, including the potential for selection bias and confounding, the statistical power of the study, and the generalizability of the results. The source of the study population is the underlying population from which the subjects were drawn. For example, the underlying population of a hospital-based case–control study is the catchment area of the hospital. Cases and controls will be comparable and confounding will be reduced if the catchment areas (and underlying populations) for cases are similar to those for controls. Furthermore, the source population and actual study population greatly influence to whom the study results are applicable.

The process of subject selection should be carefully examined for evidence of selection bias, which is described in more detail below. The sample size and ratio of propositi to comparison subjects provides information on the statistical power of the study—that is, the ability of the study to detect an association that is truly present. The ratio of propositi to comparison subjects is the ratio of exposed to unexposed subjects (for example, for a cohort study) or the ratio of cases to controls (for a case–control study). These ratios are often one to one, but they may be as high as one to three or one to four. High ratios and a large sample size improve the statistical power of the study.

COULD THERE HAVE BEEN BIAS IN THE SELECTION OF THE STUDY SUB-JECTS? HOW LIKELY WAS THIS BIAS? Selection bias is an error that arises from systematic differences in selecting the study groups. These differences lead to an effect estimate among subjects in the study that is different from the estimate obtainable from the entire underlying population. Selection bias can cause the true measure of association to be either over- or underestimated. As described in Chapter 10, selection bias is more likely in case–control and retrospective cohort studies because both the exposure and disease have occurred by the time of subject selection.

When reviewing an article, the reader should look for evidence of the specific types of selection bias including control selection bias in case–control studies; the healthy-worker effect in occupational cohort studies; self-selection bias; and differential surveillance, diagnosis, and referral of subjects according to exposure and disease status. It is particularly important to consider selection bias when different criteria are used to select cases and controls or exposed and unexposed subjects, and these criteria are related to the other axis; when participation rates are low and different across compared groups; when diagnostic practices and referral patterns are not taken into account; and when self-referrals are accepted into a study.

COULD THERE HAVE BEEN BIAS IN THE COLLECTION OF INFORMATION?
HOW LIKELY WAS THIS BIAS? Information bias is an error that arises from systematic differences in the way that information on the exposure and disease is obtained from the study groups. It results in incorrect classification of participants as either exposed or unexposed or as diseased or not diseased. This type of bias arises after the subjects have been selected for study. When reviewing an article, the reader should look for evidence of the specific types of information bias including recall bias, interviewer bias, loss to follow-up, and differential and nondifferential misclassification. Except for nondifferential misclassification of a dichotomous exposure and nondifferential loss to follow-up, these biases can pull the measure of association either toward or away from the null.

Recall bias can occur when individuals with particular adverse health events remember or report their previous exposure differently than do individuals who are not affected. Thus, recall bias can only occur in retrospective studies that gather data from study subjects. When evaluating a study, the reader should look for methods that may have been used to avoid recall bias, such as development of a carefully designed questionnaire, use of closed-ended questions, comparison of diseased cases to diseased controls (in case–control studies), use of a prospective study, collection of study data that is not based upon interviews and questionnaires, or use of participants who are blinded to the study hypothesis. The reader should also note if the investigators undertook a direct assessment of recall bias, such as asking participants about their knowledge of the hypothesis and stratifying the results on the basis of their responses.

Interviewer bias occurs when there are systematic differences in soliciting, recording, or interpreting information from in-person and telephone interviews. This bias can occur when interviewers lack training in appropriate interview techniques (such as nondirective probing), when they are aware of the study hypothesis and the disease or exposure status of subjects, or when questionnaires are unstructured. Epidemiologists can request to receive the study questionnaire from the corresponding author in order to assess its structure.

Loss to follow-up occurs when subjects can no longer be located or when they no longer want to participate in the study. It is problematic because it can reduce statistical power and can bias the study results. The latter arises when subjects who are lost differ from those who remain with respect to the exposure and outcome. When evaluating a study, the reader should note the proportions and any available demographic information on subjects lost to follow-up. Losses greater than 20%, especially if they occur among different types of subjects than those who remain, call the validity of the study into question.

Misclassification occurs when the subject's exposure or disease status is erroneously classified. Misclassification can be either nondifferential or differential. Nondifferential misclassification means that inaccuracies with respect to disease are independent of exposure, or that inaccuracies with respect to exposure are independent of disease. This type of misclassification, which is probably the most common form of bias in epidemiologic research, biases the results toward the null if the misclassified exposure variable is dichotomous. Differential misclassification means that inaccuracies with respect to disease are dependent on exposure status and vice versa. When evaluating a study for misclassification, the reader should carefully examine the operational exposure and disease definitions. Misclassification should be considered when single (instead of multiple) measurements are used to define the exposure or disease, when data are not validated using alternate information sources, or when subjects are required to recall information from long ago.

WHAT PROVISIONS WERE MADE TO MINIMIZE THE INFLUENCE OF CONFOUNDING FACTORS PRIOR TO THE DATA ANALYSIS? WERE THESE PROVISIONS SUFFICIENT? Confounding is a bias in the crude measure of association between an exposure and disease that is the result of a third factor that is associated with the exposure and is an independent risk factor for the disease. Confounding can bias results either toward or away from the null. The methods to control for confounding prior to data analysis include randomization, restriction, matching, and use of the same source population for the compared groups. Collecting information on potential confounders is an important provision to control for confounding prior to data analysis, because—except for randomization—it is impossible to control for a confounder at any stage without data. When evaluating a study, the reader should review the information on confounders that was collected. If data on key confounders are missing, residual confounding may have occurred.

It is also important to determine the methods used to address confounding. Randomization is the "act of assigning or ordering that results from a random process."[15(p220)] Random methods include flipping a coin, using a random number table or a computerized random number generator. A unique advantage of randomization is that it will control for variables that the study investigator is unable to measure if the sample size is sufficient. Restriction means that admissibility criteria for study subjects are limited. Thus, a study that is restricted to women has no confounding by gender. Restriction limits the generalizability of the findings. Matching means that the investigator selects study subjects so that the potential confounders are distributed in an identical manner. Closer matches control for confounding better than broader matches. For example, matching by age within 2 years will control for confounding better than matching within 10 years. Note that matching in the design phase of a case–control study requires a matched analysis. If this analysis is not done, the measure of association will be biased toward the null.

Analysis of Data

WHAT METHODS WERE USED TO CONTROL CONFOUNDING DURING THE DATA ANALYSIS? WERE THESE METHODS SUFFICIENT? During analysis, the main ways to control for confounding are standardization, stratification, matched analysis (for case–control studies), and multivariate analysis. Standardization involves taking weighted averages of the relevant measures of disease frequency. The weights typically come from the exposed group in the study population. This method is commonly used to control for demographic characteristics such as age. Stratification is "the process of or result of separating a sample into several subgroups according to specific criteria."[12(p161)] Thus, it enables the investigator to evaluate an association within homogeneous categories of a variable. The narrower the category, the better the control of confounding. Multivariate analysis involves the construction of a mathematical model that describes the association between the exposure, disease, and confounders. Commonly used methods of multivariate analysis include multiple linear regression, logistic regression, Poisson regression, and Cox proportional hazard models. The main advantage of multivariate models is that they allow investigators to control for many confounders simultaneously.

WHAT MEASURES OF ASSOCIATION WERE REPORTED IN THIS STUDY? Commonly used measures of association in epidemiologic studies are rate ratios, risk ratios, rate differences, risk differences, odds ratios, standardized mortality ratios, and standardized proportional mortality ratios. Note that the alternative terms—attributable and relative risk and rate—are also commonly used. Other measures of association such as mean differences are used if the data are continuous. It is important to distinguish the measure of association from the measure of statistical stability, described below. Sometimes authors incorrectly interpret the measure of statistical stability as the measure of association.

WHAT MEASURES OF STATISTICAL STABILITY WERE REPORTED IN THIS STUDY? Hypothesis testing and interval estimation are used to assess the precision of study findings and to evaluate the role of chance in epidemiologic studies. Chance refers to the likelihood that an unrepresentative sample was drawn due to "the luck of the draw." P values and confidence intervals are the two main ways to assess the role of chance in epidemiologic research. The null P value and 95% confidence interval are most commonly used. The P value is defined as the probability of observing the study results or more extreme results, given that the null hypothesis is true. Thus, it measures the compatibility of the data with the null hypothesis. The 95% confidence interval is defined as follows: If one repeats a study 100 times, the true measure of association will lie inside the confidence interval in 95 out of 100 studies. Although incorrect from a statistical viewpoint, a 95% confidence interval can also be conceptualized as follows: One has 95% confidence or assurance that the true measure of association lies somewhere inside the interval. A statistically significant result has been arbitrarily defined as a P value less than 0.05 or a 95% confidence interval that does not include the null. Statistical significance has been overemphasized in epidemiologic research.

Interpretation of Data

WHAT WERE THE MAJOR RESULTS OF THIS STUDY? A critique should describe the main results of the study using numbers. Qualitative statements such as "the study found a relationship between the exposure and disease" are inadequate because it is necessary to know how strong the relationship was.

HOW IS THE INTERPRETATION OF THESE RESULTS AFFECTED BY INFOR-MATION BIAS, SELECTION BIAS, AND CONFOUNDING? DISCUSS BOTH THE DIRECTION AND MAGNITUDE OF ANY BIAS. The reader should gather all of the relevant information from the other sections of the critique to determine the net effect of any information bias, selection bias, and confounding that may be present in the study. It is important to assess: the likelihood of bias and confounding, their magnitude, and their direction. A small amount of bias or confounding will usually not have a major impact on the study results, but a large amount of bias or residual confounding could completely alter the findings. The impact of bias and confounding will also depend on the true size of the association. They can account entirely for a weak association, but they are unlikely to account entirely for a strong one.

It may be useful to conduct a "sensitivity analysis" in order to determine the magnitude of the bias. This analysis determines the robustness of the results by examining the extent to which they are affected by assumptions about the amount of bias.[12(p154)] Both likely and extreme scenarios should be considered. For example, how would the results be altered if one assumed that 0%, 20%, and 100% of the people lost to follow-up had the disease of interest?

HOW IS THE INTERPRETATION OF THESE RESULTS AFFECTED BY NON-DIFFERENTIAL MISCLASSIFICATION? DISCUSS BOTH THE DIRECTION AND MAGNITUDE OF THIS MISCLASSIFICATION. Nondifferential misclassification is a common form of bias that pulls the results toward the null under certain circumstances. Null results need to be carefully examined for nondifferential misclassification to determine if mismeasurement caused the findings. In addition, mismeasurement causes positive results to be weaker than they otherwise would have been.

DID THE DISCUSSION SECTION ADEQUATELY ADDRESS THE LIMITATIONS OF THE STUDY? A self-critical examination of the study methods and findings should be included in the discussion section of the article. For example, the discussion section of the article on breast cancer risk associated with tetrachloroethylene-contaminated drinking water made the following statements:

> Because the exposures occurred many years ago, it was not possible to determine with certainty the exact PCE [an abbreviation for tetrachloroethylene] levels to which the women were exposed. Our exposure estimates were based on the Webler-Brown model. Any false assumptions about the model or errors determining the model variables would have led to errors in estimating the RDDs [relative delivered dose, an ordinal estimate of the amount of pollutant that entered the home]. Even if the PCE concentration of the drinking water that entered the house was correctly estimated, women were likely to ingest and come into contact with differing amounts of water at home depending on their personal habits. Furthermore, no information was available on possible workplace exposures.[14(p951)]

WHAT WERE THE AUTHORS' MAIN CONCLUSIONS? WERE THEY JUSTIFIED BY THE FINDINGS? The conclusions are a brief summary of the findings and their implications. In addition, the authors sometimes include recommendations for future research and public health policy. All conclusions should be supported by the study findings. For example, the conclusion of the breast cancer and tetrachloroethylene-contaminated drinking water article was as follows: "The results of this study suggest that women with high relative delivered doses of PCE-contaminated drinking water have an increased risk of breast cancer, particularly when the cancers occurred during the postmenopausal years." The authors went on to say: "Firm conclusions on the relationship between PCE-contaminated drinking water and breast cancer in our study were limited by the small proportion of exposure subjects, particularly when long latent periods were considered."[14(pp951–952)]

TO WHAT LARGER POPULATION CAN THE RESULTS OF THIS STUDY BE GENERALIZED? The internal validity of a study must be established before the study results can be generalized to populations beyond the study subjects. If a study is invalid, its results cannot be generalized to any population. The evaluation of generalizibility or "external validity" requires review of the study methods (for example, was restriction used to control for confounding?), the composition of the study population (for example, were minorities included?), and subject matter knowledge such as the biological basis of the association (for example, would the same results be expected among men and women?).

Sample Critiques of Epidemiologic Studies

This section provides critiques for three published articles. The first article deals with the risk of HIV infection among household contacts of AIDS patients[16] (see Exhibit 14–2), the second deals with the long-term effects of lead exposure on the central nervous system[17] (see Exhibit 14–3), and the third evaluates therapies for premenopausal breast cancer[18] (see Exhibit 14–4). Because each of these studies presents interesting issues regarding their quality and interpretation, they provide useful examples for practicing the critique process.

Critique of a Study on the Prevalence of HIV in Household Contact of AIDS Patients in Kinshasa, Zaire

A. Collection of data
 1. *What was the context of the study?* At the time of the study, the virus that causes AIDS (HTLV-III/LAV, now known as HIV) was known

---

EXHIBIT 14–2

ABSTRACT OF "PREVALENCE OF HTLV-III/LAV IN HOUSEHOLD CONTACTS OF PATIENTS WITH CONFIRMED AIDS AND CONTROLS IN KINSHASA, ZAIRE"

Household members of 46 patients with confirmed acquired immuno-deficiency syndrome (AIDS) and 43 human T-cell lymphotropic virus type III/lymphadenopathy-associated virus (HTLV-III/LAV)-seronegative controls from Kinshasa, Zaire were identified and sought for serologic testing for evidence of HTLV-III/LAV infection. Twenty (9.8%) of 204 case-household members and three (1.9%) of 155 control-household members were HTLV-III/LAV seropositive (relative risk = 5.1; 95% confidence interval, 1.7 to 15.2). Eleven (61.1%) of 18 spouses of patients with AIDS were HTLV-III/LAV positive, compared with one (3.7%) of 27 control spouses (relative risk = 16.5, 95% confidence interval, 3.7 to 75.0). Except for spouses, the rate of HTLV-III/LAV seropositivity did not differ significantly between cases and control households. Furthermore, for adults in case households who were not spouses, the number seropositive for HTLV-III/LAV was identical to that predicted from sex- and age-specific HTLV-III/LAV seroprevalence rates. These data from Zaire confirm the results of U.S. and European studies of household contacts of infected hemophiliacs and pediatric patients with AIDS.

Source: Reprinted from Mann JM, et al. Prevalence of HTLV-III/LAV in household contacts of patients with confirmed AIDS and controls in Kinshasa, Zaire. *JAMA.* 1986;256:721.

to be transmitted sexually, through contact with blood and blood products, and pre- and perinatally from infected mothers to infants. However, epidemiologists were concerned that it could also be transmitted in close-contact settings through other fluids. This study of household contacts appears to be the first of its kind in Zaire, where the epidemiologic pattern of AIDS is considerably different from that in the United States and Europe.

2. *What were the objectives of the study?* The purpose of the study was to "examine the possibility of household transmission of HTLV-III/ LAV in Kinshasa, Zaire."

3. *What was the primary exposure of interest? Was this accurately measured?* The exposed subjects were household members of AIDS patients who were diagnosed at Mama Yemo Hospital and met a modified Centers for Disease Control definition of AIDS based on clinical criteria and laboratory tests, including repeated testing by ELISA (enzyme-linked immunosorbent assay) and Western blot. Unexposed subjects were household members of HTLV-III/LAV seronegative individuals who were the same sex and age as the AIDS patients. Seronegative individuals were selected from patients in the orthopedic and surgical wards of Mama Yemo Hospital, or they were identified as former Mama Yemo patients by four Zairian physicians. A household member was defined as a person who lived in the same household as the AIDS patient or the seronegative patient for at least 6 months during 1983 or 1984. The exposure appears to be accurately measured through the use of clinical symptoms, multiple laboratory tests, and sensitive and specific definitions.

4. *What was the primary outcome of interest? Was this accurately measured?* The primary outcome was a positive antibody test to HTLV-III/LAV. It was accurately measured because it was based on two positive ELISA results and one positive Western blot assay.

5. *What type of study was conducted?* A cross-sectional study was conducted. The authors' use of the terminology "case-households" and "control-households" is misleading because a case–control study was not conducted.

6. *Describe the source of the study population, process of subject selection, sample size, and ratio of propositi to comparison subjects.* The source population consisted of household members of AIDS patients and seronegative patients from Mama Yemo Hospital in Kinshasa, Zaire. The study enrolled 46 patients with AIDS and 45 apparently seronegative patients. Two "seronegative" patients were subsequently excluded when they were found to be seropositive. The authors provided no information on the number of AIDS patients

and seronegative patients who were approached but refused to participate. The authors attempted to enroll all household members who met the eligibility criteria (see A3). They enrolled 204 household members of AIDS patients and 155 household members of seronegative patients. This represented 65% and 54% of the household contacts of AIDS and seronegative patients, respectively, who were approached. The ratio of propositi to comparison subjects was 204 to 155, or 1.3 to 1.

7. *Could there have been bias in the selection of the study subjects? How likely was this bias?* Although similar selection criteria for exposed and unexposed subjects minimized the possibility of certain types of selection bias, self-selection bias is possible given the low and slightly different participation rates among exposed and unexposed subjects (65% and 54%, respectively). However, this would have led to bias only if the decision to participate was related both to the exposure (being a household member of an AIDS or seronegative patient) and to the outcome (being seropositive or seronegative). The authors stated: "Not all household members participated in this study. If HTLV-III/LAV infections in case-household members led to failure to participate because of ill health or death, a bias against detection of household clusters would have occurred."

8. *Could there have been bias in the collection of information? How likely was this bias?* The investigators obtained the outcome data through laboratory tests, and so recall bias and interviewer bias were not possible. The authors did not state if the laboratory personnel who performed the serological tests were aware of the exposure status of subjects, but these tests are fairly objective and so it is unlikely that this knowledge would have influenced the serologic test results. Exposure data were obtained through interviews and laboratory tests. For example, the interviews identified the household members and each household member's relationship to the index patient (for example, spouse, parent, child). The authors did not state if the interviewers were masked, but it is unlikely that the key interview data were influenced by interviewer or recall bias. There was no loss to follow-up because this was a cross-sectional study.

9. *What provisions were made to minimize the influence of confounding factors prior to the analysis of the data? Were these provisions sufficient?* The AIDS and seronegative index patients came from the patient population of Mama Yemo Hospital. These two groups were selected to be of similar age and sex, so it appears that some matching occurred. However, it is unknown if the catchment areas are exactly the same for these two groups of patients. The

authors collected information on some confounders. For example, they collected information on household size, age, gender, religion, marital status, educational level, and occupation. Patients with AIDS and seronegative patients were similar for almost all demographic variables. The only difference between AIDS and seronegative patients was that the former were more likely to have a high-level occupation. No differences were seen among household contacts for length of residence and total household size. However, the household contacts of AIDS patients were more likely to be women than were the household contacts of seronegative patients. No information was collected on many other risk factors for infection, including sexual practices, blood transfusions, scarifications, or medical injections, and so residual confounding by these unmeasured factors may be present.

B. Analysis of data

1. *What methods were used to control confounding bias during data analysis? Were these methods sufficient?* Investigators used no methods to control for confounding in the analysis, and so residual confounding may be present.

2. *What measures of association were reported in this study?* The study reported prevalence ratios.

3. *What measures of statistical stability were reported in this study?* The study reported 95 percent confidence intervals.

C. Interpretation of data

1. *What were the major results of this study?* The prevalence of seropositivity among household contacts of AIDS patients and seronegative patients was 9.8% (20/204) and 1.9% (3/155), respectively (relative risk = 5.1; 95% confidence interval, 1.7 to 15.2). When these data were stratified by the relationship to the index patient, the prevalence of seropositivity was 61.1% (11/18) among spouses of AIDS patients and 3.7% (1/27) among spouses of seronegative patients (relative risk = 16.5; 95% confidence interval, 3.7 to 75.0). In addition, 4.8% (9/186) of nonspousal household contacts of AIDS patients and 1.6% (2/128) of nonspousal contacts of seronegative patients were seropositive (relative risk = 3.1; 95% confidence interval, 0.7 to 13.3). Although the prevalence of seropositivity was higher among parents, children, and sibling household contacts of AIDS patients than among household contacts of seronegative patients, the number of seropositive household contacts was quite small and so the relative risk estimates were highly imprecise.

2. *How is the interpretation of these results affected by information bias, selection bias, and confounding? Discuss both the direction and magnitude of any bias.* Information bias is unlikely in this study; however,

selection bias and confounding were quite possible. Selection bias probably resulted from the low and slightly differential participation rates of exposed and unexposed subjects. In fact, the authors presented the results of a 1984 seroprevalence study from Kinshasa that suggested that the seroprevalence rate among exposed subjects was as expected but that the rate among unexposed subjects was less than expected. Missing data on key confounders (such as other sources of infection) also make the results difficult to interpret because the magnitude of the residual confounding may be large and its direction is difficult to predict.

3. *How is the interpretation of these results affected by nondifferential misclassification? Discuss both the direction and magnitude of this misclassification.* Although nondifferential laboratory errors were possible, they were not likely given that two ELISA and one Western blot were used to define seropositive subjects. Furthermore, these tests are known to have a high level of sensitivity and specificity. In addition, interview data on subjects' relationship to the index patients were objective and easy to determine. Thus, nondifferential misclassification of exposure and outcome were unlikely to have affected the study results.

4. *Did the discussion section adequately address the limitations of the study?* The authors acknowledged the possibility of selection bias and residual confounding.

5. *What were the authors' main conclusions? Were they justified by the findings?* The authors concluded that the data do not support the hypothesis that nonsexual transmission occurs among household members. However, the authors' conclusions are not justified by their findings. Although the numbers were small, the risk of infection was 3.1 times higher among nonspousal household contacts of AIDS patients than among nonspousal contact of seronegative patients. The 95% confidence interval for this association ranged from 0.7 to 13.3, and so the data are consistent with a wide range of values for the relative risk, not just the null value. The main error that the authors made was "equating the lack of statistical significance with the lack of effect."[19]

6. *To what larger population can the results of this study be generalized?* If valid, the study results could be generalized to persons in other developing countries with living conditions similar to those in Zaire (for example, crowded housing, lack of modern sanitary systems, and substantial numbers of mosquitos). However, given the possibility of selection bias and confounding and the low level of precision, it would be unwise to generalize these results to any population.

Critique of a Study on the Long-Term Effects of Low-Level Lead Exposure in Childhood

A. Collection of data

1. *What was the context of the study?* Low doses of lead exposure are known to have toxic effects on the central nervous system of infants and children; however, it is unknown if these effects persist into young adulthood. Three follow-up studies had previously been published on this topic but the longest length of follow-up was 5 years. The average length of follow-up in the current study is 11 years.

2. *What were the objectives of the study?* The purpose of the study was to evaluate the neuropsychological and academic performance in

---

EXHIBIT 14–3

ABSTRACT OF "THE LONG-TERM EFFECTS OF EXPOSURE TO LOW DOSES OF LEAD IN CHILDHOOD. AN 11-YEAR FOLLOW-UP REPORT"

To determine whether the effects of low-level lead exposure persist, we reexamined 132 of 270 young adults who had initially been studied as primary school children in 1975 through 1978. In the earlier study, neurobehavioral functioning was found to be inversely related to dentin lead levels. As compared with those we restudied, the other 138 subjects had had somewhat higher lead levels on earlier analysis, as well as significantly lower IQ scores and poorer teachers' ratings of classroom behavior. When the 132 subjects were reexamined in 1988, impairment in neurobehavioral function was still found to be related to the lead content of teeth shed at the ages of six and seven. The young people with dentin lead levels > 20 ppm had a markedly higher risk of dropping out of high school (adjusted odds ratio, 7.4, 95 percent confidence interval, 1.4 to 40.7) and of having a reading disability (odds ratio, 5.8, 95 percent confidence interval, 1.7 to 19.7) as compared with those with dentin lead levels < 10 ppm. Higher lead levels in childhood were also significantly associated with lower class standing in high school, increased absenteeism, lower vocabulary and grammatical-reasoning scores, poorer hand-eye coordination, longer reaction times, and slower finger tapping. No significant associations were found with the results of 10 other tests of neurobehavioral functioning. Lead levels were inversely related to self-reports of minor delinquent activity. We conclude that exposure to lead in childhood is associated with deficits in central nervous system functioning that persist into young adulthood.

Source: Reprinted from Needleman HL, Schell A, Bellinger D, Leviton A, allred EN. The long-term effects of exposure to low doses of lead in childhood. An 11-year follow-up report. *N Engl J Med*. 1990;332:83.

young adulthood of a sample of first- and second-grade children who were first studied in 1975 to 1978.

3. *What was the primary exposure of interest? Was this accurately measured?* The primary exposure was the dentin lead level from children ages 6 and 7 years. Children provided at least one shed primary tooth; these teeth were analyzed for their lead content. The details of this analysis, including its level of accuracy, were not described. Investigators computed the arithmetic mean lead level for each subject using all collected teeth. Current blood lead measurements were also taken for the first 48 subjects tested in the study. This practice was discontinued because blood lead levels were quite low.

4. *What was the primary outcome of interest? Was this accurately measured?* The investigators examined numerous outcome measures of neuropsychological and academic performance based on an automated battery of tests, including hand-eye coordination, simple visual reaction time, pattern memory, vocabulary, and grammatical reasoning. A single examiner who was masked to the lead levels of the subjects administered the tests. The testing time lasted about 2 hours. This battery of tests is considered an accurate representation of neuropsychological functioning. Self-reports of delinquency were obtained using a structured questionnaire from the National Youth Survey. School records were also reviewed for attendance and class rank. The delinquency self-reports may not have been accurate, but the school record data should have been reliable.

5. *What type of study was conducted?* A retrospective cohort study was conducted.

6. *Describe the source of the study population, process of subject selection, sample size, and ratio of propositi to comparison subjects.* This study re-examined children who were initially studied in 1975 to 1978. The initial source population consisted of 3329 students who were enrolled in the first and second grade in Chelsea, Massachusetts, from 1975 through 1978. Of this population 70% (n = 2335) provided at least one tooth for analysis. For the initial study, investigators selected 270 children who lived in English-speaking homes and whose dentin lead levels were either greater than 24 ppm or less than 6 ppm. These subjects were traced for the current study. Of these, 177 were located; 132 agreed to be retested in 1988, and 45 refused. About equal numbers of participants had low, moderate, and high lead levels and so the ratio of propositi to comparison subjects was roughly 1 to 1.

7. *Could there have been bias in the selection of the study subjects? How likely was this bias?* The authors state that selection bias occurred in

the current study. However, according to our definitions, we would term this problem differential loss to follow-up. See item A. 8.

8. *Could there have been bias in the collection of information? How likely was this bias?* The individual performing the neuropsychological tests was blinded to exposure status and so observer bias (which is akin to interviewer bias) was eliminated. It is unknown if subjects themselves were aware of their exposure status, but it is unlikely that they would purposely alter their test performance on the basis of this information. Nondifferential or differential underreporting of delinquency was possible, but this was only one of many outcome variables. However, this study does suffer from differential loss to follow-up. Those who were retested in 1988 tended to have lower dentin lead levels, fewer head injuries, higher IQ scores, better 1979 teacher ratings, and more highly educated mothers and fathers than did those who could not be located or refused to participate in the follow-up study.

9. *What provisions were made to minimize the influence of confounding factors prior to the analysis of the data? Were these provisions sufficient?* All subjects came from the same source population of first- and second-grade students from Chelsea, Massachusetts, from 1975 through 1978. The study population's racial composition was homogeneous—almost all were white. In addition, investigators collected data on numerous confounders.

B. Analysis of data

1. *What methods were used to control confounding bias during data analysis? Were these methods sufficient?* Multiple linear regression and logistic regression analyses were used to control for 10 confounders simultaneously. These confounders included mother's age at the subject's birth, mother's educational level, mother's IQ, family size, socioeconomic status, sex, age at testing, birth order, alcohol use, and whether the mother and subject were discharged together following the subject's birth. Five of these variables were shown to be confounders on the basis of analyses conducted on the study population. The other five variables were known to influence the results of neuropsychological tests based on prior knowledge.

2. *What measures of association were reported in this study?* Odds ratios and mean differences in test scores, reading levels, and class standing were used as the measures of association.

3. *What measures of statistical stability were reported in this study?* P values and 95% confidence intervals were reported.

C. Interpretation of data

1. *What were the major results of this study?* Impairment in neurobehavioral functioning in young adults was related to dentin lead

levels from the first and second grade. In particular, there was a 7.4-fold increased risk of dropping out of high school (95% confidence interval, 1.4 to 40.7), and a 5.8-fold increased risk of having a reading disability (95% confidence interval, 1.7 to 19.7) among children with dentin levels greater than 20 ppm as compared to children with dentin levels less than 10 ppm. Higher lead levels were also associated with lower class standing in high school (average percentile 45th versus 60th), lower vocabulary scores (14.6 versus 18.0 correct words), and poorer hand-eye coordination (6.2 versus 5.1 errors). These were no differences between children with high and low dentin lead levels for 10 of the other tests.

2. *How is the interpretation of these results affected by information bias, selection bias, and confounding? Discuss both the direction and magnitude of any bias.* The results were mainly influenced by differential loss to follow-up. Because children with high lead levels and adverse outcomes were less likely to participate in this follow-up study, the magnitude of the association was underestimated. Thus, the results would have been stronger if these children had been included.

3. *How is the interpretation of these results affected by nondifferential misclassification? Discuss both the direction and magnitude of this misclassification.* Nondifferential misclassification of exposure and outcomes was possible but unlikely to be large because exposure and outcome measurements were fairly accurate (for example, laboratory measurements of dentin levels). Nondifferential misclassification probably biased associations for the continuous measures toward the null. The direction of the bias for the categorical analyses is more difficult to predict because there were three to four exposure categories.

4. *Did the discussion section adequately address the limitations of the study?* The discussion section acknowledges the presence of bias stemming from differential loss to follow-up, which the authors termed selection bias. The problem is real, regardless of what it is called.

5. *What were the authors' main conclusions? Were they justified by the findings?* The authors concluded that the associations reported earlier between lead exposure in childhood and academic success and cognitive functioning persist into young adulthood. These conclusions are justified by the numerous findings. Although bias was present, it served only to underestimate the detrimental effects of lead exposure.

6. *To what larger population can the results of this study be generalized?* These results can be generalized to other children in developed countries of similar socioeconomic status and with similar lead levels.

Critique of a Study on Adjuvant Radiotherapy and Chemotherapy in Premenopausal Women with Breast Cancer

A. Collection of data

1. *What was the context of the study?* Adjuvant chemotherapy has been the standard treatment for high-risk premenopausal breast cancer since the late 1970s. Adjuvant radiotherapy has been used infrequently because it does not appear to improve survival and it can cause immune suppression and cardiac complications. However, the authors state that adjuvant radiotherapy should be reconsidered in certain situations such as for bulky disease and residual locoregional tumors.

2. *What were the objectives of the study?* The purpose of the study was "to test the hypothesis that adding radiation to adjuvant systemic therapy improves the outcome in patients with breast cancer."

EXHIBIT 14–4

ABSTRACT OF "ADJUVANT RADIOTHERAPY AND CHEMOTHERAPY IN NODE-POSITIVE PREMENOPAUSAL WOMEN WITH BREAST CANCER"

Radiotherapy after mastectomy to treat early breast cancer has been known since the 1940s to reduce rates of local relapse. However, the routine use of postoperative radiotherapy began to decline in the 1980s because it failed to improve overall survival. We prospectively tested the efficacy of combining radiotherapy with chemotherapy. From 1978 though 1986, 318 premenopausal women with node-positive breast cancer were randomly assigned, after modified radical mastectomy, to receive chemotherapy plus radiation or chemotherapy alone. Radiotherapy was given to the chest wall and locoregional lymph nodes between the fourth and fifth cycles of cyclophosphamide, methotrexate, and fluorouracil. After 15 years of follow-up, the women assigned to chemotherapy plus radiotherapy had a 33 percent reduction in the rate of recurrence (relative risk, 0.67; 95 percent confidence interval, 0.50 to 0.90) and a 29 percent reduction in mortality from breast cancer (relative risk 0.71; 95 percent confidence interval, 0.51 to 0.99), as compared with the women treated with chemotherapy alone. Radiotherapy combined with chemotherapy after modified radical mastectomy decreases rates of locoregional and systemic relapse and reduces mortality from breast cancer.

Source: Reprinted from Ragaz J, Jackson SM, Le N, Plenderleith IH, Spinelli JJ, Basco VE, et al. Adjuvant radiotherapy and chemotherapy in node-positive premenopausal women with breast cancer. *N Engl J Med.* 1997;337:956.

3. *What was the primary exposure of interest? Was this accurately measured?* The experimental treatment group received adjuvant chemotherapy plus locoregional radiotherapy. The comparison group received only chemotherapy. Chemotherapy in both groups consisted of cyclophosphamide, methotrexate, and fluorouracil given intravenously every 21 days for either 12 months (for the first 80 patients) or 6 months (for subsequent patients). Radiation therapy consisted of 16 daily treatments to five fields over a 3- to 4-week period between the fourth and fifth cycles of chemotherapy. Patients with estrogen-positive tumors were also treated with radiation-induced ovarian ablation. These exposures were accurately measured, given the objective nature of the treatments.

4. *What was the primary outcome of interest? Was this accurately measured?* The investigators studied several end points including any recurrence of breast cancer, a locoregional and/or systemic recurrence of breast cancer, death from breast cancer, and death from any cause. Death from any cause is obviously the most accurate end point, and the authors provided no operational definitions of the other end points. In addition, they did not state how differences of opinion were resolved, or if physicians assessing end points were masked. However, the remaining end points are usually clear-cut, so it is likely that they were accurately measured in most instances.

5. *What type of study was conducted?* A randomized clinical trial was conducted.

6. *Describe the source of the study population, process of subject selection, sample size, and ratio of propositi to comparison subjects.* From 1979 through 1986, 318 premenopausal women with newly diagnosed stage I or II breast cancer were enrolled after undergoing a modified radical mastectomy if their axillary node dissection revealed at least one positive lymph node. The surgery was done by specialists in the Vancouver, British Columbia area. All patients were subsequently referred to the British Columbia Cancer Agency for enrollment, randomization, and treatment planning. Therefore, the source population consisted of the patient populations of the referring physicians. No information was given on the number and characteristics of women who refused to participate. Of the participants, 164 women were randomized to chemotherapy plus radiation, and 154 women were randomized to chemotherapy alone. Thus, the ratio of propositi to comparison subjects was approximately one to one.

7. *Could there have been bias in the selection of the study subjects? How likely was this bias?* Selection bias was not possible because a

prospective study was conducted, and the outcomes were unknown at enrollment.

8. *Could there have been bias in the collection of information? How likely was this bias?* The article does not mention if individuals assessing the end points were masked to treatment group. However, even if they were unmasked, the end points were objective and so it is unlikely that this type of observation bias influenced the results. The authors did not indicate that any data were collected using interviews or questionnaires, and so interviewer bias and recall bias did not occur. Although losses to follow-up were different between the two groups (4.9% for the experimental group and 1.9% for the comparison group), only 11 women were lost and so this was unlikely to have affected the results. In fact, all 11 women were alive and had experienced no recurrences at the time that they were lost to follow-up. Noncompliance with the assigned treatment regimen was also fairly low. Of the 164 patients who were assigned to chemotherapy and radiotherapy combined, 12 did not receive radiotherapy, and 8 of the 154 patients assigned to chemotherapy alone received additional radiotherapy.

9. *What provisions were made to minimize the influence of confounding factors prior to the analysis of the data? Were these provisions sufficient?* Randomization was used to control for confounding. It appears to have been successful because the prognostic variables at baseline were quite similar between compared groups. These variables included age, mean number of nodes studied, number of positive nodes, nodal size, and tumor grade. The investigators collected data on these prognostic factors to determine if the randomization was effective. Data on race or socioeconomic status were not given.

B. Analysis of data

1. *What methods were used to control confounding bias during data analysis? Were these methods sufficient?* An intent-to-treat analysis was performed. This type of analysis preserves the benefits of randomization. Stratified analyses were also conducted according to the number of positive lymph nodes.

2. *What measures of association were reported in this study?* Relative risks were reported.

3. *What measures of statistical stability were reported in this study?* The authors reported 95% confidence intervals and *P* values.

C. Interpretation of data

1. *What were the major results of this study?* Of the 164 patients in the group assigned to chemotherapy and radiation, 79 had recurrences (48%) as compared to 97 of the 154 patients assigned to chemotherapy alone (63%). Thus, compared to women who were assigned to

chemotherapy alone, there was a 33% reduction in the rate of breast cancer recurrence (relative risk, 0.67; 95% confidence interval, 0.5 to 0.9) among women who were assigned to chemotherapy plus radiotherapy. In addition, 62 deaths resulting from breast cancer occurred in the group assigned to chemotherapy and radiation, and 76 breast cancer deaths occurred in the chemotherapy alone group. This translates to a 29% reduction in breast cancer mortality (relative risk, 0.71; 95% confidence interval, 0.51 to 0.99). These results were based on 15 years of follow-up.

2. *How is the interpretation of these results affected by information bias, selection bias, and confounding? Discuss both the direction and magnitude of any bias.* These results do not appear to be influenced by selection bias or confounding. It is unlikely that information bias from possibly unmasked outcome assessment had a meaningful impact on the findings.

3. *How is the interpretation of these results affected by nondifferential misclassification? Discuss both the direction and magnitude of this misclassification.* A low and similar level of noncompliance occurred in the two groups (7.3% among the chemotherapy and radiotherapy group and 5.2% among the chemotherapy only group, n = 20 patients). It is possible that the findings would have been slightly stronger had these individuals received their assigned treatments. The authors chose to conduct an intent-to-treat analysis to preserve the benefits of randomization and to determine the effectiveness of the treatment under everyday practice conditions. They also could have conducted an efficacy analysis to determine the effects of treatment under ideal conditions. The efficacy analysis would have excluded the noncompliers.

4. *Did the discussion section adequately address the limitations of the study?* The discussion section did not describe any study limitations. However, the authors attempted to reconcile the results of the current study with those of earlier ones. This was done mainly by citing differences between the study populations, treatment regimens, and so forth.

5. *What were the authors' main conclusions? Were they justified by the findings?* The authors concluded that locoregional radiation therapy reduced the rates of locoregional and systemic recurrence and the chance of dying from breast cancer among premenopausal women with node-positive breast cancer. These conclusions were justified by the results seen in this population.

6. *To what larger population can the results of this study be generalized?* These results can be generalized to other premenopausal women with stage I and II breast cancer who are at high risk for locore-

gional and distant recurrences. These women would need to receive the same treatments as those in the study: a modified radical mastectomy with axillary node dissection for the initial treatment of the breast cancer, and similar doses and schedules of chemotherapy and radiotherapy. Apparently, the chemotherapy given to the study patients is not the classical treatment regimen.[20] In fact, some clinicians consider it a suboptimal treatment.

Summary

The ability to evaluate critically the results of published epidemiologic studies is an important skill for public health professionals. The critique outline presented in this chapter is a useful framework for conducting such an assessment. The outline helps the reader to assess: (1) whether the methods used to select the study subjects and collect and analyze the data were comparable across groups; (2) whether any errors were committed in the design, conduct, and interpretation of the study; and (3) what impact these errors had on the reported findings.

The critique outline is divided into three sections that address data collection, analysis, and interpretation. The section on data collection poses questions about the context and objectives of the study, the primary exposure and outcome definitions, the study design, selection of the study population, and likelihood for selection bias, information bias, and confounding. The section on data analysis deals with the methods for handling confounding and the measures of association and statistical stability. The section on data interpretation covers the major results and how the interpretation of the results might be influenced by bias, confounding, and nondifferential misclassification. This section closes with questions about the authors' conclusions and whether they were justified by the study data and a question on the generalizability of the findings.

References

1. Chiu W-T, Kuo C-Y, Hung C-C, Chen M. The effect of the Taiwan motorcycle helmet use law on head injuries. *Am J Public Health*. 2000;90:793–796.

2. Steering Committee of the Physician's Health Study Research Group. Final report on the aspirin component of the ongoing Physician's Health Study. *N Engl J Med*.1989;321:129–135.

3. Seage GR, Mayer KH, Horsburgh CR, Holmberg SD, Moon MW, Lamb GA. The relation between nitrite inhalants, unprotected receptive anal intercourse, and the risk of human immunodeficiency virus infection. *Am J Epidemiol*. 1992; 135:1–11.

4. Aschengrau A, Ozonoff D, Paulu C, Coogan P, Vezina R, Heeren T, et al. Cancer risk and tetrachloroethylene-contaminated drinking water in Massachusetts. *Arch Environ Health*. 1993;48:284–292.

Whenever possible, the hypothesis should quantify the relationship between the exposure and disease. For example, a reduction of 1000 ppm or more of lead in soil accessible to children will decrease their blood lead levels by at least 3 µg/dL.[13] Specific hypotheses are easier than nonspecific ones to test and refute.

WHAT WAS THE PRIMARY EXPOSURE OF INTEREST? WAS THIS ACCU-RATELY MEASURED? The exposure of interest is the factor that either causes, prevents, or treats the outcome. It is important to consider whether the exposure was accurately defined and measured because exposure mis-classification stems from broad definitions and inaccurate measurements. Thus, when evaluating the accuracy of exposure data, one should also compare the exposure's conceptual and operational definitions. For example, the conceptual exposure definition in a study conducted to investigate the cancer risk associated with tetrachloroethylene-contaminated drinking water was simply "exposure to tetrachloroethylene-contaminated drinking water." The operational definition was as follows: An ordinal estimate of exposure to tetrachloroethylene-contaminated water was defined as "the estimated mass of tetrachloroethylene that entered the home through the drinking water during a specified time period."[4] Exposure to contaminated water was estimated using an algorithm based on information about the water pipe that supplied each subject's home. This information included the pipe length, diameter, installation date, and number of loads. Note that the operational definition omits important behavioral data on water use, and so it may lead to exposure misclassification.

When reviewing an article, the reader should look for steps that were taken to ensure the accuracy of the exposure data such as use of exposure biomarkers, use of sensitive and specific exposure definitions, and verification of one information source with another. Also, it is important to note how broadly the exposure categories were defined. For example, several exposure categories were compared in the tetrachloroethylene-contaminated drinking water study: ever versus never exposed, low versus never exposed, and high versus never exposed.[4] Clearly, the ever-exposed category was quite broad, and the two exposure level categories were narrower. It is possible to get different results with different exposure definitions. For example, investigators in the contaminated drinking water study reported much greater increases in the risk of bladder cancer among highly exposed individuals (odds ratio = 4.0) than among ever-exposed individuals (odds ratio = 1.4).[4]

WHAT WAS THE PRIMARY OUTCOME OF INTEREST? WAS THIS ACCU-RATELY MEASURED? The outcome of interest is the end point being studied such as a precursor of disease; disease incidence, prevalence, and recurrence; symptom improvement; side effects; length of survival; and

5. Frigoletto FD Jr, Lieberman E, Lang JM, Cohen A, Barss V, Ringer S, et al. A clinical trial of active management of labor. *N Engl J Med.* 1995;333:745–750.

6. Park YK, Sempos CT, Barton CN, Vanderveen JE, Yetley EA. Effectiveness of food fortification in the United States: the case of pellagra. *Am J Public Health.* 2000;90:727–738.

7. Manson JL, Barkley SE, Kappelman MM, Carter DE, Beachy WV. Evaluation of a self-instructional method for improving doctor–patient communication. *J Med Educ.*1988;63:629–635.

8. Rothman KJ. Policy recommendations in epidemiology research papers. *Epidemiology.* 1993;4:94–95.

9. Monson RR. *Occupational Epidemiology.* 2nd ed. Boca Raton, FL: CRC Press; 1990.

10. Walker AM. Reporting the results of epidemiologic studies. *Am J Public Health.* 1986;76:556–560.

11. Zierler S, Rothman KJ. Congenital heart disease in relation to maternal use of Benedectin and other drugs in early pregnancy. *N Engl J Med.* 1985;313: 347–352.

12. Last JM. *A Dictionary of Epidemiology.* 3rd ed. New York, NY: Oxford University Press; 1995.

13. Weitzman M, Aschengrau A, Bellinger D, Jones R, Hamlin JS, Beiser A. Lead-contaminated soil abatement and urban children's blood lead levels. *JAMA.* 1993;269:1647–1654.

14. Aschengrau A, Paulu C, Ozonoff D. Tetrachloroethylene-contaminated drinking water and the risk of breast cancer. *Environ Health Perspect.* 1998;106: 947–953.

15. Meinert CL. *Clinical Trials Dictionary, Terminology and Usage Recommendations.* Baltimore, MD: The Johns Hopkins Center for Clinical Trials; 1996.

16. Mann JM, Quinn TC, Francis H, Nxilambi N, Bosenge N, Bila K, et al. Prevalence of HTLV-III/LAV in household contact of patients with confirmed AIDS and controls in Kinshasa, Zaire. *JAMA.* 1986;256:721.

17. Needleman HL, Schell A, Bellinger D, Leviton A, Allred EN. The long-term effects of exposure to low doses of lead in childhood. An 11-year follow-up study report. *N Engl J Med.* 1990;332:83.

18. Ragaz J, Jackson SM, Le N, Plenderleith IH, Spinelli JJ, Basco VE, et al. Adjuvant radiotherapy and chemotherapy in node-positive premenopausal women with breast cancer. *N Engl J Med.* 1997;337:956.

19. Rothman KJ. Zaire: nonsexual household transmission of AIDS (letter). *JAMA.* 1986;256:3091.

20. Goldhirsch A, Coates AS, Colleoni M, Gelber RD. Radiotherapy and chemotherapy in high-risk breast cancer (letter). *N Engl J Med.* 1998;338: 330–331.

15

The Epidemiologic Approach to Causation

LEARNING OBJECTIVES

By the end of this chapter, the reader will be able to:

- Define and state the important characteristics of a cause.
- Describe the historical development of disease causation theories including the germ theory and the web of causation.
- Discuss the causal guidelines proposed by Hill, including their limitations.
- Distinguish between a risk factor and a cause.
- Describe the key elements of the sufficient–component cause model.
- Discuss why most scientists believe that the human immunodeficiency virus (HIV) is the cause of acquired immune deficiency syndrome (AIDS).

Introduction

In his book *When Bad Things Happen to Good People*, Rabbi Harold Kushner tries to explain why God allows ordinary people to face extraordinary pain and tragedy.[1(pp1-5)] The idea for the book originated with Kushner's own attempt to make sense of the death of his 14-year-old son. Kushner states that sometimes there is no reason, and that it is just a case of bad luck. To those who ask "Why did this happen to me?" Kushner answers that it was not part of God's fixed plan but rather that "randomness" from the "corners of the universe where God's creative light has not yet penetrated" is accountable.[1(p53)]

Whether randomness or a fixed plan causes events—good and bad—is a matter of debate among theologians and epidemiologists. Some epidemiologists, called probabilists, believe that randomness or chance is an explanation for events; others, known as determinists, think that everything has a cause and that chance is merely a term that we use when we cannot explain something because of limitations in our knowledge.[2(p116)]

At times Kushner also seems to support the deterministic view. For example, he states: "I don't know why one person gets sick, and another does not, but I can only assume that some natural laws which we don't understand are at work. . . . As we have learned more about how the human body works, as we understand more of the natural laws built into the world, we have some answers. . . . The man who smokes two packs of cigarettes a day for twenty years and develops lung cancer faces problems which deserve our sympathy but he has no grounds for asking 'How could God do this to me?'"[1(p60,65)]

Certainly, epidemiologists, probabilists and determinists alike, would agree that their goal is to learn about what causes and prevents disease. How epidemiologists determine causative and preventive factors involves a process known as causal inference. The scientific philosophy of causal inference began in ancient times and has changed considerably over the centuries. First, the doctrine of rationalism predominated. This philosophy states that knowledge accumulates through reason rather than observation.[3(p278)] For example, if the statements "all robins have red breasts" and "this bird is a robin" are correct, then the rationalist would conclude that "this bird has a red breast" without looking at any birds.

The philosophy of empiricism has prevailed since the scientific revolution of the 1700s. Empiricism emphasizes inductive inference—the formulation of explanatory hypotheses from making observations.[3(pp97–98)] For example, if the empiricist observes 100 robins and finds that they all have red breasts, he would hypothesize that all robins have red breasts, thereby making a generalization from a set of observations.

In the early 1930s, Karl Popper challenged the inductivist philosophy with his proposal that knowledge accumulates by deductive reasoning and by falsifying hypotheses that are already in one's mind.[4] According to Popper's hypothetico-deductive approach, hypotheses are formed using creativity and imagination, and no data are needed. Predictions are made on the basis of these hypotheses, and observations are collected and compared with predictions. If the observations are incompatible with the predictions, the hypothesis is falsified. Otherwise, the hypothesis remains a reasonable explanation until a better one comes along. According to this philosophy, the scientific value of a hypothesis increases with the degree to which testable and falsifiable predictions can be made from it.[5] Falsifiability increases with the empirical content of the hypothesis. For example, it is easier to falsify the following precise hypothesis: "Children living in homes with floor and window well dust lead levels above 1000 part per million have five times the risk of becoming lead poisoned as compared with children who do not live in such conditions" than it is to falsify the following general hypothesis: "Lead-contaminated dust causes childhood lead poisoning."

Today, most practicing epidemiologists use a combination of inductive and deductive reasoning to learn about the factors that cause and prevent disease. However, many have adopted Popper's thesis that causal relationships can never be proven. Instead, they acknowledge that causal inference involves judgments that are made using accumulated knowledge. This knowledge comes from many fields of study in addition to epidemiology, including medicine, biology, physics, chemistry, and toxicology.

Because causal inference is a judgment, epidemiologists often have different views about the causality of certain relationships. In fact, disagreement is the rule rather than the exception. For example, even though most scientists now believe that the human immunodeficiency virus (HIV) is the cause of acquired immunodeficiency syndrome (AIDS), virologist Peter Duesberg thinks that HIV is harmless. Instead, he believes that AIDS can be caused by many different agents such as illicit drug use, the anti-AIDS drug called AZT, and noninfectious contaminants of the clotting factor given to hemophiliacs.[6]

This chapter further develops the concepts of causation and causal inference by providing the definition and characteristics of a cause, the historical development of disease causation theories, the popular model of assessing causation proposed by Sir Austin Bradford Hill, and a more recent conceptual model of causation known as the sufficient–component cause model. The chapter concludes with a description of why mainstream scientists believe that HIV is the cause of AIDS.

Definitions of a Cause

According to the *American Heritage Dictionary*, a cause is that which produces "an effect, result, or consequence" or "the one, such as a person, event, or condition, that is responsible for an action or result."[7(p296)] The dictionary's synonyms for cause include "reason" and "occasion." For example, the reason for the car accident was the icy road conditions, or the occasion for the robbery was the absence of the night watchman. This present-day dictionary's definitions of causation follow the canons of causation first proposed by the 19th-century philosopher John Stuart Mill. One of his tenets, known as "the method of difference," states that A causes B if, all else being held constant, a change in A is accompanied by a subsequent change in B.[3(p215)]

Modern epidemiologists have restated this definition in several ways. For example, Rothman and Greenland have defined a cause as "an event, condition, or characteristic that preceded the disease event and without which the disease event either would not have occurred at all or would not have occurred until some later time."[2(p8)] In contrast, Susser has opted for the following simple, pragmatic definition "something that makes a difference."[8(p637)]

How do we know when something makes a difference? How can we tell the difference between real causes and their imposters?[8] The principles of epidemiologic research provide some answers. Epidemiologic research involves generating and testing specific hypotheses about factors that cause and prevent disease. A hypothesis is defined as "a tentative explanation for an observation, phenomenon, or scientific problem that can be tested by further investigation."[7(p866)] Epidemiologists test hypotheses by making comparisons, usually within the context of a formal study. For example, an epidemiologist might compare the death rate among people exposed to high levels of air pollution to the rate among people exposed to low levels. In this setting, the epidemiologist is starting with the potential cause and searches for its effects. On the other hand, an epidemiologist could start with the disease and search for its causes. For example, he or she might compare prenatal cocaine use among women who gave birth to an infant with a congenital malformation to those who gave birth to a normal infant.

As described in detail in Chapter 3, these types of comparisons are usually quantified in terms of absolute and relative measures of comparison. For example, people exposed to high levels of air pollution might have death rates from lung diseases that are twice the rates of people exposed to low levels of pollution. This increased death rate in the highly exposed group indicates that there is a modest association between air pollution levels and mortality.

However, the presence of an association does not necessarily imply that there is a causal relationship between the two factors. For example, there is an association between roosters crowing at dawn and the rising of the sun. This does not mean that the rooster causes the sun to rise. Thus, there are both causal and noncausal associations, and the art of causal inference is a method for distinguishing between the two.

Epidemiologists typically follow a two-step process when practicing causal inference. First, they determine if the observed result is valid or true. As described in earlier chapters, an association is considered valid only if three alternative explanations have been eliminated: bias, confounding, and random error. Bias is a systematic error in the way that the study subjects were selected or the data were gathered. For example, diseased people who live in highly polluted areas may be less willing to participate in studies than those living in less polluted areas. Confounding is a distortion in the results that arises from comparing dissimilar groups. For example, the association between air pollution and mortality may not be due to the air pollution but to a higher prevalence of cigarette smoking among the people living in highly polluted areas as compared to those living in less polluted areas. Random error is the probability that the observed results are due to "chance." Thus, the twofold increase in deaths due to lung disease among people living in highly polluted areas may be due to "the luck of the draw."

If systematic bias, confounding, and random error have been ruled out as alternative explanations of an association, epidemiologists believe that the association is real and so they begin the second step in the process of causal inference: assessing whether the exposure has actually caused the outcome. Causal inference is a complicated process with no hard and fast rules. In fact, there is considerable disagreement among epidemiologists about the appropriate way to make causal inferences, ranging from the use of causal "criteria" to the evaluation of competing hypotheses with "crucial" observations.

Characteristics of a Cause

According to Susser, true causes have three essential attributes: association, time order, and direction.[8] *Association* means that "a causal factor *(X)* must occur together with the putative effect *(Y)*." In other words, there must be a "statistical dependence" between the causal factor and effect. If no association is found, causality can be rejected. As described in Chapter 3, epidemiologists quantify associations by making absolute or relative comparisons between two or more groups.

Time order means that the cause must precede the effect. A cause may antedate the effect by either a long or short period of time. The former is termed a distant cause, and the latter is called a proximate cause. For chronic diseases such as cancer, distant causes often precede the cancer diagnosis by decades and proximate causes precede it by months or years. For example, diethylstilbestrol (DES) exposure in utero is considered a distant cause of adenocarcinoma of the vagina because this exposure occurs on average 20 years before the cancer diagnosis among the affected women.[9] In contrast, hormone replacement therapy is considered a proximate cause of breast cancer because only exposures within 5 years of the cancer diagnosis carry an increased risk.[10]

Direction, the third essential attribute of a cause, means that there is an asymmetrical relationship between the cause and effect. In other words, one must demonstrate that "a change in an outcome is a consequence of change in an antecedent factor" so a symmetrical relationship is noncausal.[8] For example, there is an asymmetrical relationship between exposure to cigarette smoke during pregnancy and the occurrence of low birthweight in the offspring. Prenatal exposure to cigarette smoke causes low birthweight[11] but low birthweight does not cause prenatal smoke exposure. This type of relationship can be diagramed as follows:

$$X \longrightarrow Y$$

TABLE 15–1 Key Characteristics of Causes

■ Essential attributes include association, time order, and directionality.
■ Causes include host and environmental factors.
■ Causes include active agents and static conditions.
■ Causes may be either positive (presence induces disease) or negative (absence induces disease).

Several other characteristics of a cause are also worth noting. First, causes include both host and environmental factors. Host characteristics include a person's genetic makeup, gender, age, immunity level, diet, behaviors, and existing diseases. These factors typically affect a person's susceptibility to disease. Environmental factors pertain to determinants that are external to the individual, and thereby encompass a wide range of natural, social, and economic events and conditions. For example, the presence of infectious agents, reservoirs in which the organism multiply, vectors that transport the agent, poor and crowded housing conditions, and political instability are environmental factors that cause communicable diseases.

Causes can also be characterized as being active or passive. According to Susser: "If the determinant is an active agent, it produces a change; the determinant is an intended or unintended intervention or a natural force or an accident, or the removal or absence of something needed, like vitamins. If the determinant is a static condition, it is an unchanging antecedent in a given set of circumstances: outcomes differ as the nature or quality of the condition differs. Usually, conditions are fixed attributes or circumstances like sex, heritage, or geography."[8(p637)]

Causes can be considered positive or negative. The presence of a positive cause results in disease, and the absence of a negative cause (which is also known as a preventive exposure) causes disease. Examples of positive causes include cigarette smoking, exposure to DES, hormone replacement therapy, and ionizing radiation. Negative causes include vitamins, vaccines, a nutritious diet, and adequate exercise. The key characteristics of causes are summarized in Table 15–1.

Risk Factors versus Causes

Epidemiologists often use the term *risk factor* instead of cause. Although this term partially reflects epidemiologists' cautiousness about making causal inferences, it is useful to discuss its meaning in the context of causal inference. Consider, for example, the following well-known factors that increase a woman's risk of breast cancer: living in North America, having a high socioeconomic status, never marrying, and being Jewish (see Table 15–2). Are these direct causes of breast cancer or something else? The answer is "something else." As epidemiologists have learned about the eti-

TABLE 15–2 Risk Factors for Breast Cancer

Characteristic	High-risk group	Low-risk group
Country of birth	North America, Northern Europe	Asia, Africa
Socioeconomic status	High	Low
Marital status	Never married	Ever married
Religion	Jewish	Seventh Day Adventist, Mormon

Source: Adapted from Kelsey JL. Breast cancer epidemiology. *Epidemiol Rev* 1993;15:256–263.

ology of breast cancer, they have come to understand that these factors are not direct causes but rather serve to identify more proximate causes. For example, never married women are at increased risk of breast cancer because they are more likely to be childless. Childlessness, in turn, is associated with less differentiated breast tissue that is more susceptible to carcinogens.[12] Note that risk factors such as these are often a few steps removed from the direct causes of disease.

In contrast, consider the causes of an automobile fatality. The direct causes include the speed of the car, presence of hazardous road conditions, the time of day, level of traffic, and mental state of the driver. These factors are more proximate to "that which produces an effect, result, or consequence" than the previously described breast cancer risk factors.

Historical Development of Disease Causation Theories

During ancient times, concepts of causation were influenced mainly by people's religious beliefs. For example, people believed that illnesses occurred because of divine retribution for committing sins. Around the fourth century B.C., Hippocrates introduced the idea that people became ill because of an imbalance in the four body humors—phlegm, yellow bile, blood, and black bile.[13(pp767–768)] He hypothesized that these imbalances were caused by changes in season, air, winds, water, and stars, as well as personal habits.

Although Hippocrates had many ideas that were correct, his misconceptions about disease causation predominated for the following 2000 years. Even in the 1800s, people thought that disease arose spontaneously or from foul clouds called miasmas. In the mid 1800s Louis Pasteur, Miles Berkeley, and others revolutionized the concept of causality with the germ theory of disease.[14(pp5–6)] This theory states that specific transmissible pathogens are responsible for disease.

In the mid- to late 1800s, Jakob Henle and his student Robert Koch developed a set of postulates of disease causation that were based on the germ theory. These postulates are summarized as follows. (1) The microorganism will occur in every case of the disease and can explain the pathology and clinical changes associated with the disease. (2) The microorganism must be shown to be distinct from any others that might be found with the disease. and (3) If the microorganism is isolated and repeatedly grown in culture, it will induce a new case of disease in a susceptible animal.[15] The first postulate is particularly important because it embodies the idea of causal specificity—that is, the one-to-one relationship between a microorganism and the occurrence of disease. This is a concept that works well for infectious diseases but not for noninfectious diseases. It is important to note that Henle and Koch did not consider these rigid criteria for causation.[16]

In the 1960s another causal paradigm—the web of causation—gained popularity because it was more useful than the Henle–Koch postulates for understanding the causes of noninfectious diseases. Consider, for example, lead poisoning—a disease that is defined by an elevated blood lead level and affects the brain, kidney, and blood-forming tissues.[17(pp7–9)] The causal web shows that its occurrence can be explained by a complex web of many interconnected factors, including both host and environmental determinants (see Figure 15-1). It illustrates that there are many ways to become lead poisoned, and that these pathways or causes may differ from person to person. For example, a young child may become lead poisoned by ingesting dust that has been contaminated with lead from crumbling paint, industrial pollution, or automobile traffic. On the other hand, an adult may become lead poisoned from workplace exposures such as bridge work, or a hobby such as stained glass work. Thus, the causal web paradigm represented a fundamental shift in thinking about disease causation, because it incorporates the idea of multiple causes of disease. In addition, the paradigm implies that cases of disease can be prevented by cutting a few strands of the web. Usually those factors that are closest to the disease are targeted.

In 1994, Krieger criticized the use of the web because of its "hidden reliance on biomedical individualism to guide the choice of factors incorporated in the web." She proposed an alternative approach that incorporates an ecosocial framework.[18] This approach focuses on the origins of the web, including the social, political, and economic determinants of health instead of individual-level determinants. Thus, for lead poisoning, such an approach would focus research questions on the reasons for particular web components such as substandard housing, lack of day care, workplace exposure to lead, and so forth.

During the 1950s and 1960s epidemiologists also developed a new set of postulates for causal inferences regarding noninfectious diseases of entirely unknown etiology.[8] They were first proposed after the discovery of the association between smoking and lung cancer. From the start, many established scientists debated whether this association was causal. Thus, it

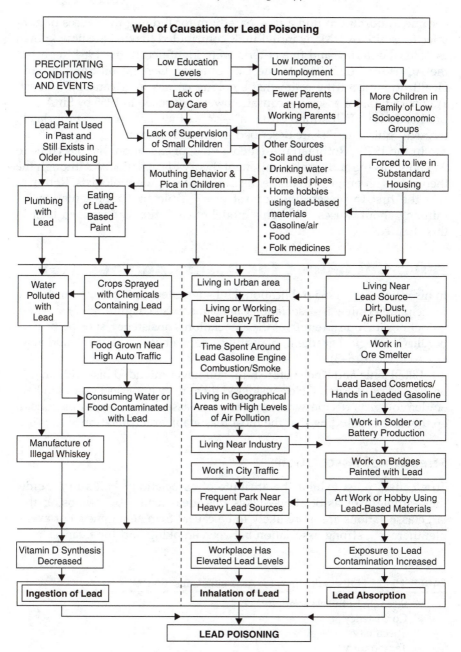

FIGURE 15–1. Example of a Web of Causation For Lead Poisoning

Source: Reprinted from Timmreck TC. *An Introduction to Epidemiology*, p. 337. Boston, MA: Jones and Bartlett Publishers;1994.

became important to find a new paradigm for judging the causes of non-infectious diseases. Many individuals contributed to what are now known as "causal criteria," and five criteria were identified in the 1964 Report of the Advisory Committee to the U.S. Surgeon General on Smoking and Health to support the claim that smoking causes lung cancer. The best-known criteria for assessing causation were proposed in 1965 by Sir Austin Bradford Hill.[8] Hill's nine "criteria"—or, as they are more appropriately termed, "guidelines"—are described in the next section.

In the 1970s, Rothman presented a view of causation that has come to be known as the sufficient–component theory of causation.[19] Although the theory was an outgrowth of the ideas of earlier epidemiologists, Rothman was the first to present the "causal pies," a pictorial representation for thinking about causes.[20(p39)] This model of causation is described later in this chapter.

Hill's Guidelines for Assessing Causation

In his much-cited 1965 publication, Hill suggested a set of nine guidelines to help determine if associations are causal (see Figure 15–2).[21] These guidelines include strength of the association, consistency, specificity, temporality, biological gradient, plausibility, coherence, experiment, and analogy (see Table 15–3).

Like Henle and Koch before him, Hill never intended his guidelines to be used as rigid criteria. He considered them to be imperfect guides to help epidemiologists decide what aspects of an association should be considered before concluding that the most reasonable interpretation is causal.

Strength of Association

True causes must exhibit the attribute of association.[8] Hill's first guideline—strength of association—takes this idea further by proposing that large associations are more likely to be causal than small ones. For example, there is a strong association between smoking and lung cancer mor-

---

TABLE 15-3 Hill's Guidelines for Assessing Causation

- Strength of the association
- Consistency
- Specificity
- Temporality
- Biological gradient
- Plausibility
- Coherence
- Experiment
- Analogy

FIGURE 15-2. Sir Austin Bradford Hill Suggested Guidelines for Assessing Causation

Source: Reprinted from *Statistics in Medicine.* 1982;1(no 4):overleaf. With permission from John Wiley and Sons, Ltd. Sussex, England.

tality. The risk of dying from lung cancer among smokers is about 10 times greater than that among nonsmokers.[22(pvi)] In addition, the risk of dying from lung cancer among heavy smokers is about 15 to 25 times higher than among nonsmokers. These strong associations are likely to be causal because they are unlikely to be accounted for entirely by alternative explanations such as bias and confounding.

Even though he emphasized this guideline, Hill stated: "We must not be too ready to dismiss a cause–effect hypothesis merely on the grounds that the observed association appears to be slight. There are many occasions in medicine when this is in truth so."[21(p296)] Thus, it is quite possible for weak associations to be causal. However, it is harder to rule out the impact of undetected biases on these associations. For example, a study found that children who were exposed to prenatal x-rays have about 1.4 times the risk of developing childhood leukemia as children without such exposures.[23] Although many believe that this association is causal, it is quite possible that it resulted from bias or confounding.

Consistency

Hill asserted that associations are more likely to be causal if they are observed repeatedly "by different persons, in different places, circumstances and times." This is because replication increases our confidence that the association is not due to an error or fallacy. For example, one of the reasons that epidemiologists believe that smoking causes lung cancer is that this association has been observed in so many different studies conducted by different investigators, in different locations, with different types of populations, and in different time periods.

However, Hill also stated: "There will be occasions when repetition is absent or impossible and yet we should not hesitate to draw conclusions."[21(p297)] In fact, there may be reasonable explanations for differing study results. For example, one study may have examined low-level exposures while another examined high-level exposures. Or, one study may have enrolled only men while another enrolled only women. Given the numerous biological and cultural differences between the sexes, it is perfectly reasonable to think that the strength of an association differs by gender. Thus, it is important to remember that, although the presence of consistency may provide evidence of causality, its absence does not preclude causation.

Specificity

The concept of specificity, which was first developed for infectious diseases, means that a cause should lead to a single effect and vice versa. Although Hill stated that specific associations enabled investigators to draw conclusions about causation without hesitation, he also acknowledged that the lack of specificity did not necessarily leave investigators "sitting irresolutely on the fence." In fact, most practicing epidemiologists consider this guideline useless because it has so many well-known exceptions. For example, smoking is a cause not only of cancer of the lung but also cancer of the larynx, oral cavity, esophagus, bladder, kidney, and pancreas, as well as many noncancerous conditions.[24(p67-72)] Furthermore, many diseases have more than one cause. For example the causes of lung cancer include tobacco smoke (both active and passive exposure), radon, asbestos, and ionizing radiation.[24(pp158-162)]

Temporality

Time order or temporality means that the cause must precede the disease. Temporality is the only one of Hill's guidelines about which there is complete agreement among epidemiologists. Prospective study designs are best for providing evidence of temporality because epidemiologists are usually sure that the cause preceded the occurrence of the disease in this type of study.

Biological Gradient

Hill stated, "If the association is one which can reveal a biological gradient, or dose–response curve, then we should look most carefully for such evidence."[21(p298)] In other words, an association is more likely to be causal if its strength increases as the exposure level increases. Hill gives as an example the linear rise in lung cancer death rates with the number of cigarettes smoked, stating that this evidence "adds a very great deal to the simpler evidence that cigarette smokers have a higher death rate than nonsmokers."[21(p298)]

However, even Hill acknowledged that there may be other or more complex dose–response relationships between a particular exposure and disease (see Figure 15–3). For example, it is possible for an exposure to exhibit, a "threshold effect" below which there are no adverse outcomes. In a 1998 study on the risk of miscarriage among pregnant women exposed to trihalomethanes (common contaminants of chlorinated drinking water that form when chlorine reacts with naturally occurring compounds in the raw water), investigators found no meaningful increase in the risk of miscarriage until contaminant levels reached 75 µg per liter, when the risk began to increase.[25] These results support the idea of a threshold effect at this exposure level. It is also possible that there is a curvilinear relationship between an exposure level and the risk of disease. For example, diets that have either too few or excessive amounts of certain vitamins can lead to illness. The absence of a particular dose–response relationship (such as linear, threshold, or curvilinear) means only that the causal hypothesis that predicts that specific dose–response curve has been disputed.[2(p26)]

Plausibility

Hill asserted that there should be an existing biological or social model to explain the association. For example, it is biologically plausible that smoking causes lung cancer because cigarettes contain many carcinogenic substances. On the other hand, Hill conceded: "This is a feature I am convinced we cannot demand. . . . In short, the association we observe may be one new to science or medicine and we must not dismiss it too lightheartedly as just too odd."[21(p298)] In fact, many epidemiologic studies

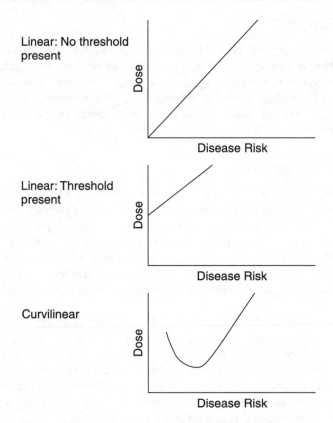

FIGURE 15-3. Possible Forms of Dose–response Relationships

have identified cause–effect relationships before biological mechanisms were identified. For example, researchers discovered the carcinogenic substances in cigarette smoke many years after the initial epidemiologic studies linking smoking to cancer.

Despite Hill's reservations, many practicing epidemiologists believe that biological plausibility is an important consideration when judging the nature of an association. Consider, for example, a study that compared the outcomes of hospitalized cardiac patients, half of whom were prayed for by strangers, Christians who volunteered for the study.[26] In this double-masked experiment, the prayed-for patients had fewer heart attacks and contracted pneumonia less often than those who were not prayed for. Many epidemiologists have difficulty believing that this association was causal because of the lack of a biological model to explain it. Instead they speculate that factors other than divine powers were at work, such as baseline differences in the level of illness between the two groups.

Coherence

Coherence is very close to biological plausibility. According to Hill, it means that "the cause-and-effect interpretation of our data should not seriously conflict with generally known facts of the natural history and biology of the disease."[21(p298)] For example, Hill found that the association between cigarette smoking and lung cancer is coherent with several diverse facts: (1) the temporal rise in both smoking and lung cancer over several decades, (2) the different temporal pattern in lung cancer between men and women because women began smoking later than men, (3) the histopathological evidence from the bronchial epithelium of smokers, and (4) the carcinogenic action of cigarette smoke in laboratory animals. Still, he stated: "The lack of such evidence cannot nullify the epidemiologic observations." For example, biological differences between species may account for differences between man and laboratory animals.

Experiment

Experiment is not a causal guideline in its strictest sense. Rather, it is a method for testing a causal hypothesis. This guideline is a reprise of John Stuart Mill's "method of difference" canon, which states that *A* causes *B* if, all else being held uniform, a change in *A* leads to a subsequent change in *B*.[3(p215)] In the context of epidemiologic research, this guideline suggests that an intervention initiated by the investigator that modifies the exposure through prevention, treatment, or removal should result in less disease or no disease at all. For example, a study of smoking cessation methods should result in lower lung cancer rates among former smokers, assuming the intervention is effective.

If available, well-designed and well-conducted experimental studies provide strong evidence for or against causation. Unfortunately, as described in Chapter 7, it is often infeasible and unethical to conduct experimental studies, and so observational studies provide most of the epidemiologic data for judging whether an association is causal. Consequently, the absence of experimental evidence should not be taken as evidence against causation.

Analogy

Hill suggested that epidemiologist use analogies or similarities between the observed association and any other associations. Hill gave the following example: "With the known effects of the drug thalidomide and the disease rubella we would be ready to accept slighter but similar evidence with another drug or another viral disease in pregnancy."[21(p299)] Critics of this guideline state that the absence of an analogy implies only that the investigator is unimaginative, not that the association is noncausal.[2(p27)]

Use of Hill's Guidelines by Epidemiologists Today

Note that the guidelines offered by Hill have many exceptions and uncertainties. Even Hill concluded: "Here then are nine different viewpoints from all of which we should study association before we cry causation. . . . None of my nine viewpoints can bring indisputable evidence for or against the cause-and-effect hypothesis and none can be required as a sine qua non. What they can do, with greater or lesser strength, is to help us make up our minds on the fundamental question—is there any other way of explaining the set of facts before us, is there any other answer equally, or more, likely than cause and effect?"[21(p299)] We agree with the essence of Hill's conclusion. However, we think that one part of his statement is incorrect—temporality *is* a requirement for causality.

Some epidemiologists support the use of Hill's guidelines for causal inference,[8] and others oppose it—particularly those who follow the Popperian philosophy of falsification.[27(pp153–162)] Some have proposed an alternative approach: testing competing causal theories using "crucial" observations.[2(pp23–24)] This process involves formulating competing hypotheses as specifically as possible, making predictions on the basis of each hypothesis, collecting observations that test each hypothesis, and assessing the compatibility of the observed data with each hypothesis. Ideally, the investigator will find a "crucial" observation that will be compatible with one hypothesis and will refute the others.

How is causal inference currently practiced in the epidemiologic community? Weed and Gorelic addressed this question in their study of review papers published on the association between alcohol consumption and the risk of breast cancer.[28] The authors found that the investigators in these studies selectively used Hill's causal guidelines: the investigators frequently excluded some of the guidelines and altered others. The most commonly used criteria were consistency, strength of association, biological plausibility, and biological gradient. The criteria of temporality, experiment, and specificity were used infrequently, and coherence and analogy were almost never used. In addition, bias and confounding were frequently considered.

Interestingly, Weed and Gorelic found that none of the review papers claimed that the association between alcohol consumption and breast cancer was causal. However, many authors made public health recommendations either for or against changes in policy or practice. This custom follows Hill's advice that public health actions may be taken even when there is insufficient evidence to definitely conclude causation. According to Hill: "All scientific work is incomplete—whether it be observational or experimental. All scientific work is liable to be upset or modified by advancing knowledge. That does not confer upon us a freedom to ignore the knowledge that we already have, or to postpone the action that it appears to demand at a given time."[21(p300)] As Weed recently stated: "Professional epidemiologists who profess (i.e. promise) to prevent disease have a *moral obligation* to consider public health recommendations when examining evidence for causality."[29(p1139)]

Sufficient–Component Cause Model

In 1976, Rothman outlined the conceptual model of causation known as the sufficient–component cause model.[19] He viewed the model as a way to bridge the gap between theoretical ideas of causation and the practice of epidemiology. He defined a *sufficient cause* as a "complete causal mechanism" that "inevitably produces disease."[2(p8)] A fundamental feature of this model is that a sufficient cause is not a single factor but rather a minimal set of factors that unavoidably produce disease. For example, a sufficient cause for AIDS may be composed of the following factors: exposure to a person who is infected with HIV, participation in a risky activity with that infected person (such as unprotected anal intercourse, shared injection equipment), susceptibility to HIV, and the absence of antiretroviral drugs (drugs that reduce HIV viral load and may reduce the risk of transmission). Thus, the set of factors may include the presence of causative exposures and the lack of preventive ones.

Each participating factor in a sufficient cause (such as susceptibility to HIV) is termed a *component cause*. In fact, most "causes" of interest to epidemiologists are actually components of sufficient causes. Note that a single component cause or a subset of component causes does not result in disease—the entire constellation is needed. For example, a person cannot get AIDS unless he or she is susceptible, *and* is exposed to HIV, *and* has unprotected intercourse, and so on. Merely being exposed to HIV is insufficient to cause AIDS.

Another important tenet of the sufficient–component cause model is the idea is that a disease can originate from several different sufficient causes. Thus, there may be several different causal constellations for AIDS. For example, one sufficient cause may include exposure to contaminated blood transfusions and another may include practicing unsafe sex with an infected partner. Different sufficient causes may or may not have causal components in common. A causal component that is a member of every sufficient cause is termed a *necessary cause*. For example, exposure to HIV (by whatever route) is a necessary cause of AIDS.

Most component causes are neither necessary nor sufficient causes of a disease. For example, smoking is neither a necessary nor sufficient cause of lung cancer. Not all smokers get lung cancer, and some nonsmokers get lung cancer. Other causal components, such as susceptibility to the carcinogenic effects of cigarette smoke, must be present for an individual to succumb to this disease.

The "causal pies" first presented by Rothman help to illustrate the concepts of sufficient, component, and necessary causes. Figure 15–4 shows a disease with three sufficient causes. In this example, there are three "pathways" for getting the disease. Each sufficient cause, in turn, has five component causes labeled A through J. Component cause A is regarded a necessary cause because it appears as a member of each sufficient cause. In contrast, none of the other component causes (B through J) are considered necessary causes because they do not appear in all three sufficient causes.

The sufficient–component cause model has several important attributes. First, blocking the action of a single causal component stops the completion of the sufficient cause and thereby prevents the disease from occurring by that pathway. This means that it is not necessary to identify all component causes of a particular sufficient cause in order to prevent the disease. For example, an effective HIV vaccine will prevent cases of AIDS, even though many causal components remain unknown.

Second, the completion of a sufficient cause is synonymous with the biological onset of disease. Thus, the disease begins when the last component cause "falls into place." Note that the biological onset of the disease process is not necessarily synonymous with the onset of symptoms or the clinical diagnosis. The latter events may occur long after biological onset. For example, the natural progression from HIV infection to full-blown AIDS often takes more than a decade, during which the virus is invading and destroying CD4 lymphocytes and damaging the immune system.[30]

The third important feature of the sufficient–component cause model is that component causes may act far apart in time. Thus, some causal components may be distant causes and others may be proximate causes. For example, consider the following possible causal components of breast cancer: carrying the BRCA1 gene, having an early age at menarche, giving birth at a late age, and taking hormone replacement therapy during

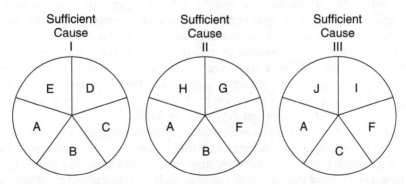

FIGURE 15–4. Conceptual Scheme for the Causes for a Hypothetical Disease

Source: Reprinted from Rothman KJ. Causes. *Am J Epidemiol.* 1976;104:589.

FIGURE 15-5. Temporal Relationship Between Induction and Latent Periods

menopause. The action of these causal components spans nearly a woman's entire lifetime.

The length of time from the action of a causal component until disease initiation is termed the *induction period*.[2(pp14-15)] For example, assume that the component causes in sufficient cause I of Figure 15-4 act in alphabetical order. Thus, the induction period for A is longer than that for B, which is longer than that for C, and so on. The induction time is zero for E, the component cause that acts last. This is because the disease process begins the instant that the last component cause acts.

Diseases themselves should not be characterized as having either a short or long induction period.[2(pp14-15)] For example, some epidemiologists would say that salmonellosis has a short induction period because it occurs within 3 days of ingesting contaminated food. However, even though the induction period for one causal component—eating contaminated food—is only a few days, the induction period for other causal components (such as the presence of low immune function) may be weeks, months, or even years.

The *latent period*, which is defined as the interval from disease onset to detection, follows the induction period.[2(p15)] This period is commonly known as the preclinical phase of a disease. Diseases are detected either when abnormal signs and symptoms appear or when screening tests such as mammograms are administered. The temporal relationship between the induction and latent periods is depicted in Figure 15-5.

Why Most Scientists Believe that HIV is the Cause of AIDS

AIDS is an illness that causes the collapse of the immune system, which—in turn—makes the body vulnerable to numerous deadly infections that the body would otherwise have little difficulty handling. Although the majority of scientists believe that HIV causes AIDS, a small group of scientists, including virologist Peter Duesberg, believe that AIDS is a behavioral rather than an infectious disease. Duesberg and his followers believe that

HIV is a harmless virus and that AIDS is caused by the use of recreational drugs, noninfectious contaminants of factor VIII (the clotting factor used to treat hemophilia), and antiretroviral drugs in the United States and Europe; and by protein malnutrition, poor sanitation, and subsequent parasitic infection in Africa.[6]

As a way of summarizing the concepts of causal inference described earlier in this chapter, let us examine the evidence that mainstream scientists use to counter Duesberg's claims. First, scientists state that HIV has fulfilled the Henle-Koch postulates for causation for infectious microbes.[31] Several papers from the early 1980s provided the evidence to support the first two postulates, particularly the one-to-one correspondence between HIV and AIDS. For example, Gallo and colleagues routinely found HIV in people with AIDS symptoms and failed to find HIV among those who lacked either AIDS symptoms or AIDS-associated risk factors.[32]

Henle and Koch's third postulate, which states that the microorganism must be isolated from a diseased host and must induce a new case of disease when given to a susceptible animal, took longer to fulfill because there are no good animal models for AIDS. Evidence to support this postulate finally emerged in the early 1990s from the accidental infection of three laboratory workers with a pure molecularly cloned strain of HIV.[33] None of the lab workers had any of the typical AIDS behavioral risk factors such as a history of intravenous drug use or homosexual sex, and so these factors could not explain their disease. One worker developed *Pneumocystis carinii* pneumonia, an AIDS-defining disease, 68 months after showing evidence of infection. This individual did not receive any antiretroviral drugs until 83 months after infection and so these drugs, as Duesberg claims, could not have caused his disease. The other two laboratory workers showed severe declines in immune function over time but no AIDS-defining diseases, and one of them eventually received antiretroviral drugs. Duesberg was not convinced by these data because only one worker developed an AIDS-defining disease. However, Anthony Fauci, the head of the National Institute of Allergy and Infectious Diseases (the federal agency that conducts and funds most research on AIDS) stated: "As far as I'm concerned, the laboratory workers prove causation."[33(p1647)]

Several other lines of evidence have also convinced the general scientific community that HIV causes AIDS. This evidence typically fulfills one of Hill's guidelines for causation. Some evidence comes from prospective epidemiologic studies that have followed large numbers of initially healthy individuals. These studies have shown a consistent relationship between HIV antibody levels and the eventual development of AIDS. (HIV antibodies develop only in response to HIV infection.) For example, a Canadian study followed a group of 715 homosexual men for almost 9 years. The investigators found 136 cases of AIDS among men with preexisting HIV antibody and no cases of AIDS among men who were antibody negative.[34] Another prospective study that followed 1027 men from San Francisco for 8 years found 215 cases of AIDS among the men who were antibody positive and no cases of AIDS among the antibody-negative men.[35]

There are two principal reasons why studies such as these provide persuasive causal evidence. First, the associations are very strong (no AIDS cases among HIV-negative men versus hundreds of cases among HIV-positive men). Second, the prospective study designs provide evidence that the HIV infection preceded the development of AIDS. In other words, they provide evidence of a clear temporal relationship between the cause and the effect.

Many epidemiologic studies have also found a dose–response relationship between measures of infection severity such as plasma HIV levels and the risk of AIDS progression and death. For example, Mellors and colleagues found that only 0.9% of men with low baseline HIV levels died of AIDS, while 18.1% of men with moderate HIV levels and 69.5% of men with high HIV levels died during the 10-year follow-up period.[36] Another study among HIV-infected hemophiliacs found that each (log 10) unit increase in baseline viral load was associated with a 2.4-fold increase in AIDS-related illness during the follow-up period.[37]

The absence of a dose–response relationship between factor VIII (the clotting factor used to treat hemophilia) and the risk of dying has been used to counter Duesberg's claim that noninfectious contaminants of factor VIII cause AIDS. For example, a study following 2000 individuals with hemophilia in the United States and Europe found that HIV-infected hemophiliacs who received low, medium, and high cumulative doses of factor VIII had similar death rates during the follow-up period (34.5% for low, 39.0% for medium, and 38.8% for high).[38] Most scientists believe that if exposure to contaminants in factor VIII were the cause of AIDS and subsequent deaths, the death rates would be higher for those who received higher doses of factor VIII.

Many studies have disproved Duesberg's claim that antiretroviral medications cause AIDS. In fact, these studies support the hypothesis that HIV causes AIDS because many of these drugs work by attacking unique aspects of HIV replication. Prospective studies of antiretroviral drugs have been shown to treat AIDS by suppressing HIV levels, causing clinical symptoms to disappear, and improving survival. For example, one study following more than 49,000 participants has found that all antiretroviral therapies improve survival in comparison to no treatment, and that the more intensive treatments produce the greatest improvements in survival rates.[39] The fact that many studies have shown similar results despite using different methodologies, different types of patients, and different investigators has been cited as evidence for their credibility. These data support Hill's guidelines on experiment and consistency.

Other evidence supporting Hill's guideline on coherence rebuts the idea that antiretroviral drugs cause AIDS. First, people died of AIDS before antiretroviral drugs were available, and so these drugs could not have caused these deaths. Second, there has been a sharp decline in AIDS deaths beginning in 1996 when antiretroviral drugs were introduced. In particular, the Centers for Disease Control and Prevention has reported that deaths from AIDS in the United States peaked at 49,992 in 1995, and then fell to 36,930 in 1996, 20,945 in 1997, 16,432 in 1998, and 10,198 in 1999 (the lowest number of deaths since 1986).[40] In addition, the number of new cases of AIDS has declined dramatically since protease inhibitors, a particular type of antiretroviral drug, became the standard of care for treating HIV-infected people.[40] Most scientists believe that these temporal trends are consistent with the idea that antiretroviral drugs control rather than cause AIDS.

Other studies have rebutted Duesberg's claim that the use of illicit drugs causes AIDS. For example, the San Francisco Men's Health Study has followed 812 homosexual/bisexual men and 215 heterosexual men for the development of AIDS.[35] Heavy drug use involving marijuana, cocaine, and amphetamines was equally common among both groups of men, yet the 215 cases of AIDS that occurred during the 8 years of follow-up were restricted to homosexual participants. Thus, there is strong evidence that these drugs did not have a role in the occurrence of AIDS among these men.

However, the use of one of the drugs—amyl nitrites—was restricted to homosexual/bisexual participants, and so the investigators performed additional analyses to determine if use of this drug could have caused the AIDS cases. They found that amyl nitrite use by itself was not associated with AIDS. Cases occurred only among amyl nitrite users who were HIV positive. No cases occurred among either heavy or light amyl nitrite users who were HIV negative.

Additional evidence that AIDS is not caused by recreational drugs comes from the National Household Survey on Drug Abuse. The survey has charted substantial increases in the use of many of the drugs that Duesberg claims causes AIDS including heroin, cocaine, and inhalants.[41] It is counterintuitive for purported causes of AIDS to be increasing while the number of AIDS cases and deaths is declining.

Duesberg's theory has another important shortcoming. Its narrowly defined risk groups do not account for everyone who develops AIDS. For example, this theory does not account for the fact that 40% of reported AIDS cases among women are among those who have no risk factors other than heterosexual contact with an HIV-infected man.[40] Nor does his theory account for the HIV-infected children born to infected mothers who develop AIDS in contrast to their HIV-negative siblings who remain healthy.

How can Duesberg maintain his views in light of all of this evidence? According to one science writer: "Mainstream AIDS researchers argue that

Duesberg's arguments are constructed by selective reading of the scientific literature, dismissing evidence that contradicts his theses, requiring impossibly definitive proof, and dismissing outright studies marked by inconsequential weaknesses."[31] Duesberg's unscientific approach contradicts the tenets of epidemiologic research and causal inference as practiced by most scientists. However, it serves to emphasize the notion that causation is ultimately in the eyes of the beholder.

Summary

A cause may be defined as "an event, condition, or characteristic that preceded the disease event and without which the disease event either would not have occurred at all or would not have occurred until some later time,"[2(p8)] or more simply, as "something that makes a difference."[8(p637)] The three essential attributes of a cause are association, time order, and direction. Causes include host and environmental factors, active agents and static conditions, and positive and negative factors.

Disease causation theories have changed considerably over time from divine retribution for committing sins, to foul clouds called miasmas, to imbalances in body humors. In the 1800s a revolutionary concept called the germ theory was proposed that states that specific transmissible pathogens are responsible for disease. During this period, Jakob Henle and Robert Koch developed a set of postulates of disease causation based on the germ theory. In the 1960s, an important causal paradigm known as the web of causation was developed. This paradigm incorporates the idea of multiple causes of disease and so is useful for noninfectious diseases.

During the 1960s, Hill described a set of nine guidelines to help determine if associations are causal. These guidelines include strength of association, consistency, specificity, temporality, biological gradient, plausibility, coherence, experiment, and analogy. These guidelines have many exceptions and uncertainties, and Hill never meant them to be used as rigid criteria. Both the Henle–Koch postulates and Hill's guidelines have been used by mainstream scientists to support the idea that HIV is the cause of AIDS.

A more recently developed conceptual model of causation that bridges theoretical ideas of causation with the practice of epidemiology is known as the sufficient–component cause model. In this model, a sufficient cause is a "complete causal mechanism" that "inevitably produces disease."[2(p8)] A sufficent cause includes at least one minimal set of factors (called component causes) that unavoidably cause disease. Blocking the action of a single component cause stops the completion of the sufficient cause and prevents the disease from occurring by that mechanism. This means that it is not necessary to identify all component causes of a sufficient cause in order to prevent the disease.

References

1. Kushner H. *When Bad Things Happen to Good People.* New York, NY: Avon Books; 1981.
2. Rothman KJ, Greenland S. *Modern Epidemiology.* 2nd ed. Philadelphia, PA: Lippincott-Raven Publishers; 1998.
3. Flew A. *A Dictionary of Philosophy.* Aylesbury, Great Britain: Laurence Urdang Associates Ltd; 1979.
4. Popper KR. *The Logic of Scientific Discovery.* New York, NY: Basic Books; 1959 (reprint of the 1935 ed).
5. Buck C. Popper's philosophy for epidemiologists. *Int J Epidemiol.* 1975;4: 159–168.
6. Duesberg P. AIDS acquired by drug consumption and other noncontagious risk factors. *Pharmacol Ther.* 1992;55:201–277.
7. Pickett JP, exec ed. *The American Heritage Dictionary of the English Language.* 4th ed. Boston, MA: Houghton Mifflin; 2000.
8. Susser M. What is a cause and how do we know one? A grammar for pragmatic epidemiology. *Am J Epidemiol.* 1991;133:635–648.
9. Herbst AL, Ulfelder H, Poskanzer DC. Adenocarcinoma of the vagina: association of maternal stilbestrol therapy with tumor appearance in young women. *N Engl J Med.* 1971;284:878–881.
10. Collaborative Group on Hormonal Factors in Breast Cancer. Breast cancer and hormone replacement therapy: collaborative reanalysis of data from 51 epidemiologic studies of 52,705 women with breast cancer and 108,411 women without breast cancer. *Lancet.* 1997;350:1047–1059.
11. Windham GC, Hopkins B, Fenster L, Swan SH. Prenatal active or passive tobacco smoke exposure and the risk of preterm delivery or low birth weight. *Epidemiology.* 2000;11:427–433.
12. Russo J, Russo IH. Toward a physiological approach to breast cancer prevention. *Cancer Epidemiol Biomarkers Prev.* 1994;3:353–364.
13. *Dorland's Illustrated Medical Dictionary.* Philadelphia, PA: WB Saunders; 1994.
14. Brock TD, Brock KM. *Basic Microbiology with Applications.* 2nd ed. Englewood Cliffs, NJ: Prentice-Hall Inc; 1978.
15. Carter KC. Koch's postulates in relation to the work of Jacob Henle and Edwin Klebs. *Med Hist.* 1985;29:353–374.
16. Evans AS. Causation and disease: a chronological journey. The Thomas Parran lecture. *Am J Epidemiol.* 1978;108:249–258.
17. Centers for Disease Control and Prevention. *Preventing Lead Poisoning in Young Children: A Statement by the Centers for Disease Control.* Atlanta, GA: Public Health Service; 1991.
18. Krieger N. Epidemiology and the web of causation: has anyone seen the spider? *Soc Sci Med.* 1994;39:887–903.
19. Rothman KJ. Causes. *Am J Epidemiol.* 1976;104:587–592.
20. Greenland S, ed. *Evolution of Epidemiologic Ideas: Annotated Readings on Concepts and Methods.* Chestnut Hill, MA: Epidemiology Resources Inc; 1987.
21. Hill AB. The environment and disease: association or causation? *Proc Royal Soc Med.* 1965;48:295–300.

22. US Department of Health and Human Services. Office of Smoking and Health. *The Health Consequences of Smoking. Cancer. A Report of the Surgeon General.* Washington, DC: US Department of Health and Human Services; 1982.

23. MacMahon B. Pre-natal x-ray exposure and childhood cancer. *J Natl Cancer Inst.* 1962;28:1173–1191.

24. US Department of Health and Human Services. *Cancer Rates and Risks.* 4th ed. Washington, DC: US Department of Health and Human Services; 1996

25. Waller K, Swan SH, DeLorenze G, Hopkins B. Trihalomethanes in drinking water and spontaneous abortion. *Epidemiology.* 1998;9:134–140.

26. Byrd RC. Positive therapeutic effects of intercessory prayer in coronary care unit population. *South Med J.* 1988;81:826–829.

27. Poole C. Induction does not exist in epidemiology, either. In: Rothman KJ, ed. *Causal Inference.* Chestnut Hill, MA: Epidemiology Resources Inc; 1988.

28. Weed DL, Gorelic LS. The practice of causal inference in cancer epidemiology. *Cancer Epidemiol Biomarkers Prev.* 1996;5:303–311.

29. Weed DL. On the use of causal criteria. *Int J Epidemiol.* 1997;26:1137–1141.

30. Coffin JM. HIV viral dynamics. *AIDS.* 1996;10(suppl 3):S75–S84.

31. Cohen J. The Duesberg phenomenon. *Science.* 1994;266:1642–1649.

32. Gallo RC, Salahuddin SZ, Popovic M, et al. Frequent detection and isolation of cytopathic retroviruses (HTLV-III) from patients with AIDS and at risk for AIDS. *Science.* 1984;224:500–503.

33. Cohen J. Fulfilling Koch's postulates. *Science.* 1994;266:1647.

34. Schechter MT, Craib KJP, Gelmon KA, et al. HIV-1 and the aetiology of AIDS. *Lancet.* 1993;341:658–659.

35. Ascher MS, Sheppard HW, Winkelstein W Jr, Vittinghoff E. Does drug use cause AIDS? *Nature.* 1993;362:103–104.

36. Mellors JW, Munoz A, Giorgi JV, Margolick JB, Tassoni CJ, Gupta P, et al. Plasma viral load and CD4+ lymphocytes as prognostic markers of HIV-1 infection. *Ann Intern Med.* 1997;126:983–985.

37. Engels EA, Rosenberg PS, O'Brien TR, Goedert JJ. Plasma HIV viral load in patients with hemophilia and late- stage HIV disease: a measure of current immune suppression. Multicenter Hemophilia Cohort Study. *Ann Intern Med.* 1999;131:256–264.

38. Goedert JJ, Kessler CM, Aledort LM, Biggar RJ, Andes WA, White GC II, et al. A prospective study of human immunodeficiency virus type 1 infection and the development of AIDS in subjects with hemophilia. *N Engl J Med.* 1989;321: 1141–1148.

39. McNaughten AD, et al. Effects of antiretroviral therapy and opportunistic illness primary chemoprophylaxis on survival after AIDS. *AIDS.* 1999;13: 1687–1695.

40. Centers for Disease Control and Prevention. *HIV/AIDS Surveillance Report. Year-End 1999 Edition* 1999;11(no 2).

41. Substance Abuse and Mental Health Services Administration. *2001 National Household Survey on Drug Abuse.* Available at: hppt://www.samhsa.gov. Accessed February 2003.

EXERCISES

1. What is the definition of each of the following terms?
   A. Cause of disease
   B. Sufficient cause
   C. Necessary cause

2. Describe the temporal relationship between the induction period and latent period.

3. Indicate whether the following statements are true or false.
   A. Hill's guideline of temporality is more easily established in a prospective than a retrospective study.
   B. Strong associations are more likely to be causal than weak ones because they are less likely to be due to alternative explanations.
   C. A causal relationship between an exposure and a disease cannot be established unless all of Hill's guidelines are met.
   D. Hill's guideline of specificity means that an exposure can cause only one disease.
   E. Exposure to HIV is a necessary cause of AIDS.
   F. Exposure to HIV is a sufficient cause of AIDS.

4. Suppose that an article was published on the relationship between caffeine consumption during pregnancy and the risk of low birthweight. Caffeine is in a wide variety of beverages, foods, and drugs, including coffee, tea, and colas. Suppose that the following statements were taken from the introduction and results section of this article.
   A. Caffeine has a similar molecular structure to that of other chemicals that are known to affect human cell division and growth.
   B. Caffeine exposure during pregnancy could have a harmful effect because caffeine may interfere with cell division, metabolism, and growth.
   C. Several animal studies have shown an association between caffeine and lower fetal weight.
   D. Seven previously published epidemiologic studies of caffeine intake during pregnancy have shown an increased risk of low birthweight offspring among women who consumed high levels of caffeine.
   E. In the current study, the risk of low birthweight increased as caffeine consumption increased. Compared to women who did not consume any caffeine during pregnancy, women who had low caffeine consumption had a 40% increased risk of giving birth to a low

birthweight infant, women who had moderate caffeine consumption had a 90% increased risk, and women who had high caffeine consumption had a 150% increased risk. State which of Hill's guidelines is supported by each of the statements above. For example, statement A supports Hill's guideline on analogy.

16

Screening in Public Health Practice

LEARNING OBJECTIVES

By the end of this chapter, the reader will be able to:

- Describe the general features of the natural history of disease.
- Distinguish between primary, secondary, and tertiary prevention.
- List the key characteristics of diseases appropriate for screening.
- Describe the important features of a screening test.
- Define and calculate sensitivity, specificity, predictive value positive, and predictive value negative.
- Discuss the outcome measures and study designs for evaluating the effectiveness of a screening program.
- Define lead-time bias, length-bias sampling, and volunteer bias.

Introduction

Screening is defined as follows: "The presumptive identification of an unrecognized disease or defect by the application of tests, examinations or other procedures which can be applied rapidly. Screening tests sort out apparently well persons who probably have a disease from those who probably do not. . . . Persons with positive or suspicious findings must be referred to their physicians for diagnosis and treatment."[1(pp152–153)] A diagnostic test typically carries more risk and is more expensive than a screening test. People who are found to have the disease are then treated. Screening is used mainly to identify asymptomatic individuals at an earlier stage than if they waited for symptoms to arise. An important assumption is that earlier diagnosis will lead to earlier, more effective treatment

FIGURE 16–1. The Screening Process

that, in turn, will decrease the adverse effects of a disease and improve survival. The screening process is described in Figure 16–1.

Screening programs are currently popular in medicine and public health and will continue to grow as new technologies are developed to identify biological markers of early disease. In fact, policy makers have often responded too quickly to emerging public health problems by prematurely instituting screening programs. For example, mandatory screening for the human immunodeficiency virus (HIV) was instituted among blood donors, immigrants, and premarital couples in order to stop the spread of HIV before effective treatments were available and evaluation programs were in place.[2]

Many new students of public health and even seasoned policy makers think that it is appropriate to screen for most diseases. However, screening is a complex activity with both beneficial and detrimental effects. Consequently, it is important for all public health practitioners to have a thorough understanding of screening principles. These concepts, which are described in this chapter, include the natural history of a disease; primary, secondary, and tertiary prevention; the hallmarks of a disease that make it appropriate for screening; the performance characteristics of screening tests and programs; and the methods and biases involved in evaluating the effectiveness of screening programs.

Natural History of Disease

The natural history of a disease is defined as the course of a disease from its inception to its resolution.[1(p110)] It begins with the pathological onset of disease (point A, Figure 16–2), such as the transformation of a normal breast epithelial cell into a cancerous one or the infection of CD4 lymphocytes with HIV. It continues with the preclinical stage, which lasts from the pathological onset to the first appearance of signs and symptoms (point A to point B). Thus, the person is unaware that he has a disease during the preclinical stage. The clinical stage lasts from the first appearance of symptoms to the end of the disease (point B to point E). Although the person usually seeks medical attention when symptoms develop, the actual time of diagnosis is a function of the availability of medical care and the individual's

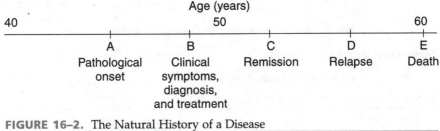

FIGURE 16–2. The Natural History of a Disease

level of awareness. Once the diagnosis is made, treatment usually begins. Depending on the disease, the clinical stage may progress to death (point E), include remissions and relapses (Points C and D, respectively), or regress either spontaneously or from successful treatment and cure (not shown in Figure 16–2). There is substantial variation in the length of each phase. Some individuals progress rapidly, and others progress slowly.

Definition of Primary, Secondary, and Tertiary Prevention

The central goal of public health is to protect and promote health—in other words, to prevent disease, disability, and premature death. Prevention activities are customarily divided into three levels: primary, secondary, and tertiary. The main distinction between the levels is the stage at which they are implemented.

Primary Prevention

Primary prevention is defined as the maintenance of health through individual or community efforts so that the disease process never starts. Thus, primary prevention activities occur before pathological onset (point A in Figure 16–3) and reduce the incidence of disease. Examples of primary prevention activities include a healthy diet; regular exercise; avoidance of smoking; sunscreen use; immunizations against infectious diseases; policies to maintain a clean supply of water, air, and food; and safe home and work environments. Public and medical education campaigns at the individual and community levels and governmental legislation are among the many ways the general public becomes aware of and adopts behaviors and policies to prevent disease.

Although most primary prevention efforts target the general population, some focus on special subgroups within the population. For example, only women with a family history or other breast cancer risk factors are being targeted to take the drug tamoxifen to prevent the occurrence of

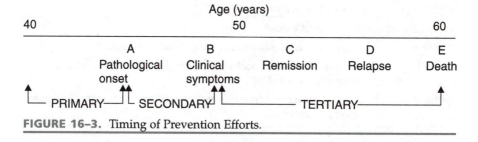

FIGURE 16-3. Timing of Prevention Efforts.

breast cancer,[3] and only groups at high risk of HIV infection have been targeted for intervention programs that reduce risky behaviors such as needle sharing and unsafe sex.

All primary prevention activities assume that the action taken will reduce the occurrence of disease and its after effects. For example, behavioral interventions for men who have sex with men assume that reducing the frequency of unsafe sex will, in turn, reduce the incidence of HIV infection and subsequent acquired immune deficiency syndrome (AIDS) diagnosis and death.[4]

Secondary Prevention

Secondary prevention is defined as delaying the onset of the symptomatic or clinical phase of disease. Secondary prevention efforts do not prevent disease occurrence, but instead they identify asymptomatic individuals during the window between the pathological onset and the occurrence of clinical symptoms (between points A and B in Figure 16-3). Secondary prevention activities assume that early detection will lead to prompt and effective interventions that will ultimately improve survival. For many diseases, secondary prevention reduces disease prevalence by delaying the onset of clinical disease (point B) and by decreasing disease duration (points B to E). For example, screening for HIV infection, combined with the early use of highly active antiretroviral therapies, may substantially delay the onset of clinical symptoms, immune dysfunction, and mortality associated with AIDS.[5]

For some diseases, secondary prevention may increase the disease incidence and prevalence (at least temporarily), because asymptomatic cases are identified at an earlier stage. For example, a portion of the increased incidence of breast cancer from the 1970s through the mid-1990s has been attributed to widespread use of mammography screening in the U.S. population. This phenomenon is described in greater detail at the end of this chapter.

Secondary prevention of infectious diseases may have the added benefit of reducing or halting the spread of disease. For example, early screening,

TABLE 16–1 Levels of Prevention

Prevention level	Impact on disease
Primary	Prevents disease from occurring. Goal is to reduce incidence.
Secondary	Delays onset and duration of clinical disease. Goal is to improve survival.
Tertiary	Slows disease progression; reduces disease sequelae. Goal is to improve survival.

accompanied by counseling and drug therapies, may reduce the spread of HIV by reducing risky behaviors and virus levels in semen.

Tertiary Prevention

The goal of tertiary prevention is to slow or block the progression of a disease, thereby reducing impairments and disabilities, and improving the quality of life and survival among diseased individuals. It is implemented after a clinical diagnosis has been made (any time after point B in Figure 16–3) and may include prompt treatment, proper follow-up and rehabilitation, and patient education. A typical example of tertiary prevention is the use of drugs to prevent opportunistic infections among HIV-infected individuals. Fewer life-threatening infections and fewer difficult-to-follow treatment regimens and hospitalizations substantially improve the quality of life and survival among HIV-infected people. Another example of tertiary prevention is careful control of insulin levels and patient education to prevent retinopathy and other circulatory complications among patients with diabetes. The three levels of prevention and their impact on disease are summarized in Table 16–1.

Appropriate Diseases for Screening

A disease must have certain characteristics in order to be appropriate for screening (see Table 16–2). First, the disease must be serious and have important consequences. Given the high cost and possible adverse consequences of screening, it is only justifiable to screen for major diseases, such as cancer of the cervix, breast, colon-rectum, prostate, and skin; noncancerous diseases such as diabetes, hypertension, and glaucoma; and infectious diseases such as HIV infection and tuberculosis.

Second, the disease must be progressive, and early treatment must be more effective than later treatment. This is because screening is carried out in the belief that the natural history of the disease can be altered by earlier treatment. Thus, breast cancer is a suitable disease for screening because its treatment is more effective (at least among women aged 50 to 69 years)

TABLE 16–2   Characteristics of Diseases Appropriate for Screening

■ Disease is serious with severe consequences.
■ Treatment is more effective at an earlier stage.
■ Disease has a detectable preclinical phase (DPCP).
■ DPCP is fairly long and prevalent in the target population.

when the cancer is discovered at an earlier stage by mammography than at a later stage by physical exam.[6] On the other hand, lung cancer is a serious disease that is not suitable for screening because mortality is high even with early treatment.

Third, an appropriate disease must have a preclinical phase (from point A to B in Figure 16–1) that can be identified by a screening test. This phase is known as the detectable preclinical phase or DPCP. The DPCP is a function of both the natural history of the disease and the technical capabilities of the screening test. When a disease process begins, abnormalities occur in the body, such as the division and shedding of abnormal cells, abnormal bleeding, or the production of compounds such as antigens and antibodies. A screening test is designed to identify these initial biological abnormalities so the affected individual comes to medical attention earlier. For example, breast cancer starts with the transformation of a single normal breast cell into a cancerous one. Over the next decade or so, the cancer cell and its progeny divide enough times to form a tumor large enough to be detectable by currently available screening methods. Presently, the smallest tumor detectable by screening mammography is one half centimeter in diameter; the smallest tumor detectable by physical examination alone is 1 centimeter.[7(p210)]

Finally, an appropriate disease must have a DPCP that is fairly prevalent and has a long duration in the screened population. The prevalence of the DPCP in a population depends on three factors: the incidence of the disease, the average length of the preclinical phase, and any prior screening activities. Higher incidence and longer preclinical phases lead to a higher DPCP prevalence. Any prior screening activities will reduce the prevalence during the DPCP, particularly if the screening was recently conducted.

If the prevalence of the DPCP is high enough in the general population, mass screening—that is, screening of the entire population—is both feasible and cost-effective. If the prevalence is not sufficiently high in the general population, screening efforts are targeted to high-risk groups such as individuals over a certain age or with a family history of the disease. Screening at frequent intervals is recommended in very high-risk populations.

It is not efficient or cost-effective to screen for diseases with a low DPCP prevalence, because thousands of people would need to be screened to detect only a few cases. For the same reason, it is inefficient to screen for acute infectious diseases with a short DPCP (lasting hours to weeks).

HIV infection is an example of an appropriate disease that meets all the criteria for targeted screening. It is a severe disease with very dire consequences: The case-fatality rate among all reported adult AIDS cases during the period 1981 to 1999 was 58.7.%[8] It has a long and a highly prevalent DPCP in certain populations, such as intravenous drug users. In fact, the seroprevalence of HIV among intravenous drug users without clinical symptoms can be as high as 39%.[9] Finally, there are many treatments that are effective at reducing the disease sequelae of HIV/AIDS when given at an early stage.

Figure 16–4 illustrates the natural history of a typical HIV infection. Transmission occurs when viruses from one person's infected cells enter another person and infect some of that person's cells. In most cases, the primary HIV infection is asymptomatic. However, for some, nonspecific symptoms of the acute HIV syndrome occur within a few days or weeks. (These symptoms are often attributed to a severe cold or influenza.) During the first few weeks after infection, HIV can only be detected using a sophisticated and expensive test called polymerase chain reaction or PCR test. This test is not used for screening because it is costly and difficult to perform.

By 6 weeks, most immune systems produce HIV antibodies in response to the infection, which is now detectable by the HIV antibody screening test.[10] This simple, inexpensive test is the predominant screening test for HIV infection around the world. Once antibody production is

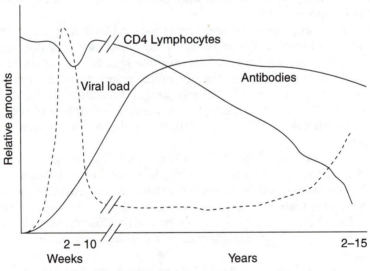

FIGURE 16–4. Natural History of HIV Infection

detectable by the screening test, the person has entered the DPCP. This phase is often quite long—its median length is 10 years. Even though the person has no symptoms during the DPCP, the virus is invading and destroying CD4 lymphocytes and damaging the immune system. When CD4 lymphocyte levels fall to 200 per cubic millimeter, the person meets the official case definition of AIDS. By this time, the individual's immune system is unable to respond to pathogens, and severe symptoms and life-threatening infections and malignancies may occur. The first occurrence of any symptoms marks the end of the preclinical phase.

The time course and clinical manifestations of HIV infection vary widely. Some individuals progress rapidly, and others move slowly. Some have a life-threatening illness as the first manifestation of AIDS, and others experience subtle cognitive deficits. Thus, the first time a population is screened for HIV, the individuals identified are at varying stages of pre-clinical illness. The effectiveness of screening varies from one population to another, because effectiveness depends on the relative proportions of individuals identified at the early, middle, and late stages of the preclinical phase. The AIDS diagnosis is delayed and survival is better when treatment is started when CD4 lymphocyte counts drop below 350 per cubic millimeter.[5]

The only way to treat HIV infection as early as possible is to screen as early as possible. But who should get screened for HIV? Currently, mass screening for HIV is not recommended. Rather, epidemiologists advise targeted screening of high-risk populations. These groups include men who have sex with men (particularly those who have unprotected anal intercourse), men and women with a history of injecting drug use, women who have ever had an infected partner, and women who have had a sexually transmitted disease or more than five sexual partners in the last year. Recommendations aside, the decision to get screened is also a function of the person's awareness of the risk factors for infection, perceptions about the severity of this health threat and the effectiveness of screening, and access to health care.

Substantial decreases in AIDS incidence and mortality have been noted over the last few years.[5] In the United States, it is believed that these changes have resulted from the availability of confidential HIV counseling and testing (primary and secondary prevention), an increased awareness of high-risk behaviors among individuals and health care professionals (primary prevention), and knowledge about the effectiveness of highly active antiretroviral therapy (secondary prevention). The effectiveness of this therapy in the secondary prevention of AIDS diagnoses and death has been clearly established. The precise role of screening and early treatment in primary prevention of HIV transmission and incidence has been more difficult to ascertain.

Characteristics of a Screening Test

In order for screening to be successful, the screening test must be economical, convenient, relatively free of risk and discomfort, acceptable to a large number of individuals, and highly valid and reliable. Currently screening tests that meet these criteria include serology tests for markers for HIV, hepatitis B, and tuberculosis; mammograms for the detection of breast cancer; PAP smears for cervical cancer; blood pressure monitoring and cholesterol screening for heart disease; stool guaiac tests for colorectal cancer; and vision tests for glaucoma. The following section describes in more detail the characteristics of a suitable screening test.

Validity

The purpose of a screening test is to identify correctly individuals who do and do not have preclinical disease. Those who have preclinical disease should test positive, and those who do not have it should test negative. The ability of a screening test to successfully separate these two groups is a measure of its validity, which is expressed by its sensitivity and specificity. These two measures are described in more detail later in this chapter.

Reliability

The reliability of a test is its ability to give the same result on repeated testing. Reliability is influenced by the stability of the physiologic state being measured (for example, blood pressure varies by time of day and recent activities), the technical characteristics of the test method (such as the instrument being used), and interobserver and intraobserver agreement among the technicians conducting the test. Interobserver agreement refers to reliability between different technicians, and intraobserver agreement refers to reliability for the same technician over time. Although a valid test is always reliable, a reliable test is not always valid. A reliable test can incorrectly classify individuals as diseased or disease free with great consistency.

Source of Test Errors

All screening tests currently in use are affected by measurement errors. Mismeasurement may occur through sloppiness such as mislabeling specimens, poor training of screening technicians, or poor equipment. Whatever the source, the outcome of mismeasurement is usually an incorrect test result. Although errors can often be corrected by performing a second test, a false-positive result and subsequent retesting can cause great distress for the patient. In addition, when a more invasive procedure is needed to follow-up a false-positive result, there may be morbidity from the procedure. For example, maternal serum alpha-fetoprotein is a prenatal blood test that is used to screen for birth defects known as neural tube defects (such as spina bifida). A positive result may be followed up with an amniocentesis that carries a small but real risk of miscarriage. In addition, false-negative results are harmful because the undetected disease continues to progress.

Criterion of Positivity

Even when test errors are minimized, the decision to term certain test results "positive" and others "negative" is somewhat arbitrary. The criterion of positivity is a point on a continuum that extends from clearly normal results (for healthy people) to clearly abnormal results (for people who have preclinical disease) (see Figure 16–5). Questionable results that may occur for some people with and without preclinical illness fall into a gray zone in the middle of the continuum. For example, the criterion of positivity may be the presence of dysplastic cells on a PAP smear test for cervical cancer, the presence of calcifications on a mammogram for breast cancer, or a diastolic blood pressure reading of 90mm Hg for hypertension. A particular criterion of positivity is selected in order to maximize the validity of the screening test. If the criterion is set high (point B, Figure 16–5), then only very abnormal results will be considered positive and slight abnormalities will be missed. Thus, there will be more false-negative results. If the criterion is set low (point A), then any slight abnormality will be considered positive and there will be more false-positive results.

Figure 16–6 illustrates the use of the criterion of positivity for the enzyme immunoassay (EIA)—the standard test for detecting antibodies to HIV antigen—in a population with HIV infection and a population without HIV infection. The EIA is performed by incubating a person's serum with recombinant HIV antigens. If HIV antibodies are present in the serum, they will bind to the antigen-covered walls and turn yellow. The degree of the yellow color is measured by a laboratory instrument called a spectrophotometer. The amount of color in a sample is compared to the colors in the control samples.

Note from Figure 16–6 that there is overlap between the two populations in the way they react to the EIA. Although most uninfected people

Clearly Negative	Gray Zone	Clearly Positive
– – – – – – – – – – – – – – ??????????????????????????????+++++++++++++++++++++++++		
A	B	
LOW	HIGH	

FIGURE 16–5. Criterion of Positivity

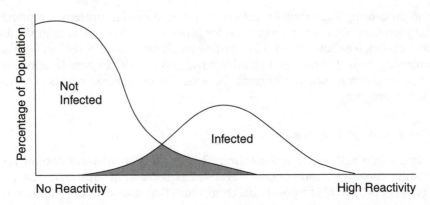

FIGURE 16–6. Schematic Representation of HIV EIA result in Two Populations

have no reactivity, some uninfected individuals have a low degree of reactivity. Likewise, although most infected people have a high degree of reactivity, some infected individuals have a low degree of reactivity. (The area of overlap in Figure 16–6 is analogous to the gray area in Figure 16–5.) The criterion of positivity for this screening test is generally set at a low level (see point A in Figure 16–5) because of the severe consequences of a false-negative result. The EIA was first used to screen donated blood. Any donated blood that tested positive was discarded, and the individual who donated this blood was retested with a second EIA and another test called a Western blot that does a better job weeding out false-positive results. The individual was notified only if both follow-up tests were also positive.

Sensitivity and Specificity

Sensitivity and specificity are measures of the validity of a screening test—that is, its ability to determine the "truth" about the presence or absence of preclinical disease. Sensitivity is the probability that a test correctly classifies as positive individuals who have preclinical disease. Sensitivity is expressed as a percentage; the number of individuals with preclinical disease who test positive is in the numerator, and the total number of individuals with preclinical disease is in the denominator.

$$\frac{\text{Number of individuals with preclinical disease who test positive}}{\text{Number of individuals with preclinical disease}} \times 100$$

Specificity is the probability that a test correctly classifies individuals without preclinical disease as negative. Specificity is also expressed as a percentage, the number of individuals without preclinical disease who test

TABLE 16–3   Calculating Sensitivity, Specificity, and Predictive Value Using a Two-by-Two Table

Screening test result	Disease present		
	Yes	*No*	*Total*
Positive	a	b	$a + b$
Negative	c	d	$c + d$
Total	$a + c$	$b + d$	$a + b + c + d$

negative is in the numerator, and the total number of individuals without preclinical disease is in the denominator.

$$\frac{\text{Number of individuals without preclinical disease who test negative}}{\text{Number of individuals without preclinical disease}} \times 100$$

Table 16–3 presents the results of a screening test in a population in the form of a two-by-two table. The sensitivity is equal to $a/(a + c)$ and the specificity is equal to $d/(b + d)$.

Denominator data for determining the sensitivity $(a + c)$ and specificity $(b + d)$ are usually determined in one of two ways. First, a gold-standard diagnostic procedure (that is, a very accurate and commonly used procedure) can be used to make a definitive diagnosis and to determine the total number of individuals with and without the disease. Second, when the gold-standard procedure is too invasive or expensive, the population is followed for a period of time to determine who develops the disease. For example, the sensitivity and specificity of physical examination and mammography for the detection of breast cancer were determined by following a group of study participants for about 10 years.[11(pp74–80)] Any woman who developed clinical symptoms of breast cancer within a year of a negative screening test was considered a false negative.

Lead Time

Lead time is the amount of time that the disease diagnosis is advanced by screening. In other words, it is the length of time from disease detection by screening to the time that the diagnosis would have been made on the basis of symptoms.[12] For example, suppose that a person's disease is detected by screening at age 50, and that this person would have been diagnosed at age 60 when symptoms developed (see Figure 16–7). The lead time for this individual is 10 years. Note that lead time varies from one person to another, depending on the stage of preclinical disease at screening and the duration of preclinical disease in the individual.[11(pp11–12)] The

FIGURE 16-7. Lead Time in a Hypothetical Individual

lead time will be longer if detection by screening occurs in the early part of the preclinical phase and shorter if detection occurs close to the onset of symptoms.

Because we can never know when the disease would have been diagnosed as a result of symptoms, it is impossible to determine the actual lead time in a screened individual. However, it is possible to estimate the distribution of lead times in a screening program by comparing the rate of clinical disease over time in the screened group and comparable unscreened group.[11(p12)]

Predictive Value: A Measure of Screening Program Feasibility

A screening program is defined as "a set of procedures for early detection and treatment of a disease that is available to a population." It includes both diagnostic and therapeutic components, and includes the screening test and the follow-up evaluations for people with positive test results.[11(pp5–6)] The therapeutic component consists of treatment of confirmed cases of disease. Thus, a screening program is much more than just a screening test. Furthermore, the feasibility and success of a screening program depend a great deal on the population in which it is applied.

The predictive value is the main way to measure a screening program's feasibility. Predictive value has two components: predictive value positive (PVP) and predictive value negative (PVN). The PVP is the proportion of individuals with a positive test who have preclinical disease. It is calculated as a percentage; the number of individuals with preclinical disease who test positive is in the numerator, and the total number of individuals who test positive is in the denominator.

$$\frac{\text{Number of individuals who test positive and have preclinical disease}}{\text{Number of individuals who test positive}} \times 100$$

The PVN is defined as the proportion of individuals without preclinical disease who test negative. It is calculated as a percentage; the number of individuals without the disease who test negative is in the numerator, and the total number of individuals who test negative is in the denominator.

$$\frac{\text{Number of individuals who test negative and do not have preclinical disease}}{\text{Number of individuals who test negative}} \times 100$$

Note from the two-by-two table presented in Table 16–3 that the PVP equals $a/(a + b)$ and the PVN equals $d/(c + d)$. The key components of PVP are the number of true positive cases detected (a) and the number of false positives (b), and the key components of PVN are the number of true negatives (d) and the number of false negatives (c).

A high PVP is essential for a successful screening program. It implies that the screening program is effective because the program detects a large proportion of actual cases among individuals with positive re-sults. A low PVP implies that resources are being wasted on diagnostic follow-ups of false-positive results. A low PVP can have additional consequences if a positive screening test is followed by a potentially harmful diagnostic evaluation, as was described earlier for the maternal serum alpha-fetoprotein test.

PVP is influenced by the sensitivity and specificity of the screening test and by the prevalence of the DPCP in the screened population. PVP is influenced more by specificity than sensitivity because the specificity determines the number of false-positive results.

The following paragraphs describe two hypothetical HIV screening programs in order to illustrate the validity and feasibility measures described. Suppose that an EIA screening test for HIV infection is being evaluated by a private company who hopes to market the test for use in the population. The company tries out the test on 1000 HIV-infected control samples. Of these, 980 react sufficiently to be declared positive, establishing the sensitivity at 98% ($a/(a + c) = 980/1000$). The company uses the same EIA to test 1000 samples from individuals known to be uninfected. Of these samples, 998 are nonreactive (true negatives) and 2 are reactive (false positives). Thus, the specificity of the test is established at 99.8% ($d/(b + d) = 998/1000$). The test is licensed for commercial and research use on the basis of this information.

Two public health officials decide to institute an HIV-screening program using the EIA described above, with the intention of identifying HIV-infected individuals in the DPCP and initiating highly active antiretroviral therapy. They plan to follow up all positive EIA results with the Western blot, which separates truly positive screening test results from false-positive ones. One public health official decides to screen a low-risk population and the other decides to screen a high-risk population. They both decide to use the same laboratory to analyze the screening test so that the results of the two programs can be compared.

The public health official interested in screening a low-risk population sets up a program in the general population of Massachusetts, where the estimated prevalence of clinical HIV infection is 2 per 1000 (or 0.2%). He screens 40,000 randomly selected Massachusetts residents. The results of his efforts are described in Table 16–4.

Among the 80 individuals in the DPCP (80/40,000 = 0.2% prevalence), 78 are identified as positive and 2 are missed. This result reflects that the sensitivity of the EIA is 98% (78/80 = 97.5%). The two who are missed show clinical symptoms of HIV infection a few months after testing and so are considered false negatives. Among the 39,920 disease-free individuals, 39,840 test negative and 80 test positive. This result reflects that the specificity of the EIA is 99.8% (39,840/39,920 = 99.8%). Of the 39,842 individuals who test negative, 39,840 are truly not infected, and so the PVN is 99.99% (39,840/39,842 = 99.99%). Of the 158 individuals who test positive, 78 have HIV infection as confirmed by the Western blot test, and so the PVP is 49.4% (78/158 = 49.4%). Thus, the net result of screening this low-risk population is that 78 HIV-infected individuals in the DPCP are identified. On the other hand, 80 individuals have a false-positive EIA upon follow-up with a Western blot test.

The second public health official is concerned about the low PVP associated with screening a low-risk population, so she sets up her screening program in a high-risk community in Massachusetts. High-risk individuals are identified using behavioral criteria such as injecting drug use and having sex with an HIV-infected partner. The estimated prevalence of HIV infection in this high-risk population in Massachusetts is 250 per 1000 or 25%. She proceeds to screen 40,000 randomly selected high-risk individuals using the EIA followed by a Western blot. The results of her efforts are described Table 16–5.

Among the 10,000 individuals in DPCP (10,000/40,000 = 25% prevalence), 9800 are identified as positive and 200 are missed, given that the sensitivity of the EIA is 98% (9800/10,000 = 98%). The 200 who are missed show clinical symptoms of HIV infection a few months after testing and so are considered false negatives. Among the 30,000 disease-free individuals, 29,940 test negative and 60 test positive, given that the specificity of the test

TABLE 16–4   Results of a Hypothetical HIV Screening Program in a "Low-Prevalence" Population

| EIA | HIV infection | | |
	Yes	No	Total
Positive	78	80	158
Negative	2	39,840	39,842
Total	80	39,920	40,000

TABLE 16–5   Results of a Hypothetical HIV Screening Program in a "High-Prevalence" Population

EIA	HIV infection		
	Yes	*No*	*Total*
Positive	9,800	60	9,860
Negative	200	29,940	30,140
Total	10,000	30,000	40,000

is 99.8% (29,940/30,000 = 99.8%). Of the 30,140 individuals who test negative, 29,940 are truly not infected, and so the PVN is 99.3% (29,940/30,140 = 99.3%). Of the 9860 individuals who test positive, 9800 have HIV infection, and so the PVP is 99.4% (9860/9800 = 99.4%). Thus, the net result of screening this high-risk population is that 9800 HIV-infected individuals in the DPCP are identified. Note that there is a much higher yield from screening the high-risk population, even with identical tests. In addition, a high-risk individual with a positive test result is much more likely to be infected than a low-risk individual with a positive test result.

Evaluating a Screening Program

Formal evaluation of a screening program may be unnecessary in certain circumstances, such as when the intervention is simple and highly effective.[11(pp12–13)] For example, it is not necessary to evaluate screening for eye and hearing problems among children, and failure to screen would be considered unethical.

Formal evaluations are not conducted when policy makers believe, often without objective evidence, that early detection and treatment are beneficial and prematurely institute mandatory screening programs. For example, compulsory HIV screening was instituted among blood donors, immigrants, and premarital couples before effective treatments were available and evaluation programs were in place.[2] These programs quickly became the standard of care, and now there is great resistance to conducting formal evaluations.

When public health officials conduct a formal evaluation of screening programs, they look at several features of the program including the potential for bias and outcome measures.

Bias

Lead-Time Bias

The customary way to evaluate the success of a screening program is to compare the survival experience of a screened population to that of a similar unscreened population. Survival is assessed either as the percentage of patients alive as of a certain time after diagnosis (for example, the percentage surviving 5 years after diagnosis) or by the average number of years that a patient lives after diagnosis. Note that survival is measured from the time of diagnosis to the time of death, and that the diagnosis time is—by definition—different for screened individuals (shortly after screening) and unscreened individuals (at the onset of symptoms) (see Figure 16–7). Thus, survival may appear longer among screened individuals simply because their diagnoses were made earlier, not because they actually lived longer. This phenomenon, which is known as lead-time bias, overestimates the benefit of screening and needs to be taken into account when evaluating a screening program.

Figure 16–8 illustrates lead-time bias using three hypothetical men with prostate cancer. The first man was an unscreened case of prostate cancer.

Case 1

Age (years)

40	50	65	80
A	B	C	D
Biologic onset	Becomes detectable (but not screened)	Symptoms (diagnosis made)	Death

Case 2

Age (years)

40	50	65	80
A	B	C	D
Biologic onset	Becomes detectable (found at screen)	Symptoms (if not screened)	Death

Case 3

Age (years)

40	50		78	83
A	B		C	D
Biologic onset	Becomes detectable (found at screen)		Symptoms	Death

FIGURE 16–8. The Natural History of Three Men with Prostate Cancer: An Illustration of Lead-time Bias

Biological onset of disease began at age 40 years (A), but the man underwent no screening during the detectable preclinical phase (B to C). He was diagnosed with cancer only when symptoms occurred at age 65 (C), and although he was treated he died from prostate cancer at age 80 (D). There was no lead time in his case because there was no screening. This man's survival time was 15 years—from diagnosis at age 65 to death at age 80.

The second man was a screen-detected case who was diagnosed at age 50 years (B). He would have been diagnosed at age 65 (C) if he had waited for symptoms to occur, and so his lead time was 15 years (B to C). He died at age 80 (D), and so his survival time was 30 years (B to D). Screening appears to be effective because survival was longer for case 2 than case 1 (30 versus 15 years). However, early treatment was not effective in postponing his mortality. Both men died at exactly the same age. The apparent survival benefit for case 2 results from lead-time bias.

The third man was also a screen-detected case. He was diagnosed by screening at age 50 years (B), and early treatment delayed the onset of symptoms to age 78 (C) and death to age 83 (D). His survival time is 33 years from age 50 to age 83. Case 3 lived 3 years longer than the first two men, and so he illustrates the benefit of screening—the postponement of morbidity and mortality.

Length-Bias Sampling

Length-bias sampling is another bias that should be considered when evaluating a screening program. This bias occurs because screening tends to identify cases with less aggressive forms of the disease.[11(p14)] Screening tends to detect cases with a long preclinical course, which—in turn—should have a long clinical course and better survival.

Figure 16–9 illustrates length-bias sampling using two hypothetical men with prostate cancer. The first man experiences biological onset of disease at age 40 years. He is identified by screening at age 50 years when his DPCP begins. He undergoes treatment, but symptoms develop at age 60. Death from prostate cancer occurs at age 70, because the treatment is ineffective. Thus, his DPCP is 10 years, and his survival time is 20 years. This man is considered a slow progressor because his entire disease course lasts 30 years (A to D), and his DPCP (B to C) and clinical phase (C to D) last 10 years each.

Case 2 has a very different natural history because his disease course is quite rapid. Like case 1, his biological onset is at age 40 years. However, his DPCP starts at age 45, his symptoms appear and he is diagnosed at age 50 (C), and death occurs at age 55 (D). The entire disease course lasts 15 years—half of that of case 1.

Which type of case is a typical screening program more likely to identify? The answer is case 1, simply because his DPCP is twice as long as that

Case 1

Age (years)

40	50	60	70
A	B	C	D
Biologic onset	Becomes detectable, diagnosed by screening	Symptoms	Death

Case 2

Age (years)

40	45	50	55
A	B	C	D
Biologic onset	Becomes detectable, but not screened	Symptoms (diagnosed)	Death

FIGURE 16-9. The Natural History of Two Men with Prostate Cancer: Illustration of Length Bias Sampling

of case 2. Thus, length-bias sampling makes a screening program appear to have a beneficial effect on survival because people who are destined to have a favorable course are selectively identified.

Volunteer Bias

The third type of bias to consider when evaluating a screening program is called volunteer bias. This type of bias occurs only in observational studies of screening efficacy. It means that the decision to be screened is influenced by a person's health awareness, which—in turn—may be related to his or her subsequent morbidity and mortality.[11(p17)] One could argue either that healthy people are more likely to volunteer for screening than sick people, or that sick people are more likely to be screened than healthy people. (The former would overestimate the benefit of the screening program, and the latter would underestimate it.) In either case, the results are confounded by patient characteristics that are difficult to assess and control.

Selecting an Outcome

Epidemiologists use several outcome measures to evaluate the success of a screening program, including: (1) process measures, (2) survival, (3) shift in stage distribution, (4) overall mortality, and (5) cause-specific mortality. Process measures include the number of people who have been screened and the number of cases of disease that have been detected by screening. These measures are simple to obtain, but they do not gauge screening effectiveness—that is, they do not indicate if the screening program has decreased the adverse effects of disease and improved survival.

A more direct way of assessing screening effectiveness is to compare the survival of screen-detected cases with that of unscreened cases. Survival is commonly assessed in terms of the percentage of individuals alive as of a certain time after diagnosis. Screen-detected cases may appear to survive longer than unscreened cases as a result of lead-time bias, length-biased sampling, or volunteer bias. Thus, using survival as an outcome measure may give a false impression of the benefit of screening.

An alternative assessment measure is the comparison of disease stage distribution among individuals identified by screening versus those identified by other methods. If screening is effective, the stage distribution should shift toward earlier cases of disease. For example, one study found that from 63 to 71% of screen-detected cases of prostate cancer had clinically or pathologically localized disease, and 43% of unscreened cases did so.[13] Nevertheless, it is difficult to determine if such shifts result from a real screening benefit or from confounding caused by volunteer bias or length-bias sampling.

Another way to assess the effectiveness of screening is to compare the overall mortality rate among screened and unscreened populations. If the overall mortality rate is lower in the screened population, then one may conclude that the combination of screening and early treatment has been effective in postponing death. Although the total mortality rate is not influenced by lead-time bias or length-biased sampling, it may be an insensitive end point if the disease of interest only accounts for a small proportion of deaths. For example, even though prostate cancer is the most common cancer among U.S. men, it only accounts for about 2% of deaths among males.[14] Thus, disease-specific mortality rate is considered the best outcome measure for evaluating a screening program. However, even disease-specific mortality is not appropriate for outcomes that do not lead to death. For example, the occurrence of blindness is the best outcome for assessing the effectiveness of glaucoma screening. It does not make sense to use glaucoma mortality to measure the effectiveness of screening, because blindness does not usually cause death.

Study Designs to Evaluate Screening Programs

The effectiveness of a screening program can be evaluated using the analytic study designs described in Chapters 6 through 9. These designs are briefly recounted here in the context of screening. Recall that the designs fall into two major categories, experimental and observational. The experimental approach for evaluating screening programs consists mainly of randomized, controlled clinical trials. Observational studies include cohort, case–control, and ecologic studies.

Experimental Studies

In an experimental study, the investigator randomly assigns individuals to be screened or not screened, and then follows the two groups for the outcomes of interest (such as mortality, survival, and morbidity). Experimental studies can only be performed when there is a state of equipoise regarding screening effectiveness within the medical community. There must be genuine confidence that screening is worthwhile in order to administer it to some individuals, and genuine reservations in order to withhold it from others.

The main advantage of experimental studies is that, if the study size is sufficiently large, both known and unknown confounders will be balanced between compared groups. A second advantage is the elimination of confounding from volunteer bias. Thus, an experimental evaluation will provide the most rigorous data on the effectiveness of screening. In addition, it can give estimates of lead time and evaluate the impact of length-bias sampling.

Although experimental designs have strong methodologic appeal, they also have some important drawbacks. First, several thousand participants are typically needed to demonstrate a relatively modest level of efficacy. Second, follow-up may take many years, and much time and effort must be expended to keep losses to a minimum. These issues make experimental evaluations of screening programs very expensive and reduce their feasibility and relevance, particularly when advances in screening technology and treatment are occurring rapidly. Swift advances in medical knowledge also reduce the acceptability of participating in long-term, randomized trials among physicians and patients, and may raise ethical concerns for the unscreened patients. Consequentially, epidemiologists usually employ observational designs to evaluate screening programs.

Cohort Studies

In cohort studies, participants decide themselves whether to be screened. Participants are followed to ascertain the outcomes of interest. Thus, they are more susceptible to confounding than experimental studies. If the confounder is known, the investigator can measure and adjust for its effect in the design or analysis. But if the confounder is unknown, adjustment is not possible. Cohort studies also suffer from one of the same problems as experimental studies—namely, a large number of subjects must be followed for a long period of time.

On the other hand, because participants choose to be screened, the ethical dilemmas present in experimental studies are avoided. Also, although experimental studies must always be prospective, cohort studies can be either prospective or retrospective. Retrospective cohort studies of screening efficacy, which are more efficient than prospective ones, are quite feasible if detailed data on screening and confounding characteristics are documented in existing data sources such as medical records.

Case–Control Studies

In a case–control study, the investigator selects cases who are individuals either with a recent diagnosis or who have died from the disease targeted by screening. Controls are selected from the population that gave rise to the cases. For example, if cases include newly diagnosed patients, controls are selected from the same geographic area or hospital from which the cases were identified. The investigator obtains information on screening status (for example, if participants were ever screened or date of last screening) and potential confounders either by interview or medical record review. The usual challenges associated with obtaining accurate exposure information and controlling for confounding apply. The main advantage of the case–control approach is efficiency; nevertheless, the study must be carefully designed to minimize observation and selection bias.

Ecologic Studies

An ecologic or correlational study can be used to evaluate the impact of a screening program. This type of study describes the relationship between screening frequency and an outcome measure among many populations at the same time or the same population at different times. Ecologic studies are efficient because they are based solely on easy-to-obtain group-level data about the screening program (such as the proportion of the population screened) and group-level outcome data (such as disease-specific mortality rates in screened and unscreened areas).

The limitations of ecologic studies include the lack of individual-level data and the resulting difficulty making inferences from the group to the individual. In addition, data on confounding variables are usually missing. Ecologic studies are most informative when a new screening program is introduced into an isolated well-defined population.[11(pp97–100)] For example, in 1964 a cervical cancer screening program targeting women aged 25 to 59 years was initiated in Iceland.[15,16] By 1977, more than 85% of the population had been screened. The cervical cancer mortality rate among women in the targeted age group rose until 1970, but then dropped by 60%. No change in cervical cancer mortality rate was observed in older women who were not specifically targeted for screening. These data strongly suggest that the introduction of the screening program in Iceland had a beneficial impact on cervical cancer mortality rates.

Examples of the Effect of Screening on Public Health

The Effect of Screening on Disease Incidence: The Case of Prostate Cancer

Prostate cancer is the most common cancer among men, accounting for about 31% of newly diagnosed cancers in 1998.[17] This form of cancer has received a great deal of attention, as many famous men have publicly acknowledged that they have been affected.[18(pp58–65)] Currently known risk factors include African-American race, increased age, family history of prostate cancer, a diet high in animal fat, and high testosterone levels. Most prostate cancer cases appear to progress slowly—that is, they have a long preclinical and clinical phase. In fact, prostate cancer is commonly diagnosed at autopsy among elderly men who never had any symptoms and died of other causes.[19]

Currently available screening methods include the prostate-specific antigen blood test and digital rectal examination.[20] The American Cancer Society recommends that both tests be offered annually, beginning at age 50 years for the general population, and at age 45 years for men in high-risk groups. Prostate cancer trends in the United States provide a real-life example of changes in incidence that occur following the widespread use of a screening program.

Note from Figure 16–10 that prostate cancer incidence increased slowly until the late 1980s, when incidence rose sharply.[21] An abrupt decline in incidence began in 1992 for whites and 1993 for African Americans. These changes are likely due, in part, to the effects of screening. When a screening test becomes widely used in a population, the incidence rate of the target disease increases at first and then declines as a result of the earlier diagnosis of cases. Further evidence of the impact of prostate cancer screening on disease incidence is that, by the late 1980s, a higher proportion of those diagnosed were at early stages and younger ages.[21]

The Effect of Screening on Mortality: The Case of Breast Cancer

Since the 1960s, investigators have conducted numerous randomized, controlled clinical trials of the effectiveness of breast cancer screening, including mammography and breast self-examination.[6,22] These studies have been conducted in Europe, Canada, and the United States, and have collectively enrolled and followed nearly 500,000 women for up to 18 years.

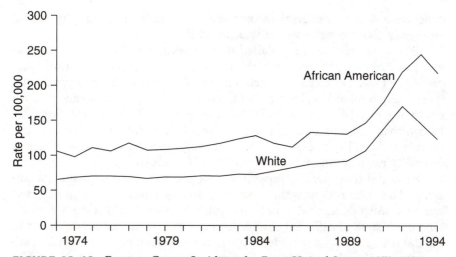

FIGURE 16-10. Prostate Cancer Incidence by Race, United States, 1973–1994

Source: Adapted from American Cancer Society. *Cancer Facts and Figures—1998,* p 22. Atlanta, GA: American Cancer Society; 1998.

In these trials, a group of women offered screening was compared to a group of women not offered screening. (The latter group received "usual care.") Women were assigned to each group using a variety of randomization methods. In some studies, population-based lists of women were compiled and individual women were randomly assigned to the study and control groups. In other studies, clusters of women (for example, all women registered in a certain medical practice) were randomly assigned to the groups.

Through the 1990s, the studies indicated that the use of screening mammography (either alone or in combination with a clinical examination) reduced the risk of dying by about 30% among women 50 to 69 years of age after 10 to 12 years of follow up.[6] Even though the risk of a false positive result in this age group was 47.3% after 10 years of mammograms, there was a widespread consensus that all women in this age group should be screened.[23]

During this period, the balance of risks and benefits appeared to be less clear for women aged 40 to 49 years. In randomized trials of mammographic screening, there was no meaningful decrease in mortality after 5 to 7 years of follow up, and only a marginal benefit after 12 to 14 years of follow up.[6] Furthermore, the risk of a false positive result in this age group was 56.2% after 10 years of screening.[23] False positive mammography results are not trivial since they lead to more outpatient appointments, mammograms, biopsies, and great emotional stress. As a result, the 1997 National Institutes of Health Consensus Development Conference concluded that a universal recommendation for mammography for all women in their forties was not warranted.[24]

Two new analyses have called these recommendations into question and have reopened the debate about the value of screening mammography. Olsen and Gotzsche conducted a meta-analysis which concluded that there was no reliable evidence that mass screening for breast cancer had a survival benefit for any women, including those 50 years and older.[25,26] In contrast, another meta-analysis by the U.S. Preventive Services Task Force's (USPSTF) concluded that mammography reduced breast cancer mortality rates among women from 40 to 74 years of age.[22]

How did these two groups of investigators reached opposite conclusions? The main reason is that two meta-analyses were based on different sets of studies. Note that a meta-analysis uses statistical methods to combine the results of different studies in order to identify an overall trend in the data. The analysis includes a qualitative component in which investigators identify all available studies and determine which ones should be excluded on the basis of poor quality. Olsen and Gotszche excluded 6 of the 8 identified trials because they considered them of poor quality or flawed, and the USPSTF investigators excluded only one trial that they rated poor quality.[22,25,26]

In response to considerable debate and confusion about the benefits of mammography, the National Cancer Institute (NCI) recently issued a statement which affirmed the value of mammography for detecting breast cancer for women aged 40 and older.[27] However, the NCI acknowledged that more data were needed to resolve the uncertainties around screening, and declared that monitoring and evaluating new data from ongoing studies would be one if its highest priorities.

Summary

Screening is defined as "the presumptive identification of unrecognized disease or defect by the application of tests, examinations or other procedures which can be rapidly applied."[1(pp152–153)] It is used mainly to identify asymptomatic individuals at an earlier stage than if they waited for symptoms to develop, under the assumption that earlier diagnosis will lead to more effective treatment and improve the consequences of disease. Lead time is defined as the amount of time that the disease is advanced by screening. It spans the length of time from disease detection by screening to the time that the diagnosis would have been made on the basis of symptoms. The actual lead time in a screened individual cannot be determined because we can never know when the disease would have been diagnosed as a result of symptoms. However, lead-time distributions can be estimated in certain settings. Screening is part of prevention activities that may deter the initial occurrence of disease (primary prevention), delay the onset and duration of clinical disease (secondary prevention), slow disease progression, and reduce disease sequelae (tertiary prevention).

In order to be suitable for screening, a disease must be serious with important consequences, and it must be progressive with an effective early-stage treatment. In addition, suitable diseases must have a detectable preclinical stage that is fairly long and prevalent in the targeted population. Examples of appropriate diseases include breast and prostate cancer, HIV infection, hypertension, and glaucoma.

The characteristics of a successful screening test, examination, or procedure include low cost, minimal risk, convenience, acceptability, and reliability. The test must also have a high degree of validity, as measured by sensitivity and specificity. Sensitivity is the probability that a test correctly classifies individuals with preclinical disease as positive; specificity is the probability that a test correctly classifies individuals without preclinical disease as negative. These two measures are influenced, in part, by the criterion of positivity—the point at which a test result is deemed positive.

A screening program is defined as "a set of procedures for early detection and treatment of a disease that is available to a population" and includes both diagnostic and therapeutic components.[11(pp5–6)] The predictive value is the principal way to assess a screening program's feasibility. Predictive value positive is the proportion of individuals with a positive test who have preclinical disease; predictive value negative is the proportion of individuals with a negative test who do not have preclinical disease. A high predictive value positive, which is crucial to the success of a screening program, is attained by increasing the sensitivity and specificity of the screening test, and by targeting a population whose detectable preclinical phase is fairly prevalent.

Outcome measures that can be used to evaluate the success of a screening program include process measures such as the number of people screened, the stage distribution of screened versus unscreened cases, and overall mortality and cause-specific mortality among screened and unscreened cases. Cause-specific mortality is the best outcome measure for diseases that are generally fatal. Analytic designs that are used to evaluate the effectiveness of screening programs include experimental, case–control, cohort, and ecologic studies.

When evaluating a screening program, one must consider three sources of bias: lead-time bias, length-biased sampling, and volunteer bias. Lead-time bias can overestimate the benefit of screening when survival is used to evaluate a screening program. It occurs because survival is measured from the time of diagnosis until death, and diagnoses occur earlier with screening even when death is not delayed. Length-biased sampling can exaggerate the benefit of a screening program because screening tends to detect less aggressive forms of disease that have a long preclinical phase. Volunteer bias occurs when observational studies are used to evaluate a screening program and stems from confounding between screened and unscreened populations.

References

1. Last JM. *A Dictionary of Epidemiology*. 3rd ed. New York, NY: Oxford University Press; 1995.
2. Cleary PD, Barry MJ, Mayer KH, et al. Compulsory premarital screening for the human immunodeficiency virus. *JAMA*. 1987;258:1757–1761.
3. Fisher B, Constantino JP, Wickerham DL, Redmond CK, Kavanah M, Cronin WM et al, and other National Surgical Adjuvant Breast and Bowel Project Investigators. Tamoxifen for prevention of breast cancer: report of the National Surgical Adjuvant Breast and Bowel Project P-1 Study. *J Natl Cancer Inst*. 1998; 90:1371–1387.
4. National Institute of Mental Health (NIMH) Multisite Prevention Trial Group. The NIMH Multisite HIV Prevention Trial: reducing HIV sexual risk behavior. *Science*. 1998;280:1889–1894.
5. Yeni PG, Hammer SM, Carpenter CCJ, Cooper DA, Fischl M, Gatell JM et al, Antiretroviral treatment for adult HIV infection in 2002. Updated recommendations of the International AIDS Society-USA Panel. *JAMA*. 2002;288:222–235.
6. Fletcher SW, Black W, Harris R, Rimer BK, Shapiro S. Report of the International Workshop on Screening for Breast Cancer. *J Natl Cancer Inst*. 1993; 85:1644–1656.
7. Love SM, Lindsay K. *Dr. Susan Love's Breast Book*. Reading, MA: Addison-Wesley Publishing Co, Inc; 1990.
8. Centers for Disease Control and Prevention. *HIV/AIDS Surveillance Report*. 1999;11(no2):1–44.
9. Freedberg KA, Samet JH. Think HIV: why physicians should lower the threshold for HIV testing. *Arch Intern Med*. 1999;159:1994–2000.
10. Horsburgh CR, Ou C-Y, Jason J, Holmberg SD, Longini IM, Schable C, et al. Defining the interval between human immunodeficiency virus infection and detection of antibody to the virus. *Lancet*. 1989;2:637–640.
11. Morrison AS. *Screening in Chronic Disease*. 2nd ed. New York, NY: Oxford University Press; 1992.
12. Hutchison GB, Shapiro S. Lead time gained by diagnostic screening for breast cancer. *J Natl Cancer Inst*. 1968;41:665–681.
13. Catalona WJ, Smith DS, Ratliff TL, Basler JW. Detection of organ-confined prostate cancer is increased through prostate-specific antigen-based screening. *JAMA*. 1993;270:948–954.
14. Kramarow E, Lentzer H, Rooks R, Weeks J, Saydah S. *Health and Aging Chartbook. Health, United States, 1999*. Hyattsville, MD: National Center for Health Statistics; 1999.
15. Johannesson G, Geirsson G, Day N. The effect of mass screening in Iceland, 1965–1974, on the incidence and mortality of cervical cancer. *Int J Cancer*. 1978; 21:418–425.

16. Johannesson G, Geirsson G, Day N, Tulinius H. Screening for cancer of the uterine cervix in Iceland 1965–1978. *Acta Obstet Gynecol Scand.* 1982;61: 199–203.

17. Ries LAG, Eisner MP, Kosary CL, Hankey BF, Miller BA, Clegg L, Edwards BK, eds. *SEER Cancer Statistics Review, 1973–1998.* Bethesda, MD: National Cancer Institute; 2001.

18. Jaroff L. The man's cancer. *Time.* April 1, 1996.

19. Gittes RF. Carcinoma of the prostate. *N Engl J Med.* 1991;324:236–245.

20. American Cancer Society. *Cancer Facts and Figures—2001.* Atlanta, GA: American Cancer Society; 2001.

21. American Cancer Society. *Cancer Facts and Figures—1998.* Atlanta, GA: American Cancer Society; 1998.

22. Humphrey LL, Helfand M, Chan BK, Woolf SH. Breast cancer screening: a summary of the evidence for the U.S. Preventive Services Task Force. *Ann Intern Med.* 2002; 3:347–360.

23. Elmore JG, Barton MB, Moceri VM, Polk S, Arena PJ, Fletcher SW. Ten-year risk of false positive screening mammograms and clinical breast examinations. *N Engl J Med.* 1998;338:1089–1096.

24. National Institutes of Health Consensus Development Panel. National Institutes of Health Consensus Development Conference Statement: breast cancer screening for women ages 40–49 years, January 21–23, 1997. *J Natl Cancer Inst.* 1997;89:1015–1020.

25. Gotzsche PC, Olsen O. Is screening for breast cancer with mammography justifiable? *Lancet.* 2000;355:129–134.

26. Olsen O, Gotzsche PC. Screening for breast cancer with mammography. *Lancet.* 2001;358:1340–1342.

27. National Cancer Institute. *NCI Statement on Mammography Screening.* Available at: http://www.cancer.gov. Accessed: March, 2003.

EXERCISES

1. Define each of the following terms:
   A. Sensitivity
   B. Specificity
   C. Predictive value of a positive test
   D. Lead time

2. State the main differences between primary, secondary, and tertiary prevention.

3. What types of diseases are appropriate for screening?

4. Suppose that 100,000 men were screened for prostate cancer for the first time. Of these, 4000 men had a positive result on the screening blood test; of those who tested positive, 800 had a biopsy indicating a

diagnosis of prostate cancer. Among the remaining 96,000 men who screened negative, 100 developed prostate cancer within the following year and were assumed to be false negatives to the screen.

A. Set up the two-by-two table for these data.

B. What is the prevalence of prostate cancer in this population?

C. Calculate and interpret the sensitivity of this screening test.

D. Calculate and interpret the specificity of this screening test.

E. Calculate and interpret the predictive value positive of this screening test.

F. There is a widespread assumption that screening a population to detect the early stages of disease is always beneficial. However, there are risks and costs that must be weighed against the benefits of screening. Briefly describe two hidden costs of screening for prostate cancer in this example.

5. Consider the following events in one woman's life. Note that some events are hypothetical and some are real.

Event	Age (years)
Birth	0
Cervical cancer begins	30
Cervical cancer is detectable by screening	40
Woman is screened, cancer is detected, treatment begins	45
If no screening, symptoms would have developed and cancer would have been detected	60
If no screening, death would have occurred	70
Death occurs	80

A. Compute the total preclinical phase of this woman's cervical cancer. Assume that she did not get screened.

B. Compute the detectable preclinical phase of this woman's cervical cancer. Assume that she did not get screened.

C. Compute the lead time for this patient.

D. Did screening increase the life span of this patient? Justify your answer.

6. Describe the three types of bias that must be considered when evaluating the results of a screening program.

Answers to Exercises
Chapters 1–16

Chapter 1, The Approach and Evolution of Epidemiology

1. A. Public health is a multidisciplinary field whose goal is to promote the health of populations through organized community efforts.
    B. Epidemiology is the study of the distribution and determinants of disease frequency in human populations and the application of this study to control health problems. Disease refers to a broad array of health-related states and events including diseases, injuries, disabilities, and death.
    C. A population is a group of people with a common characteristic.

2. Public health focuses on preventing diseases in communities, and medicine focuses on treating diseases at the individual level.

3. The main objectives of epidemiology are to study the natural course of disease, to determine the extent of disease in a population, to identify patterns and trends in disease occurrence, to identify the causes of disease, and to evaluate the effectiveness of measures that prevent and treat disease.

4. Epidemiologists quantify the frequency of disease by developing a definition of the disease, instituting a mechanism for counting cases of disease within a population, and determining the size of that population. It is only when the number of cases are related to the size of the population that we know the true frequency of disease.

5. A. John Graunt summarized the patterns of mortality in 17th-century London and discovered the regularity of deaths and births.

   B. John Snow conducted one of the first observational studies in the neighborhoods of 19th-century London and discovered that contaminated drinking water was the cause of cholera.

   C. Richard Doll and Austin Bradford Hill conducted groundbreaking studies on cigarette smoking and lung cancer in the 1950s.

Chapter 2, Measures of Disease Frequency

1. A. Cumulative incidence.
   B. Prevalence.
   C. Incidence rate.
   D. Prevalence.
   E. Cumulative incidence.

2. A. Prevalence quantifies existing cases; incidence quantifies new cases.
   B. The main similarity is that they both quantify the number of new cases of disease that develop in a population at risk during a specified period of time. The main difference is that the incidence rate is a true rate that directly integrates person-time of observation into the denominator, and cumulative incidence is a proportion whose denominator is the population at risk at the start of the observation period. Time in cumulative incidence is expressed only by words that go along with the proportion.
   C. A dynamic population is defined by a changeable state or condition, so its membership is transitory; a fixed population is defined by a life event, and so its membership is permanent.

3. No. It is also necessary to know the size of the population and the amount of follow-up time in each state.

4. A. 5/100.
   B. 0/100.
   C. $3/(100 - 5) = 3/95$. Remember that only the population at risk at the beginning of October is eligible for the denominator.

5. When the population is in steady state, $P = IR \times D$, where P is prevalence, IR is incidence rate, and D is average duration. Thus, $P = 500/100{,}000$ person-years x 3 years or $1500/100{,}000$.

6. $(20 \times 5 \text{ years}) + (10 \times 1 \text{ year}) + (70 \times 10 \text{ years}) = 100 + 10 + 700 = 810$ person-years.

7. A. City A = 25/25,000 over 1 year or 50/50,000 over 1 year.
    City B =30/50,000 over 1 year.
    B. City A has the higher cumulative incidence.

8. The following calculation assumes that everyone is followed for the entire 2 years and that all cases occurred at the end of the second year: 60/(100,000 persons x 2 years) = 60/200,000 person-years or 30/100,000 person-years. Different assumptions can be made regarding the length of follow-up for cases and noncases and the time of case occurrence.

9. A. Dynamic. This is a changeable condition; people are continually entering and leaving the city.
    B. Fixed. This is a permanent characteristic; once a man has the surgery, he is forever part of this group.
    C. Fixed. This is also a permanent characteristic; same rationale as above.
    D. Dynamic. This is a changeable characteristic. New graduates are entering practice, others are leaving by retirement, etc.

10. A1. 4/1000.
    A2. 6/996. Remember the population size has decreased by 4 because of death.
    A3. 4/994. Again the population is smaller.
    B. 6/996. Only those who do not have the disease of interest are "at risk."
    C. 6/1000. Everyone in the population is at risk of dying.

Chapter 3, Comparing Disease Frequencies

1. A. They are both ways to compare measures of disease frequency in order to assess the impact of an exposure on a disease. The ratio measure gives information on the strength of the relationship between an exposure and disease; the difference measure describes the excess number of cases of disease that are associated with the exposure.
    B. Both provide information on the absolute effect of the exposure or the excess risk of disease. However, the risk difference gives the number of cases of disease among the exposed that may be attributable to the exposure, and the population risk difference gives the number of cases of disease in the total population that may be attributable to the exposure.

2. A. 30/100,000 person-years /45/100,000 person-years = 0.67.

    B. Women who engage in regular physical activity have 0.67 times the risk of ovarian cancer (or a 33% reduced risk of ovarian cancer) compared to women who do not engage in regular physical activity.

    C. 30/100,000 person-years – 45/100,000 person-years = –15/100,000 person-years. Note that the incidence rate difference is negative.

    D. The excess rate of ovarian cancer among women who do not engage in regular physical activity is 15/100,000 person-years. Or, if regular physical activity prevents ovarian cancer, then 15 cases per 100,000 person-years of follow-up would be eliminated if the women engaged in regular physical activity.

    E. Null value for the incidence rate ratio is 1.0, and the null value for the incidence rate difference is 0.0.

3. An age-specific rate is a rate that applies only to a particular age group. For example, the incidence rate of AIDS among 15- to 24-year-olds is an age-specific rate. In contrast, an age-adjusted rate is a summary rate that accounts for the age differences between two populations. The numeric value of the age-adjusted rate depends on the particular weights used for the adjustment.

4. A. Crude heart disease death rate in developing country = (0.30 x 2/100,000 person-years) + (0.40 x 20/100,000 person-years) + (0.30 x 40/100,000 person-years) = 20.6/100,000 person-years. Crude heart disease death rate in developed country = (0.20 x 2/100,000 person-years) + (0.30 x 20/100,000 person-years) + (0.50 x 40/100,000 person-years) = 26.4/100,000 person-years.

    B. The age-adjusted rate is better because the age structures of the two populations are different.

5. A. Cumulative incidence (CI) among the delegates = $a/(a + b)$ = 125/1849 = 0.068 (in 41 days). CI among the nondelegates = $c/(c + d)$ = 3/762 = 0.004 (in 41 days).

    B. Cumulative incidence ratio = CI $_{delegates}$ / CI $_{nondelegates}$ = 0.068/0.004 = 17.0.

    C. The risk of Legionnaires' disease was 17 times greater among delegates than among nondelegates. Or, a delegate had 17 times the risk of contracting Legionnaires' disease as did a nondelegate.

    D. Cumulative incidence difference = CI $_{delegates}$ – CI $_{nondelegates}$ = 0.068 – 0.004 = 0.064 (in 41 days).

    E. If delegate status is a "cause" of Legionnaires' disease, then 64 cases per 1000 delegates would be eliminated if the delegates had been nondelegates. Note that delegate status is not the actual cause of Legionnaire's disease but reflects which part of the hotel that the individual entered during the convention. Further investigation found that the organism that causes Legionnaires' disease was present in certain air conditioners.

F. Attributable proportion = [(CI $_{delegates}$ − CI $_{nondelegates}$)/CI $_{nondelegates}$] × 100% = [(0.068 − 0.004) / 0.068] × 100% = 94%.

G. This means that 94% of the cases of Legionnaires' disease among the delegates can be attributed to their delegate status.

Chapter 5, Descriptive Epidemiology

1. A. i. There was more than a fourfold increase in the prevalence of ectopic pregnancy from 1970 through 1992.

   ii. During the period 1970 through 1989, black women aged 15 to 44 years had about 1.4 times the prevalence of ectopic pregnancy as did white women of the same age.

   iii. Among all races during the period 1970 to 1989, there was about a threefold increase in the prevalence of ectopic pregnancy among women from ages 15–24 to ages 35–44 years.

   B. If one considers prevalence in 1970 as the normal expectancy, these data suggest that there was an epidemic of ectopic pregnancy in the following years.

   C. There are many possible hypotheses. For example, the prevalence of ectopic pregnancy increased over time because risk factors for the disease (such as pelvic inflammatory disease) also increased over time.

   D. There are many possible answers. For example, these data could be used to support increased screening activities for ectopic pregnancy among black women who come to hospital emergency rooms with suggestive symptoms.

Chapter 6, Overview of Epidemiologic Study Designs

1. A. In an observational study, the investigator "watches" as subjects themselves choose which group they will be in (exposed or unexposed); in an experimental study, the investigator assigns participants to their exposure groups.

   B. Both the exposures and outcomes have already occurred at the start of a retrospective cohort study; the outcomes have not yet developed at the start of a prospective cohort study. Thus, a retrospective cohort study investigates prior outcomes and a prospective cohort study investigates future ones.

    C. A cohort study defines subjects according to their exposure level and follows them for disease occurrence; a case–control study defines cases of disease and controls and compares their exposure histories.

2. A cross-sectional study examines the relationship between diseases and other variables at one particular time. Subjects are commonly selected without regard to exposure or disease status. Its main limitation is that one cannot infer the temporal sequence between the exposure and disease.

3. An ecologic study examines the rates of disease in relation to a population-level factor. Thus, the units of analysis are populations rather than individuals. The lack of information about individuals leads to a limitation known as the "ecological fallacy," which means that the association observed on an aggregate level does not necessarily represent the association that exists on the individual level.

4. A. Case–control.
   B. Retrospective cohort.
   C. Case–control.
   D. Case–control.
   E. Prospective cohort.
   F. Case–control.

5. A. Ecologic.
   B. Cross-sectional.
   C. Case–control.
   D. Experimental.
   E. Retrospective cohort.

Chapter 7, Experimental Studies

1. A. A process by which the investigator assigns subjects to the treatment and comparison groups. Subjects have an equal chance of being assigned to either the treatment or comparison group.
   B. The group of people to whom the study results may be applied or generalized.
   C. The study subject does not know whether he or she is in the treatment or comparison group.
   D. The run-in period occurs before enrollment and randomization to determine which participants are able to comply with the study regimen. Potential participants are placed on the test or control treatment for a certain period of time to assess their tolerance to

and acceptance of the treatment and to obtain information on compliance.

E. A placebo is an inactive substance, such as a sugar-coated pill, that is given as a substitute for an active substance. A sham is a bogus procedure that is designed to resemble a legitimate one. Both placebos and sham procedures permit the study participants and caregivers to be masked.

F. Equipoise is a state of mind characterized by genuine uncertainty about the appropriate course of action—that is, to give or withhold a particular treatment. It is ethical to conduct an experimental study only when there is a state of equipoise in the expert community.

2. A. In individual trials, the treatment is allocated to particular people; in community trials, the treatment is allocated to entire communities.

B. Preventive trials investigate measures that stop or delay the onset of disease; therapeutic trials investigate measures that treat existing disease.

3. A. There are several possible answers. For example, design a simple protocol, enroll motivated and knowledgeable participants, exclude subjects who might have difficulty complying, present a realistic picture of the required tasks at enrollment, maintain frequent contact with study subjects, and use items such as pill packs to make it easier to comply with the treatment regimen.

B. Randomize a large number of study subjects.

C. Mask investigators to group assignment.

4. An intent-to-treat analysis includes all individuals who were randomly allocated to the treatment and comparison groups, regardless of whether they completed or even received their assigned regimen. This type of analysis preserves the baseline comparability and gives information on the effectiveness of the treatment under real-life conditions.

5. Unique features include random assignment of subjects to the treatment and comparison groups to control for confounding and to reduce biased allocation, and the use of placebo controls to permit masked assessment of the outcomes.

6. They are expensive to conduct, physicians and patients may be reluctant to participate, and a state of equipoise must exist.

Chapter 8, Cohort Studies

1. A. An open or dynamic cohort is conducted in a population defined by a changeable characteristic such as residence in a specific place.

Thus, its members come and go, depending on whether they have the characteristic.

B. A fixed cohort is defined by an irrevocable event, so it does not gain any new members.

C. A retrospective cohort study looks back in time and examines exposures and outcomes that have already occurred by the time the investigator begins the study.

D. A prospective cohort study looks forward in time and examines future outcomes in relation to past or current exposures.

E. A standardized mortality ratio (SMR) study is a special type of cohort study in which the mortality experience of an exposed group is compared to that of the general population. It is commonly conducted in occupational settings.

2. The main similarity is that both compare two or more exposure groups, which are followed to monitor outcome rates. The main difference is that the investigators allocate the exposure in experimental studies, and the participants choose their exposures in cohort studies.

3. Of the three types of comparison groups, the internal comparison group comes closest to the counterfactual ideal because it comes from the same source population as the exposed group and so is most comparable. However, internal comparison groups are often difficult to identify. The general population is the next best option mainly because it is stable and easy to obtain. Its limitations can include lack of comparability to the exposed group and lack of information on confounders. The comparison cohort is the least preferable option. Although it may be comparable to the exposed group, results from such a study are difficult to interpret because the comparison cohort often has other, possibly noxious exposures.

4. A. Yes.
   B. No.
   C. No.
   D. Yes.

5. Loss to follow-up decreases the number of individuals who can be included in the analysis and so reduces the statistical power of the study. Also, if those who are lost have different rates of disease than those who remain, the study results may be biased.

6. Person-time is accrued for each individual in a cohort study. It begins when the follow-up period of the study begins. It ends when one of the following occurs: the individual develops the outcome under study, dies, is lost, or the follow-up period for the study ends.

Chapter 9, Case–Control Studies

1. A. TROHOC is the word *cohort* spelled backwards. Some epidemiologists have used TROHOC as a disparaging term for case–control studies because they believe that case–control studies are inferior to cohort studies since they move from effect to cause rather than from cause to effect. The TROHOC fallacy means that it is incorrect to consider the logic of a case–control study backwards, because the key comparison is identical to that of a cohort study: between exposed and unexposed groups.

    B. The odds ratio can be defined in two ways: (1) the odds of being a case among the exposed compared to the odds of being a case among the nonexposed, or (2) the odds of being exposed among the cases compared to the odds of being exposed among the controls.

    C. A case-crossover study is a new variant of the case–control study that is used to study the acute effects of transient exposures. Here, cases serve as their own controls, and the exposure frequency during a hazard period is compared to that during a control period.

2. It is desirable to conduct a case–control study when the exposure data are difficult or expensive to obtain, when the disease is rare, when the disease has a long induction and latent period, when little is known about the disease, and when the underlying population is dynamic.

3. A.

Mother used hormones during pregnancy	Testicular cancer Yes (cases)	No (controls)
Yes	90	50
No	410	950
Total	500	1000

    B. Odds ratio = ad/bc = $(90 \times 950)/(50 \times 410)$ = 4.2.

    C. Men whose mothers took hormones during their pregnancies have 4.2 times the risk of testicular cancer than do men whose mothers did not take hormones.

    D. There are many possible answers. The basic principle is that the controls should be comparable to the cases. They should satisfy the "would criterion." That is, if they developed testicular cancer they would end up as a case in the study. For example, one could select men who were hospitalized at the same facilities as the cases. The advantages of hospital controls include easy assess, good cooperation, and recall of prior events that is similar to the cases. The difficulty lies in choosing suitable diagnoses for which the controls may be hospitalized. One should not pick diagnoses that are known to be associated with maternal hormone use or diseases whose referral pattern differs from that of the testicular cancer cases.

E. The purpose of the control group is to provide information on the exposure distribution in the source population that produced the cases.

F. Incident or newly diagnosed cases should be chosen because prevalent ones may represent a biased subset of all men who are diagnosed with testicular cancer. In other words, if prevalent cases are used, men who died from testicular cancer (and other causes) may be excluded. The results based on such a sample can be biased if death is associated with the exposure being studied.

4. *Advantages:* They usually come from the same source population as the cases and so they are likely to be comparable. *Disadvantages:* They are time consuming and expensive to identify, they are usually not as cooperative as hospital controls, and their recall of prior exposures may not be as accurate as that of cases.

5. *Advantages:* Case–control studies take less time and money to conduct than cohort and experimental studies, they are well suited for studying rare diseases and diseases with long induction and latent periods, and they can provide information on a large number of possible risk factors. *Disadvantages:* The possibility of bias is increased, and it may be difficult to establish the correct temporal relationship between the exposure and disease because the data are retrospective.

Chapter 10, Bias

1. A. Recall bias occurs when the level of accuracy differs between the compared groups. It occurs in a case–control study when cases remember or report their exposures differently (more or less accurately) from controls. It occurs in a cohort study when individuals who are exposed remember or report subsequent illnesses differently than those who are unexposed.

B. The healthy-worker effect occurs in occupational studies when disease and death rates in a working population are compared to those among the general population. The rates of disease and death among workers are typically lower than those in the general population because there is a higher proportion of ill people in the general population.

C. Control selection bias is a type of selection bias that occurs in case–control studies when the controls do not accurately represent the exposure distribution in the source population that produced the cases. It occurs when different criteria are used to select cases and controls, and these criteria are related to the exposure.

2. In nondifferential misclassification, inaccuracies that occur on one axis (exposure or disease) are *independent* of the other axis. For example, if there is an error in exposure misclassification, it occurs with equal likelihood among diseased and nondiseased individuals. In differential misclassification, inaccuracies that occur on one axis (exposure or disease) are *dependent* on the other axis. For example, if there is an error in exposure misclassification, it occurs more often in the case group than the control group. Nondifferential misclassification of dichotomous variables (that is, variables with two categories) biases the results toward the null. Differential misclassification can bias the results either toward or away from the null.

3. A. Nondifferential misclassification of the exposure. Some women who filled the health maintenance organization's prescriptions for antihistamines may not have used them, and other women may have obtained antihistamines from outside sources. This type of misclassification is as likely to occur among cases as among controls, so it is nondifferential.

   B. Recall and interviewer bias. Subjects were not asked to recall their exposures, and interviews were not used to obtain the exposure data.

4. A. Yes.
   B. Yes.
   C. No.
   D. Yes. (because it is a prospective study).

5. A. Interviewer bias: Mask interviewers to the study hypothesis and to the disease or exposure status of the study subjects, and carefully design the interview instrument.

   B. Recall bias: Mask study subjects to the study hypothesis, use diseased controls if conducting a case–control study, and carefully design an interview instrument.

   C. Conduct a prospective study and obtain high participation rates.

   D. Use the most accurate source of information, and use sensitive and specific criteria to define the exposure and disease.

Chapter 11, Confounding

1. A. Confounding is a mixing of effects between an exposure, an outcome, and a third extraneous variable that is termed the confounder.

Confounding distorts the crude relationship between an exposure and outcome because of the relationships between the confounder and the exposure, and the confounder and the disease.

B. Residual confounding means that an association remains confounded even after some confounders have been controlled. It arises from lack of information on all confounding variables, classifying confounders in overly broad categories, or mismeasuring confounders.

C. Positive confounding means that true crude association is exaggerated, and negative confounding means that the true crude association is underestimated.

2. A confounder is associated with the exposure in the source population that produced the cases and an independent cause or predictor of the outcome under study. The latter means that it is associated with the disease among both exposed and unexposed individuals. In addition, a confounder cannot be an intermediate step in the causal pathway between the exposure and disease.

3. A. Yes.
   B. Yes.
   C. No.
   D. No.

4. *Randomization* is the act of assigning or ordering using a random process. It means that everyone in the study has an equal chance of being assigned to one of the groups (such as treatment versus comparison). The main advantage of randomization is that it controls for both known and unknown confounders, if the sample size is sufficiently large. Its main disadvantage is that it can only be used in experimental studies. *Matching* is the process of making the distribution of confounders identical in the compared groups while selecting the study subjects. It is good for controlling for confounding by complex nominal variables such as neighborhood or sibship and for controlling confounding in small studies. Its main disadvantages include the difficulty and expense of finding appropriate matches. *Restriction* means that the investigator limits admission into a study to individuals who fall within a specific category or categories of a confounder. Its main advantages are simplicity and relatively low expense, and its disadvantages include difficulty in identifying a sufficient number of subjects (this depends on the number and characteristics of the restrictions) and limiting the generalizability of the study.

5. *Stratification* is the process of evaluating the association within homogeneous categories of a confounder. Its main advantages are that it is

straightforward and easy to carry out. It also allows epidemiologists to view the raw data. Its chief disadvantage is that it cannot control for numerous variables because a large number of strata are generated relative to the number of study subjects. *Multivariate analysis* is a method for controlling confounding by constructing a mathematical model that describes the association between the exposure, the outcome, and the confounders. Its main advantage is that it can control for many confounders simultaneously. Its main disadvantage is that one can no longer view the raw data.

6. Epidemiologists usually compare the crude/confounded measure of association with the adjusted measure of association. If there is an appreciable difference between the two (that is, at least a 10% difference), confounding is considered present.

7. A. Restriction.
   B. Matching.
   C. Stratified analysis.

Chapter 12, Random Error

1. A. Chance is an uncontrollable force that seems to have no assignable or predictable cause.
   B. Precision is the lack of random error. It is defined either as the state or quality of being exact or the ability of a measurement to be consistently reproduced.
   C. Statistical inference is a method for generalizing results from a sample to a parent population.

2. The main assumption is that the null hypothesis is true.

3. Its chief limitation is the use of a purely arbitrary cutoff for deciding whether or not to reject the null hypothesis.

4. *P* values are affected both by the magnitude of the association and the study size. Thus, when results are summarized only by *P* values, it is impossible to determine if a *P* value is small because the measure of association is strong or because the sample size is large. It is also impossible to determine if a *P* value is large because the association is weak or the sample size is small.

5. A. Compared to olive oil users, there was a 1.8-fold increased risk (or an 80% increased risk) of coronary heart disease among margarine users.
   B. The strict statistical interpretation is as follows: If this study were repeated 100 times and 100 point estimates and confidence intervals

were calculated, 95 of the 100 confidence intervals would contain the true point estimate. Or, we could say that we have 95% confidence that the true measure of association lies within the interval 0.8 to 4.3 or that we have 95% confidence that the results are consistent with hypotheses that the strength of the association lies between 0.8 and 4.3.

C. This confidence interval is rather wide since it extends from a small decrease in risk (0.8) to a moderate increase in risk (4.3).

D. Given that the null hypothesis is true, there is a 10% chance of seeing this result (an odds ratio of 1.8) or one more extreme (an odds ratio greater than 1.8).

6. Confidence intervals are not confounded statistics like *P* values. They do a better job separating the influence of the sample size from the influence of the strength of the association. This is because the width of the interval is influenced mainly by the sample size, and the general position of the interval reflects the magnitude of the association.

7. The normal distribution is used for continuous variables, and the binomial and Poisson distributions are used for discrete variables with two mutually exclusive outcomes. In addition, the Poisson distribution is usually reserved for rare events.

Chapter 13, Effect Measure Modification

1. A. Effect measure modification occurs when the strength of an association varies according to the level of a third variable, which is called the effect modifier. The word *measure* is a key part of the term, because effect measure modification depends on the particular measure of association that is used.

B. Heterogeneity of effect is another term for effect measure modification. Homogeneity of effect means that effect measure modification is absent.

C. Synergy is a type of effect measure modification where the excess relative risk among individuals with two factors is greater than the sum of the excess relative risks among individuals with only one factor.

D. Antagonism is a type of effect measure modification where the excess relative risk among individuals with two factors is less than the sum of the excess relative risks among individuals with only one factor.

2. Confounding is a nuisance that epidemiologists try to eliminate from their studies. Effect measure modification is a natural phe-

nomenon of scientific interest that epidemiologists try to describe and understand.

3. One can determine if a factor is an effect measure modifier in a stratified analysis by comparing the stratum-specific measures of association to one another. If they are appreciably different, either by visual inspection or a statistical test result, then effect measure modification is present. One can also determine if effect measure modification is present by examining the excess relative risks.

4. A. Yes.
   B. The excess odds ratio of having both factors (50 – 1 = 49) is much greater than the sum of the two excess odds ratios for each factor alone (excess odds ratio for smoking: 10 – 1 = 9; excess odds ratio for asbestos: 5 – 1 = 4; sum of excess odds ratios: 9 + 4 = 13). Note that the odds ratio provides an estimate of relative risk in a case–control study.

5. A. 2.8.
   B. Male odds ratio: 2.0. Female odds ratio: 2.0.
   C. Yes.
   D. No.
   E. The stratum-specific (unconfounded) odds ratios are different from the crude (confounded) odds ratio. Therefore, confounding is present. However, the stratum-specific odds ratios are identical, and so there is no effect measure modification.

Chapter 15, The Epidemiologic Approach to Causation

1. A. A cause of disease is an event, condition, or characteristic that preceded the disease and without which the disease either would not have occurred or would have occurred later.
   B. A sufficient cause is a set of conditions without any one of which the disease would not have occurred.
   C. A necessary cause is a component cause that is a member of every sufficient cause.

2. The overall induction period begins with the action of the first causal component and ends with the action of the last causal component and the simultaneous biological onset of disease. The latent period follows the induction period and so begins with the biological onset of disease and ends with the disease diagnosis.

3.   A. True.
     B. True.
     C. False.
     D. True.
     E. True.
     F. False.

4.   A. Analogy.
     B. Biological plausibility and coherence.
     C. Coherence, consistency, and experiment.
     D. Consistency and coherence.
     E. Biological gradient, strength of association.

Chapter 16, Screening in Public Health Practice

1.   A. Sensitivity is a measure of a screening test's validity. It is the probability that a screening test classifies as positive those individuals who have preclinical disease.
     B. Specificity is also a measure of a screening test's validity. The complement of sensitivity, it is the probability that a screening test classifies as negative those individuals who do not have preclinical disease.
     C. Predictive value of a positive test is a way to measure a screening program's feasibility. It is the proportion of individuals with a positive test who have preclinical disease.
     D. Lead time is the amount of time that the diagnosis of disease is advanced by screening.

2.   Primary prevention occurs before the pathological onset of disease, and its aim is to block the start of disease. Secondary prevention takes place from the pathological onset of disease to the occurrence of clinical symptoms. Its aim is to delay the onset and duration of symptomatic disease and improve survival. Tertiary prevention takes place after clinical symptoms develop. Its aim is to slow or block the progression of disease, and so reduce disease sequelae and improve survival.

3.   Serious diseases with fairly long and prevalent detectable preclinical phases for which treatment is more effective at earlier stages.

4. A.

Screening test	Prostate cancer Yes	No	Total
Positive	800	3,200	4,000
Negative	100	95,900	96,000
Total	900	99,100	100,000

B. Prevalence = 900/100,000 or 0.9%.

C. Sensitivity = 800/900 or 88.9% It means that 88.9% of men who had prostate cancer tested positive on the screening test.

D. Specificity = 95,900/96,000 = 96.8% It means that 96.8% of the men who did not have prostate cancer tested negative on the screening test.

E. Predictive value positive = 800/4000 or 20% It means that 20% of the men who tested positive truly did have prostate cancer.

F. 3200 men underwent unnecessary biopsies and 100 men were falsely reassured that they did not have prostate cancer.

5. A. Age 30 to 60 or 30 years.

B. Age 40 to 60 or 20 years.

C. Age 45 to 60 or 15 years.

D. Yes. She would have died at age 70 years if no screening had been done. Instead, she died at age 80 years.

6. The three types of bias are lead-time bias, length-biased sampling, and volunteer bias. Lead-time bias means that survival among screened individuals may appear longer than that for nonscreened individuals just because they were diagnosed earlier. Length-biased sampling means that survival among screened individuals may be longer than that for nonscreened individuals because screening tends to identify less aggressive forms of the disease. Volunteer bias is a form of confounding that occurs only in observational studies of screening programs. It means that people who get screened tend to have different characteristics than those who do not get screened. These characteristics may be related to survival.

Index